Obstetrics and Gynecology
DRUG HANDBOOK

D0288090

NOTICE

Every effort has been made to ensure that the drug dosage schedules herein are accurate and in accord with the standards accepted at the time of publication. However, as new research and
experience broaden our knowledge, changes in treatment and
drug therapy occur. Therefore readers are advised to check the
product information sheet included in the package of each drug
they plan to administer to be certain that changes have not been
made in the recommended dose or in the contraindications. This
is of particular importance in regard to new or infrequently
used drugs.

Obstetrics and Gynecology
DRUG HANDBOOK

SECOND EDITION

GERALD I. ZATUCHNI, MD, MSc
Professor Obstetrics and Gynecology
Northwestern University Medical School
Chicago, Illinois

RAMONA I. SLUPIK, MD
Assistant Professor Obstetrics and Gynecology
Northwestern University Medical School
Head, Pediatric and Adolescent Gynecology
Children's Memorial Hospital
Chicago, Illinois

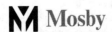

St. Louis Baltimore Boston Carlsbad Chicago Naples New York
Philadelphia Portland London Madrid Mexico City Singapore
Sydney Tokyo Toronto Wiesbaden

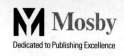

M Mosby

Dedicated to Publishing Excellence

A Times Mirror Company

Publisher: Anne S. Patterson
Editor: Susie H. Baxter
Developmental Editor: Ellen Baker Geisel
Project Manager: Linda McKinley
Production Editor: Aimee E. Loewe
Coordinator Designer: Elizabeth Fett
Manufacturing Supervisor: Dave Graybill

SECOND EDITION

Printed in the United States of America

Composition by W. C. Brown Communications, Inc.
Printing/binding by R. R. Donnelley & Sons Company

Mosby–Year Book, Inc.
11830 Westline Industrial Drive
St. Louis, MO 63146

Library of Congress Cataloging in Publication Data

Zatuchni, Gerald I., 1933–Obstetrics and gynecology drug handbook/Gerald I. Zatuchni, Ramona I. Slupik.—2nd ed. p.; cm.
Contains completely updated information and extensive revisions. Includes bibliographical references and index.
ISBN 0–8151–9894–9
1. Gynecologic drugs—Handbooks, manuals, etc. 2. Obstetrical pharmacology— Handbooks, manuals, etc. 3.Drugs—Handbooks, manuals, etc. I. Slupik, Ramona. II. Title.
RG131.Z38   1996   95–224950
618´.0461—dc20   CIP

96 97 98 99 00   /   9 8 7 6 5 4 3 2 1

Dedicated to

Bette

Tree barks, flower petals
Seeds of nature
Undiscovered secrets
Life continues . . .

PREFACE

The goal of this revision is to provide the clinician with updated information about the extensive array of pharmaceutical preparations used primarily by women. We have continued the format of drug presentation arranged into 34 chapters that has proven to be practical to use on a daily basis by obstetricians, gynecologists, nurse midwives, family practice physicians, internists, and other primary health care providers.

All selected drugs and other agents described in this volume are listed in the *Physicians' Desk Reference—1995,* and the *Physicians' Desk Reference for Generics—1995.* These reference volumes should be consulted for more detailed information.

This second edition contains completely updated information on all selected drugs and agents and includes extensive revisions of certain chapters including antibiotics, antiinfectives, antihypertensives, contraceptives, lipid-lowering drugs, psychopharmacologics, steroid hormones, tocolytics, and uterine stimulants. An Appendix has been added to indicate the recent classification of potential drug risks to the fetus.

The reader is well aware of the significant acceleration of pharmaceutical research and the increasing availability of entirely new approaches and successful modifications of pharmaceuticals. We hope that this book reflects these important advances and gives the health care provider easy access to this information.

Gerald I. Zatuchni, MD, MSc
Ramona I. Slupik, MD
Chicago, 1995

PREFACE

CONTENTS

TABLE OF TABLES

ANALGESICS

NARCOTICS (OPIOIDS)

Mechanism of Action

Bind to opioid receptors in the CNS as agonists, competitive antagonists, or mixed agents.

Indications

Acute pain of moderate to severe intensity. Obstetrical analgesia.

Classification (Table 1-1.)

Table 1-1

CLASSIFICATION OF OPIOID DRUGS AND DERIVATIVES

NATURAL ALKALOIDS
Codeine
Morphine
Opium

SYNTHETIC DERIVATIVES
Butorphanol (Stadol)
Dihydrocodeine (Synalgos)
Hydromorphone (Dilaudid)
Levorphanol (Levo-Dromoran)
Meperidine (Demerol)
Nalbuphine (Nubain)
Oxycodone (Percodan; Tylox)
Pentazocine (Talwin)
Propoxyphene (Darvon)

NARCOTIC ANTAGONIST
Naloxone (Narcan)

Precautions

1. Psychic or physical dependence and tolerance may develop (see Chapter 29).
2. Opioids cross the placenta and may cause respiratory depression in the fetus.
3. Ambulatory patients should avoid potentially hazardous activities.
4. Use of alcoholic beverages and other CNS depressants may cause additional CNS depression.
5. Drug may obscure correct diagnosis in patients with abdominal pain.
6. Overdosage can lead to coma, apnea, circulatory collapse, and cardiac arrest.

Adverse Reactions

1. Respiratory depression.
2. Nausea, vomiting, constipation.
3. Hypotension, bradycardia.
4. Somnolence.
5. Increased intracranial pressure.
6. Biliary and urinary tract spasms.
7. Miosis.
8. Pruritus.

CODEINE AND DERIVATIVES
■ Codeine Phosphate

How Supplied:
Tablet: 15, 30, 60 mg.
Solution:
    30 mg/ml in 1, 2, 20 ml vial.
    60 mg/ml in 1, 2 ml vial.

Dose: 30–60 mg q4–6h prn.

■ Codeine Phosphate in Tubex (Wyeth-Ayerst)

How Supplied:
Single-dose syringe, sterile:
    30 mg (½ gr), 25 G needle.
    60 mg (1 gr), 25 G needle.

Dose: 30–60 mg q4–6h prn.

■ Codeine Sulfate

How Supplied:
Tablet: 15, 30, 60 mg.

Dose: 30–60 mg q4–6h prn.

■ Empirin with Codeine (Burroughs Wellcome)

How Supplied:
Tablet:
   Codeine phosphate, (No. 2) 15 mg.
                    (No. 3) 30 mg.
                    (No. 4) 60 mg.
   Aspirin, 325 mg.

Dose: 1–2 tab q3–4h prn.

■ Esgic with Codeine (Forest)

How Supplied:
Capsule:
   Codeine phosphate, 30 mg.
   Butalbital, 50 mg.
   Acetaminophen, 325 mg.
   Caffeine, 40 mg.

Dose: 1–2 caps q4–6h prn, up to 6 caps/day.

■ Fiorinal with Codeine (Sandoz)

How Supplied:
Capsule:
   Codeine phosphate, (No. 1) 7.5 mg.
                    (No. 2) 15 mg.
                    (No. 3) 30 mg.
   Butalbital, 50 mg.
   Caffeine, 40 mg.
   Aspirin, 325 mg.

Dose: 1–2 caps q4h prn, up to 6 caps/day.

■ **Percocet** (Du Pont)

How Supplied:
Tablet:
    Oxycodone HCl, 5 mg.
    Acetaminophen, 325 mg.

Dose: 1 tab q6h prn.

■ **Percodan, Percodan-Demi** (Du Pont)

How Supplied:
Tablet:
    Oxycodone HCl, 4.50 mg (½ for Percodan-Demi).
    Oxycodone terephthalate, 0.38 mg (½ for Percodan-Demi).
    Aspirin, 325 mg.

Dose: 1 tab q6h prn.

■ **Phenaphen with Codeine** (Robins)

How Supplied:
Capsule:
    Codeine phosphate, (No. 2) 15 mg.
                    (No. 3) 30 mg.
                    (No. 4) 60 mg.
    Acetaminophen, 325 mg.

Dose: 1 or 2 caps q4h prn, up to 6 caps/day.

■ **Tylenol with Codeine Phosphate** (McNeil)

How Supplied:
Tablet:
    Codeine phosphate, (No. 1) 7.5 mg.
                    (No. 2) 15 mg.
                    (No. 3) 30 mg.
                    (No. 4) 60 mg.
    Acetaminophen, 300 mg.

Elixir:
    Each 5 ml:
    Codeine phosphate, 12 mg.
    Acetaminophen, 120 mg.

Dose: 1–2 tab or 15 ml q4h.

OPIUM ALKALOIDS AND DERIVATIVES
■ **Darvon** (Propoxyphene HCl; Lilly)

■ **Darvon-N** (Propoxyphene Napsylate; Lilly)

How Supplied:
Pulvule: 32, 65 mg.
Tablet (Darvon-N): 100 mg.
Suspension (Darvon-N): 50 mg/5 ml.

Dose: 65, 100 mg q4h prn.

■ **Darvon Compound** (Lilly)

How Supplied:
Pulvule:
    Propoxyphene HCl, 32 or 65 mg.
    Aspirin, 389 mg.
    Caffeine, 32.4 mg.

Dose: 1 cap q4h prn.

■ **Darvocet-N 50/N 100** (Lilly)

How Supplied:
Tablet
    Propoxyphene napsylate, 50, 100 mg.
    Acetaminophen, 325, 650 mg.

Dose: 50–100 mg q4h prn.

■ Demerol (Meperidine Hydrochloride; Winthrop)

How Supplied:
Parenteral:
   Sterile Cartridge Needle, 25, 50, 75, 100 mg.
   Uni-Amp, 25, 50, 75, 100 mg in 5% or 10% solution.
   Vials, 50, 100 mg multiple-dose vials.
Tablet: 50, 100 mg.
Syrup (banana flavored): 50 mg/ 5 ml.

Dose: 50–150 mg q3–4h prn.

■ Dilaudid (Hydromorphone HCl; Knoll)

How Supplied:
Ampule: 1, 2, 4 mg/1 ml.
Vial: 2 mg/ml, multiple dose.
Tablet: 1, 2, 3, 4 mg.
Suppository: 3 mg.

Dose: 1–2 mg q4–6h prn.

■ Fentanyl Citrate (Sublimaze; Janssen)

How Supplied:
Ampule: 50 µg/ml fentanyl base in 2, 5, 10, 20 ml ampules.

Dose: IM—must be individualized. Low dose for minor surgical procedures, 2 µg/kg; moderate dose for major surgical procedures, 2–20 µg/kg; high dose for prolonged major surgery, 20–50 µg/kg.

■ Fentanyl Oralet (Abbott)

How Supplied:
Oral transmucosal lozenge

Dose: 200, 300, 400 µg. Must be individualized. Should only be used as anesthetic premedication or for inducing conscious sedation in monitored setting.

■ Levo-Dromoran (Roche)

How Supplied:
Ampule: 2 mg/1 ml.
Vial: 2 mg/10 ml, multiple dose.
Tablet: 2 mg.

Dose: 2 mg q4h prn.

■ Meperidine HCl, USP

How Supplied:
Cartridge-Needle unit: 25, 50, 75, 100 mg/1 ml: 22, 25 G needle.

Dose: 25–100 mg q4–6h prn.

■ Mepergan (Meperidine HCl and Promethazine HCl; Wyeth-Ayerst)

How Supplied:
Vial:
    25 mg meperidine HCl/1 ml.
    25 mg promethazine HCl/1 ml.
Cartridge-Needle unit: 25 mg each drug.

Dose: 1–2 ml IM q3–4h prn.

■ Morphine Sulfate, USP

How Supplied:
Ampule: 8, 10, 15 mg/1 ml.
Vial: 5, 8, 10 mg/1 ml, multiple dose.
Cartridge-Needle unit: 2, 4, 8, 10, 15 mg/1 ml (Wyeth-Ayerst).
Soluble hypodermic tablet: 10, 15, 30 mg.

Dose: Must be individualized.

■ **Nubain** (Nalbuphine HCl; Du Pont)

How Supplied:
IV, IM, SC:
    10, 20 mg in 1 ml ampule or multidose vial.
    20 mg/ml in prefilled syringe.

Dose: 10 mg q3–6h.

■ **Numorphan** (Oxymorphone HCl; Du Pont)

How Supplied:
Suppository: 5 mg.

Dose: 1 suppos q4–6h prn.

■ **Propoxyphene HCl, Acetaminophen** (Wygesic; Wyeth-Ayerst)

How Supplied:
Tablet:
    65 mg propoxyphene HCl.
    650 mg acetaminophen.

Dose: 1 tab q4h prn up to 6/day.

■ **Stadol** (Butorphanol Tartrate; Bristol-Myers)

How Supplied:
IV, IM:
    2 mg/1 ml, 1–2 ml ampule.
    1 mg/1 ml, 1 ml ampule.
    2 mg/1 ml, multidose vial.
Nasal spray (NS): multidose bottle

Dose: 1 or 2 mg (1 mg = 1 spray in 1 nostril) q3–4h prn.

■ Talwin, Talacen (Pentazocine HCl; Winthrop)

How Supplied:
Tablet:
    Pentazocine HCl (USP), 25 mg.
    Talacen: Acetaminophen (USP), 650 mg.
Injection:
    30 or 60 mg/1 ml in Uni-Amp.
    Talwin: 30, 45, or 60 mg in cartridge-needle unit.
Vial: 30 mg/1 ml, multiple dose.

Dose:
Oral, 2 tabs q4–6h prn.
Parenteral, 30 mg q3–4h prn.

■ Talwin Compound (Winthrop)

How Supplied:
Tablet:
    Pentazocine HCl (USP), 12.5 mg.
    Aspirin (USP), 325 mg.

Dose: 2 tabs q4–6h prn.
A comparison of narcotic analgesics can be found in Table 1-2.

NARCOTIC ANTAGONISTS
■ Narcan (Naloxone HCl; Du Pont)

How Supplied (with/without paraben):
IV, IM, SC:
    0.02 mg/ml, 2 ml ampule.
    0.4 mg/ml, 1 ml ampule/syringe.
    1.0 mg/ml, 1 or 2 ml ampule/multidose.

Dose:
Adults: 0.4–2.0 mg IV at 2–3 min intervals prn for response; max 10 mg total dose.
Children: Initial dose 0.1 mg/kg body weight IV; repeat dose depending on response.

Table 1-2

COMPARISON OF NARCOTIC ANALGESICS USED IN OBSTETRICS

	Morphine	Dihydromorphone (Dilaudid)	Meperidine (Demerol)	Pentazocine (Talwin)	Fentanyl (Sublimaze)
DOSAGE					
IV	2–5 mg	1–2 mg	25–50 mg	10–20 mg	25–50 µg
IM	5–10 mg	1–2 mg	50–100 mg	20–30 mg	50–100 µg
ONSET OF ACTION					
IV (min)	3–5	3–5	3–5	2–3	1–2
IM (min)	10–20	10–20	10–20	5–15	6–8
DURATION OF ACTION					
IV (hr)	2–3	2–4	2–3	2–3	½–1
IM (hr)	3–4	3–5	3–4	3–4	1–2

Neonates: initial dose 0.1 mg/kg body weight IV, IM, or SC; repeat dose depending on response.

Indication: Complete or partial reversal of narcotic-induced depression or narcotic overdosage.

Contraindication: Naloxone should not be administered to infants of narcotic-dependent mothers; may cause withdrawal syndrome (see Chapter 22).

NONNARCOTIC ANALGESICS (Antiinflammatory, Antipyretics)

NSAIDs (Nonsteroidal Antiinflammatory Drugs)

Mechanism of Action

Inhibition of prostaglandin synthesis resulting in analgesic, antipyretic, and antiinflammatory effects. Do not bind to opiate receptors and are not included under controlled substances.

Toxicity

Inhibition of platelet aggregation may result in prolonged bleeding time, gastric ulceration, decreased renal function, and allergic syndromes including bronchospasm.

Indications

Mild to moderately severe pain (dysmenorrhea postop minor surgery) and/or used as antipyretics. Analgesic potencies are similar, although aspirin or acetaminophen may be preferred when antipyretic therapy is necessary.

■ Acetaminophen

How Supplied:
Tablet: 325, 500, 650 mg.
Capsule: 300, 500 mg.
Suppository: 120, 325, 650 mg.

Indication: Mild to moderate pain; antipyrexis. Efficacy equivalent to aspirin. Preferred over aspirin in patients with peptic ulcer or coagulation disorders.

Products Available:
Datril (Bristol-Myers), 500 mg tablet or caplet:
  Dose: 2 tab/cap q4h prn; max 8 tab/24 hr.
Phenaphen (Robins), 325 mg capsule:
  Dose: 2 caps q4h prn; max 12 tab/24 hr.
Tylenol (McNeil), 325 mg tablet or capsule:
  Dose: 1–2 cap/tab q4h prn; max 12 tab/24 hr.

◼ Ibuprofen

How Supplied:
Advil (Whitehall), 200 mg tablets or caplets.
Motrin (Upjohn), 800 mg tablets.
Nuprin (Bristol-Myers), 200 mg tablets.
Rufen (Boots), 400, 600, 800 mg tablets.

Dose: 400 mg q4h prn with food; max 3,200 mg/24 hr.

Indication: Very useful in conditions of mild to moderate or severe pain, especially in primary dysmenorrhea and inflammatory syndromes, and as antipyretic.

◼ Diclofenac Sodium (Voltaren; Geigy)

◼ Diclofenal Potassium (Cataflam; Geigy)

How Supplied:
Voltaren, 25, 50, 75 mg delayed release tablet.
Cataflam, 50 mg tablet.

Indication: Acute/chronic treatment of musculoskeletal pain, including bone/joint pain and dysmenorrhea; cataflam preferred here.

Dose: 25 mg qid-75 mg bid-tid; max 225 mg/day.

Toxicity: Similar to ibuprofen.

■ Fenoprofen Calcium (Nalfon; Dista, Lederle, Mylan)
Similar to ibuprofen.

How Supplied:
Capsules: 200–300 mg.
Caplet: 600 mg.

Dose: 200–600 mg q4–6h prn with food; max 3,200 mg/24 hr.

■ Flurbiprofen (Ansaid; Upjohn)
Similar to ibuprofen.

How Supplied:
Tablet: 50, 100 mg.

Dose: 50–100 mg q6–8h prn; max 300 mg/24 hr.

■ Indomethacin (Indocin; Merck)

How Supplied:
Capsule/Suppository: 25, 50, 75 mg.

Dose: 25 mg bid with food.

Indications: Moderate to severe pain associated with musculoskeletal system abnormalities. High potency and toxicity; limit use.

■ Ketoprofen (Orudis; Wyeth-Ayerst)
Similar to ibuprofen.

How Supplied:
Capsule: 25, 50, 75 mg.

Dose: 25–50 mg q6–8h prn; max 300 mg/24 hr.

■ Ketorolac tromethamine (Toradol: Roche)

How Supplied:
IV, IM, Oral: use oral only as continuation therapy; combined use not to exceed 5 days.

Dose:
IM, IV: 30 mg q6h; max 120 mg/day.
Oral: 2 tabs 10 mg; max 40 mg/day.
    1 tab q4–6h; max 40 mg/day.

Indication: Short-term (5 days) management of moderately severe pain.

Toxicity: Similar to ibuprofen.

Contraindication: Labor and delivery; postpartum; nursing.

■ Meclofenamate Sodium (Meclomen; Parke-Davis)
Similar to ibuprofen.

How Supplied:
Capsule: 50, 100 mg.

Dose: 50 mg q4–6h prn; max 400 mg/24 hr.

■ Mefenamic Acid (Ponstel; Parke-Davis)
Similar to ibuprofen.

How Supplied:
Capsule: 250 mg.

Dose: 500 mg q4–6h prn with food.

■ Naproxen (Naprosyn; Syntex)
Similar to ibuprofen.

How Supplied:
Tablet: 250, 375, 500 mg.

Dose: Initial dose 500 mg, then 250 mg q6–8h prn; max 1,250 mg/24 hr.

■ Naproxen Sodium (Anaprox; Syntex)

How Supplied:
Tablet: 250 mg naproxen + 25 mg sodium.

Dose: Initial dose 550 mg, then 275 mg q6–8h prn; max 1,375 mg/24 hr.

■ Salicylates

How Supplied: Various products available OTC.

Dose: 650 mg q4h prn; max 4 g/24 hr.

■ Dolobid (Diflunisal; Merck)

How Supplied:
Tablet: 250, 500 mg.

Dose: Initial dose 1,000 mg with food, then 500 mg q12h prn; max 1,500 mg/24 hr.

Indication: Mild to moderate pain; less effective than newer NSAIDs in relief of dysmenorrhea.

Adverse Effects: Gastrointestinal distress, bleeding, gastric ulcer.

ANTIMIGRAINE ANALGESICS
■ Ergotamine Tartrate

How Supplied:
Sublingual tablet: 2 mg (Ergostat; Parke-Davis).
Sublingual tablet: 1 mg (Gynergen; Sandoz).

Dose: Tab sublingually; repeat q30min prn; max 6 mg/24 hr.

Indication: Acute migraine.

Action: Peripheral vasoconstriction.

Adverse Reactions: Nausea, vomiting, diarrhea, diplopia, drowsiness, tachycardia/bradycardia, paresthesia.

Contraindication: Peripheral vascular disease, peptic ulcer, renal/hepatic disease.

■ Ergotamine Mixtures

How Supplied:
Cafergot (Sandoz), tablets, suppository:
    Ergotamine tartrate, 1 mg.
    Caffeine, 100 mg.
Cafergot P-B (Sandoz), tablets, suppository:
    Ergotamine tartrate, 1 mg.
    Caffeine, 100 mg.
    Belladonna malate, 0.125 mg.
    Pentobarbital, 30 mg.

■ Imitrex (Sumatriptan Succinate), injection-Glaxo

How Supplied: 6 mg-unit syringe/vial.

Dose: 6 mg injected subcutaneously; max two doses/24 hr.

Indication: Acute treatment of migraine attack with or without aura.

Contraindication: Pregnancy. Use only when effective contraception is being used.

Toxicity: Serotonin (5-HT) Receptor Agonist may cause increased blood pressure, tachycardia, coronary artery vasospasm.

■ Migral (Burroughs-Wellcome),

How Supplied:
Tablet:
    Ergotamine tartrate, 1 mg.
    Caffeine, 50 mg.
    Cyclizine HCl, 25 mg.

■ Wigraine (Organon),

How Supplied:
Tablet; suppository:
    Ergotamine tartrate, 1 mg.
    Caffeine, 100 mg.
    Belladonna alkaloids (Wigraine-PB), 0.1 mg.
    Phenacetin (Wigraine-PB), 130 mg.

Dose: 2 tab at onset, repeat q30min prn; max 6 tab/attack or 10 tab/wk. 1 suppos at onset, may repeat in 1 hr; max 2 suppos/attack or 5 suppos/wk.

Indication: Acute migraine.

■ Bellergal (Sandoz)
    Not for acute migraine attack.

How Supplied:
Tablet:
    Ergotamine tartrate, 0.3 mg.
    Phenobarbital, 40 mg.
    Belladonna alkaloids, 0.1 mg.
Bellergal-S: Sustained release.

Dose: 4 tab/day or 1 timed-release bid.

■ **Dihydroergotamine Mesylate** (D.H.E. 45; Sandoz)

How Supplied:
Parenteral: 1 mg/ml vial.

Dose: 1 mg IM/IV at onset; repeat hourly; max 3 mg.

Indication: Acute migraine.

β-ADRENERGIC BLOCKERS
■ **Propranolol** (Inderal; Wyeth-Ayerst)

How Supplied:
Tablet: 10, 20, 40, 80 mg.

Dose: 20–40 mg bid or tid initially; increase gradually until therapeutic effect.

Indication: Migraine prophylaxis.

Adverse Reactions: Light-headedness, insomnia, bradycardia, hypotension.

Contraindication: Asthma, cardiac disease (see Chapter 8).

CHAPTER 2

ANESTHETICS

LOCAL AND REGIONAL AGENTS

Local and regional agents are used to produce loss of sensation or prevent muscle activity in specific areas of the body (e.g., muscle relaxation during labor and delivery).

All agents (except cocaine) have an aromatic portion—a carbon ring attached to an intermediate alkyl chain by an ester or amide linkage and further connected to a tertiary amine. The ester amide linkage determines the route of metabolism. Esters are hydrolyzed by plasma cholinesterase; amides are metabolized in the liver (Table 2-1).

Local anesthetics block the generation and conduction of nerve impulses. Progression of anesthesia depends on the diameter and myelination of nerve fibers. The order of clinical loss of nerve function is pain, temperature, touch, proprioception, and skeletal muscle tone.

Onset and duration of action depends on diffusion of agent across nerve coverings, local pH, protein-binding capacity, and lipid solubility. All agents cause vasodilatation; therefore adding vasoconstrictor increases duration of effect (Table 2-2).

All local anesthetics cross the placenta and can be detected in fetal blood within 1–2 minutes of maternal IV administration. Absorption of agent is highly dependent on local vascularity; absorption from the paracervical area is much more rapid than from the epidural space.

Table 2-1
CLASSIFICATION OF LOCAL ANESTHETIC AGENTS

Amides	Esters
Bupivacaine	Chloroprocaine
Etidocaine	Procaine
Lidocaine	Tetracaine
Mepivacaine	
Prilocaine	

Table 2-2

CHARACTERISTICS OF LOCAL ANESTHETICS

	CLASS	USE	ONSET	DURATION (min)	SINGLE MAXIMUM Dose
LOW POTENCY					
Procaine (Novocain; Winthrop)	Ester	Local	Slow	60–90	800 mg* 1000 mg†
INTERMEDIATE POTENCY					
Chloroprocaine HCl (Nesacaine; Astra)	Ester	Local, nerve block, epidural	Fast	30–90	800 mg* 1000 mg†
Lidocaine (Xylocaine; Astra)	Amide	Local, nerve block, epidural, spinal	Fast	90–200	300 mg* 500 mg†
Mepivacaine (Carbocaine; Winthrop)	Amide	Local, nerve block, epidural	Fast	120–240	400 mg
HIGH POTENCY					
Tetracaine (Pontocaine HCl; Winthrop)	Ester	Spinal	Slow	180–600	200 mg
Bupivacaine (Marcaine; Winthrop; Sensorcaine; Astra)	Amide	Local, nerve block, epidural, spinal	Slow	180–160	175 mg* 225 mg†
Etidocaine (Duranest; Astra)	Amide	Nerve block, epidural	Fast	180–600	300 mg* 400 mg†

*Without epinephrine.
†With epinephrine.

Indications

- Topical (surface).
- Infiltration.
- Peripheral.
- Epidural.
- Spinal (subarachnoid).

Adverse Reactions

Hypersensitivity: Usually associated with ester-type agents (derivatives of *p*-aminobenzoic acid).

Systemic Toxicity: Usually results from inadvertent intravascular injection.

CNS: Restlessness, dizziness, circumoral paresthesias, tinnitus, difficulty focusing, tremors and convulsions, respiratory arrest and coma.

Cardiovascular: Bradycardia, hypotension, heart block, cardiac arrest.

Fetus: Diminished muscle tone, bradycardia, CNS depression, death.

Precautions

Local anesthetics should be administered only by physicians knowledgeable about their use and about diagnosis and management of drug-related toxicity, including acute emergencies. The immediate availability of oxygen, resuscitative drugs, equipment, and personnel trained in proper management of toxic reactions and related emergencies is absolutely essential.

TOPICAL ANESTHETIC AGENTS

Nonionized forms of local anesthetics penetrate unbroken skin and may be useful for the relief of burning or itching. Both nonionized and cationic forms readily penetrate abraded skin and mucous membranes (e.g., vagina, urethra, bronchi).

Representative Agents

Benzocaine (Americaine; American Critical Care):
Aerosol, cream, ointment, or lubricant.

Butesin Picrate (Abbott):
Ointment 1%.

Dibucaine (Nupercainal; CIBA):
Creams, 0.5%.
Ointment, 1%.

Hexylcaine HCl (Cyclaine; MSD):
Solution 5%.

Lidocaine (Xylocaine; Astra):
Ointment and jelly, 2.5/5.0%.

Pontocaine (Winthrop):
Cream 1%
Ointment 0.5%.
Solution 2%.

ANESTHETIC PREMEDICATION AGENTS

These drugs are administered before anesthesia to reduce anxiety, induce sedation, inhibit salivary and tracheal secretions, facilitate induction, diminish the dose of anesthetic agent required, and prevent bradycardia (Table 2-3).

Most opiates and opioids produce adequate sedation but do not lessen anxiety or cause amnesia. The incidence of postoperative nausea and vomiting is increased. Potential adverse effects include tachycardia, dizziness, sweating, restlessness, hypotension, and respiratory depression.

Barbiturates have been used to avoid adverse effects of opiates, but they may cause respiratory depression, and disorientation may develop.

Benzodiazepines are gradually replacing barbiturates for premedication because they reduce anxiety and produce amnesia. In addition, these drugs can be substituted or allow reduction in dosage of opiates, which have the potential for adverse effects.

Table 2-3

ANESTHETIC PREMEDICATION AGENTS

Agent-Manufacturer	Route	Dosage	Major Adverse Effects
ANTICHOLINERGICS			
Atropine sulfate (Astra)	Oral	2 mg	Anticholinergic effects, gastric reflux, confusion, emergence delirium, tachycardia, inhibit heat loss
	IM	0.6 mg	
Glycopyrrolate (Robinul injectable; Robins)	IM	0.0044 mg/kg	Same as atropine sulfate
Scopolamine hydrobromide (Robins)	Oral	1 mg	Same as atropine sulfate; bradycardia
	IM	04–0.6 mg/kg	
BARBITURATES			
Pentobarbital sodium (Nembutal sodium; Abbott, Wyeth-Ayerst)	IM	75–200 mg	Respiratory depression, apnea, laryngospasm, hypotension
Secobarbital sodium (Seconal sodium; Wyeth-Ayerst)	IM	75–200 mg	Same as pentobarbital sodium
BENZODIAZEPINES			
Chlordiazepoxide HCl (Librium)	Oral	50–100 mg	Hypotension, paradoxical excitement, ataxia, confusion
	IM		
Diazepam (Valium)	Oral	0.10 mg	Venous thrombophlebitis, apnea, cardiac arrest
	IV	10–20 mg	
Lorazepam (Ativan; Wyeth-Ayerst)	Oral	4 mg	CNS depression, excessive drowsiness, local irritation
	IM	0.05 mg/kg–max 4 mg	
	IV	0.044 mg/kg–max 2 mg	

Continued.

23

Table 2-3

ANESTHETIC PREMEDICATION AGENTS—cont'd

Agent-Manufacturer	Route	Dosage	Major Adverse Effects
BENZODIAZEPINES—cont'd			
Midazolam (Versed; Roche)	IV	5 mg	Laryngospasm, respiratory depression,
	IM	0.07–0.1 mg/kg	hypotension, local irritation, blurred vision
Temazepam (Restoril; Sandoz)	Oral	20–30 mg	Oversedation, dizziness, ataxia, confusion
Triazolam (Halcion; Upjohn)	Oral	0.125–0.25 mg	Drowsiness, dizziness, ataxia, confusion
NARCOTICS			
Fentanyl citrate (Sublimaze; Janssen)	IM, IV	0.05–0.1 mg	Nausea and vomiting, dizziness, bradycardia, hypotension, excitement, respiratory depression
Morphine (Morphine sulfate; Astra)	SC	5–12 mg	Same as fentanyl citrate
	IM, IV	5–12 mg	
Meperidine HCl (Demerol, HCl; Wyeth-Ayerst, Astra)	SC	50–100 mg	Same as fentanyl citrate
	IM, IV	15–100 mg	
Pentazocine lactate (Talwin lactate; Winthrop)	SC	20–40 mg	Same as fentanyl citrate
	IM, IV	20–40 mg	
NEUROLEPTICS			
Droperidol (Inapsine; Janssen)	IM, IV	2.5–10 mg	Hypotension, tachycardia, extrapyramidal symptoms, hallucinations, muscle rigidity
Droperidol and fentanyl citrate (Innovar; Janssen)	IM, IV	0.5–2 ml	Same as droperidol, respiratory depression
Hydroxyzine HCl (Vistaril; Pfizer)	IM	25–100 mg	Potentiate narcotic/barbiturate effects including respiratory depression, hypotension

CHAPTER 3

ANTIBIOTICS

SULFONAMIDES

Common sulfonamides are listed in Table 3-1.

Mechanism of Action

Structural analogues and competitive antagonists of *p*-aminobenzoic acid (PABA); thus prevent normal bacterial utilization of PABA for folic acid synthesis.

General Considerations

1. Derivatives of *p*-aminobenzene sulfonamide (sulfanilamide).
2. First effective chemotherapeutic agents to be used systemically for prevention or cure of bacterial infections in humans.
3. Usually bacteriostatic.
4. Wide range of activity against both gram-positive and gram-negative microorganisms (Table 3-2).
5. Seventy percent to 100% of an oral dose rapidly absorbed from the GI tract.
6. Distributes into pleural, peritoneal, synovial, and ocular fluids and crosses the placenta.
7. Metabolized by acetylation in the liver to inactive acetylated (conjugated) fraction.
8. Excreted in urine partly as unchanged drug and partly as metabolic products; decrements in renal function cause accumulation.

Classification

1. Agents rapidly absorbed and excreted (e.g., sulfisoxazole, sulfadiazine).
2. Agents poorly absorbed orally and thus active in bowel lumen (e.g., sulfasalazine).
3. Agents for topical use (e.g., sulfacetamide, mafenide, silver sulfadiazine).

Table 3-1
SULFONAMIDES

Chemical Name	Brand Name	How Supplied	Dose	Major Indications
WELL-ABSORBED PO				
Sulfisoxazole	Gantrisin (Roche)	500 mg	2–4 gm then 1–2 gm q4–6h	UTI; meningitis; otitis media
Sulfamethoxazole	Gantonol (Roche)	500 mg	2 gm then 1 gm q8–12h	UTI; meningitis; prophylaxis; otitis media
Sulfadiazine		500 mg	2–4 gm then 1 gm q4–8h	
Sulfamethizole	Thiosulfil Forte (Wyeth-Ayerst)	500 mg	500–1000 mg tid–qid	UTI
POORLY ABSORBED SULFONAMIDES				
Sulfasalazine	Azulfidine, Azulfidine EN-Tabs (enteric-coated) (Pharmacia Adria)	500 mg	1–3 gm/day	Inflammatory bowel disease
COMBINATION AGENTS				
Trimethoprim-sulfamethoxazole (TMP-SMX)	Bactrim (Roche); Septra (Burroughs Wellcome)	80 mg TMP + 400 mg SMX/tab	1–2 tabs bid–tid	UTI
	Bactrim DS; Septra DS	160 TMP + 800 SMX/tab	1 tab bid–tid	
	Septra IV	16 mg TMP + 80 mg SMX/ml	15–20 TMP + 75–100 SMX mg/kg/day	Pneumocystis carinii; shigellosis
Sulfisoxazole/sulfamethoxazole phenazopyridine	Azo Gantrisin (Roche)	500 mg SMX + phenazopyridine tab 50 mg	4–6 tabs then 2 tabs qid × 2 days	Acute pain phase of UTI
	Azo Gantanol (Roche)	500 mg SMX + 100 mg phenazopyridine/tab		

PO, Per os; *UTI,* urinary tract infection.

Table 3-2
ANTIBACTERIAL SPECTRUM MISCELLANEOUS ANTIBIOTICS

	Clindamycin	Erythromycin	Sulfonamide	Tetracycline	TMP-SMX	Vancomycin	Gentamicin	Quinolones
GRAM-POSITIVE								
Peptococcus	+	+	-	>	-	-	-	+
Peptostreptococcus*	+	+	-	>	-	-	-	+
Staphylococcus aureus	+	+	-	-	+	+	+	+
S. epidermidis	>	+	-	-	+	+	+	+
Streptococcus S. faecalis (enterococcus)	-	-	-	-	-	+	+	+
Other sp.	+	+	-	-	+	+	-	+
GRAM-POSITIVE BACTERIA								
Actinomyces*	-	+	-	+	-	+	>	-
Clostridium difficile*	-	-	-	+	-	+	-	-
C. perfringens*	+	-	-	+	-	+	>	+
Listeria	-	+	+	+	+	+	>	-
GRAM-NEGATIVE COCCI								
Neisseria	-	+	>	+	+	-	>	+

Continued.

27

Table 3-2
ANTIBACTERIAL SPECTRUM MISCELLANEOUS ANTIBIOTICS—Cont'd

	Clindamycin	Erythromycin	Sulfonamide	Tetracycline	TMP-SMX	Vancomycin	Gentamicin	Quinolones
GRAM-NEGATIVE BACTERIA								
Bacteroides*	+	+	–	V	–	–	–	+
Chlamydia	–	+	–	+	–	–	–	+
Enterobacter	–	–	+	V	+	–	+	+
Escherichia coli	–	V	+	V	+	–	+	+
Haemophilus influenzae	–	V	+	+	V	–	+	+
Klebsiella	–	–	+	V	+	–	+	+
Proteus	–	–	+	–	+	–	+	+
Pseudomonas	–	–	–	–	–	–	V	+
Salmonella	–	–	–	–	+	–	+	+
Serratia	–	–	V	–	+	–	+	+
Shigella	–	–	V	–	+	–	+	–

+, Sensitive; –, resistant; V, varied sensitivity.
*Anaerobic.

Indications

Most often used in management of UTI: acute and chronic cystitis, chronic infections of the upper urinary tract, asymptomatic bacilluria.

Previously used to treat bacillary dysentery, meningococcal infections, and streptococcal infections. These uses are now limited because of the high degree of resistance.

WELL-ABSORBED SULFONAMIDES
■ **Sulfisoxazole** (Gantrisin; Roche)

How Supplied:
Tablet: 500 mg.

Administration:
PO: Well absorbed.

Dose:
Loading: 2–4 gm PO
Maintenance: 4–8 gm/24 hr PO, divided q4–6h.

Elimination: 95% of single dose excreted by kidney in 24 hr.

Spectrum: (see Tables 3-1 and 3-2):
1. UTI: acute, chronic, and recurrent infections because of susceptible organisms *(E. coli, Klebsiella, Enterobacter, Proteus)*.
2. Meningococcal meningitis with susceptible organisms.
3. *H. influenzae* meningitis as adjunctive therapy with parenteral streptomycin.
4. Acute otitis media because of *H. influenzae* (with adequate doses of penicillin [PCN] or erythromycin).
5. Trachoma and inclusion conjunctivitis.
6. Nocardiosis.
7. Chancroid.
8. Toxoplasmosis (with pyrimethamine).
9. Malaria because of chloroquine-resistant strains of *P. falciparum* as adjunctive therapy.

Contraindications: Pregnancy at term, lactation (excreted in breast milk; may cause kernicterus in neonate); history of hypersensitivity to sulfonamides; group A Strep infections.

Toxicity (less than 0.1%):
1. Hematuria/crystalluria (0.2%–0.3%). Avoid by increasing fluid intake to maintain urine volume at least 1200 ml/day; alkalinize urine if necessary with sodium bicarbonate; use with caution in patients with impaired renal function.
2. Acute hemolytic anemia because of sensitization or glucose-6-phosphate dehydrogenase (G-6-PD) deficiency.
3. Agranulocytosis (direct myelotoxic effect); aplastic anemia (extremely rare); thrombocytopenia; eosinophilia.
4. Hypersensitivity reaction: vascular lesions, skin manifestations (1%–2%), serum sickness–like syndrome, anaphylaxis, drug fever.
5. Hepatocellular necrosis (less than 0.1%) because of direct drug toxicity or sensitization.
6. Miscellaneous: pancreatitis, lupuslike syndrome, neuritis, convulsions, and ataxia.

Interaction: May potentiate effects of oral anticoagulants, sulfonylurea hypoglycemic agents (tolbutamide, chlorpropamide), and hydantoin because of inhibition of metabolism or displacement from albumin; cross-sensitivity to thiazides.

■ Sulfamethoxazole (Gantanol; Roche)

How Supplied:
Tablet: 500 mg.

Administration:
PO: Well absorbed.

Dose:
Loading: 2 gm × 1.
Maintenance: 1 gm q8–12h.

Elimination: Renal excretion but slower than sulfisoxazole.

Spectrum: See Sulfisoxazole, p. 29.

Toxicity: See Sulfisoxazole, p. 29. Crystalluria more likely because of high percentage of acetylated, relatively insoluble form of the drug in urine.

■ **Sulfadiazine** (Sulfadiazene; Eon)

How Supplied:
Tablet: 500 mg.

Administration:
PO: Rapidly and well absorbed.

Dose:
Bacterial infections:
    Loading: 2–4 gm × 1.
    Maintenance: 2–4 gm/24 hr divided in 3–6 doses.
Malarial infections: No longer considered drug of choice when
used alone.

Elimination: Renal excretion.

Spectrum/Toxicity: See Sulfisoxazole, p. 29.

■ **Sulfamethizole** (Thiosulful Forte; Wyeth-Ayerst)

How Supplied:
Tablet: 500 mg.

Administration:
PO: Well absorbed.

Dose:
Loading/maintenance: 500–1000 mg, tid/qid.

Elimination/Spectrum/Toxicity: See Sulfisoxazole, p. 29.

Indication: UTI only because of lower blood concentrations
than other sulfonamides.

POORLY ABSORBED SULFONAMIDES
■ **Sulfasalazine** (Azulfidine, Azulfidine EN-Tabs;
   Pharmacia Adria)

How Supplied:
Tablet/enteric-coated tablet: 500 mg.

Administration:
PO: Poorly absorbed from GI tract. Broken down in gut to sulfapyridine (rapidly absorbed) and 5-aminosalicylate (poorly absorbed); the effective agent in inflammatory bowel disease.

Indication: Mild to moderate ulcerative colitis or as adjunctive therapy in severe ulcerative colitis. May also prolong remission periods between acute attacks. Enteric-coated form for patients with GI intolerance (nausea, vomiting) to regular Azulfidine even at lowered dose. Sometimes also used in treatment of regional enteritis.

Dose: 3–4 gm/day initially, then 500 mg qid.

Elimination:
Sulfapyridine: Hepatic metabolism and renal excretion.
5-Aminosalicylic acid: Excreted in feces.

Toxicity: Nausea, fever, arthralgias, rashes in up to 20%; desensitization may be effective. Heinz body anemia, acute hemolysis in patients with G-6-PD deficiency, and agranulocytosis rarely.

TOPICAL SULFONAMIDES
■ Sulfacetamide Sodium (Sodium Sulamyd; Schering)

How Supplied:
Ophthalmic ointment:
    100 mg/gm (10%, 3.5 gm tube).
Ophthalmic solution:
    100 mg/ml (10%, 5, 15 ml dropper bottle).
    300 mg/ml (30%, 15 ml dropper bottle).

Administration/Dose:
Topical:
    1–2 drops of 10% or 30% solution q2h for severe infections.
    1–2 drops tid or qid for chronic conditions.
Ointment: qhs if no corneal wound.

Contraindication: Known hypersensitivity to sulfonamides.

Toxicity: Local irritation (i.e., stinging, burning); rarely Stevens-Johnson syndrome or allergic reaction.

■ Silver Sulfadiazene (Boots. Par. Silvadene; Marion.)

How Supplied:
Cream, 1%: 100 mg/gm; 20, 50, 400 gm.

Administration/Dose:
Topical: Apply over burn (1/16 inch thick) bid.

Indication: Drug of choice for prevention of infection in burns. Slow release of silver from the compound is selectively toxic to microorganisms and reduces colonization.

Toxicity: Infrequently causes allergic reactions, burning, pruritus, rash, transient neutropenia/leukopenia. If used over large surface area, may be absorbed systemically (see Sulfisoxazole, p. 29).

COMBINATION SULFONAMIDES

■ Trimethoprim (TMP)-Sulfamethoxazole (SMX) (Bactrim, Bactrim DS, Bactrim Pediatric Suspension, Bactrim IV Infusion; Roche. Septra, Septra DS, Septra IV infusion; Burroughs Wellcome)

How Supplied:
Tablet: 80 mg TMP + 400 mg SMX or 160 mg TMP + 800 mg SMX (double strength [DS]).
Suspension: 40 mg TMP + 200 mg SMX/5 ml (20 ml and 1 pint bottle).
Injection: 16 mg TMP + 80 mg SMX/ml (5, 10, 20, 30 ml vial).

Administration:
IV: Dilute in D_5W for slow infusion.
PO: Well absorbed.

Mechanism of action: Trimethoprim binds dihydrofolate reductase, thereby blocking production of tetrahydrofolate from dihydrofolate; combination with sulfamethoxazole blocks two consecutive steps in biosynthesis of nucleic acids and proteins essential to many bacteria.

Dosage/Indication:
UTI: 160 mg TMP + 800 mg SMX bid (if mild) or tid (if severe) × 10 days or 320 mg TMP + 1600 mg SMX as one dose (uncomplicated UTI in adults).

Bacterial respiratory tract infections (e.g., acute exacerbation of chronic bronchitis): 240 TMP + 1200 SMX tid.

GI infection (shigellosis and typhoid fever in certain instances such as chloramphenicol-resistant strains): 160 TMP + 800 SMX bid × 15 days.

P. carinii: 15–20 mg/kg/day TMP + 75–100 mg/kg/day SMX in 3–4 divided doses.

Elimination: Renal excretion.

Spectrum: See Table 3-1.

Contraindications: Renal disease, especially if creatinine clearance less than 15 ml/min; severe hepatic impairment; allergy to sulfonamides or TMP; blood dyscrasias; pregnancy at or near term; lactation; megaloblastic anemia because of folate deficiency.

Toxicity:
1. Skin manifestations constitute 75% of untoward reactions (see Sulfisoxazole, p. 29). Severe reactions are rare (e.g., Stevens-Johnson syndrome, toxic epidermal necrolysis).
2. Nausea, vomiting, glossitis, stomatitis.
3. Megaloblastosis, leukopenia, or thrombocytopenia in folate-deficient patients.
4. Hematologic reactions (see Sulfisoxazle, p. 29).
5. Increased incidence in AIDS patients when used to treat *P. carinii* pneumonia: fever, malaise, rash, or leukopenia elevated in 45%–90%.
6. Increased risk in elderly: severe skin reactions, bone marrow suppression.

Interaction: Increased risk of elevated transaminase levels and thrombocytopenia when used with diuretics, especially in elderly patients with heart failure. May potentiate oral anticoagulants, hypoglycemics, phenytoin, methotrexate.

■ Sulfisoxazole (Azo Gantrisin)/Sulfamethoxazole (Azo Gantanol)–Phenazopyridine HCL (Roche)

How Supplied:
Tablet: 500 mg sulfisoxazole + 50 mg (Azo Gantrisin) or 100 mg (Azo Gantanol) phenazopyridine HCl (urinary analgesic).

Administration:
PO: Well absorbed.

Mechanism of Action: Addition of phenazopyridine HCl has specific analgesic effect on urinary tract, relieving pain and burning.

Dose for Acute, Painful Phase of UTI:
Azo Gantrisin:
    Loading: 4–6 tablets.
    Maintenance: 2 tablets qid for up to 2 days, then continue treatment with sulfisoxazole alone.
Azo-Gantanol:
    Loading: 4 tablets.
    Maintenance: 2 tablets bid × 2 days, then continue Rx as above.

Contraindications:
Phenazopyridine HCl: glomerulonephritis, severe hepatitis, uremia, pyelonephritis of pregnancy with GI disturbances (see Sulfisoxazole, p. 29).
NOTE: Orange-red dye (phenazopyridine HCl) will color urine.

Spectrum/Toxicity: See Sulfisoxazole, p. 29.

ANTIBIOTICS

PENICILLINS
Table 3-3 lists common penicillins (PCNs).

Mechanism of Action
Inhibits peptidoglycan synthesis in bacterial cell walls. Bacterial resistance depends on the presence of ß-lactamase

Table 3-3
PENICILLINS

Chemical Name	Brand Name (Co.)	Usual Dose Range
PENICILLIN G AND V		
Penicillin G benzathine	Bicillin L-A (Wyeth-Ayerst)	0.6–2.4 million U IM
Penicillin G potassium	Pfizerpen (Roerig)	5–30 million U/day IV or IM, divided
Penicillin G procaine	Wycillin (Wyeth-Ayerst)	0.3–4.8 million U/day divided q12–24h
Penicillin G benzathine	Bicillin C-R, 900/300 (Wyeth-Ayerst)	1.2–2.4 million U IM
Penicillin V potassium	Betapen VK (Bristol-Myers)	250–500 mg PO qid
	Ledercillin VK oral solution (Lederle)	
	Pen-Vee K (Wyeth-Ayerst)	
	Veetids (Squibb)	
PENICILLINASE-RESISTANT PCNS		
Oxacillin sodium	Bactocill (Smith-Kline Beecham)	2–4 gm/day PO divided qid
Cloxacillin sodium	Tegopen (Bristol-Myers)	250–1000 mg PO qid
Dicloxacillin sodium	Dynapen (Bristol-Myers)	125–500 mg PO qid
	Pathocil (Wyeth-Ayerst)	
Nafcillin sodium	Nafcil (Bristol-Myers)	250–500 mg PO q4–6h or
	Unipen (Wyeth-Ayerst)	500 mg–1 gm q4 h
AMINOPENICILLINS		
Ampicillin	Omnipen (Wyeth-Ayerst)	500–3000 mg IV or 500–1500 mg IM q4–6h
	Polycillin (Bristol-Myers)	or 250–1000 mg PO q6h
	Principen (Squibb)	Uncomplicated *N. gonorrhoeae*: 3.5 gm PO
		with 1 gm probenicid

Continued.

Table 3-3
PENICILLINS—cont'd

Chemical Name	Brand Name (Co.)	Usual Dose Range
AMINOPENICILLINS—cont'd		
Amoxicillin	Amoxil (Smith-Kline Beecham) Polymox (Bristol-Myers)	250–500 mg tid Uncomplicated *N. gonorrhoeae*: 3.5 gm PO with 1 gm probenicid
	Trimox (Squibb) Wymox (Wyeth-Ayerst)	
Bacampicillin	Spectrobid (Roerig)	400–800 mg po bid Uncomplicated *N. gonorrhoeae*: 1.6 gm PO with 1 gm probenicid
CARBOXYPENICILLINS		
Carbenicillin	Geopen (Roerig) Geocillin (Roerig)	1–2 gm IM or IV q6h 2–4 gm/day PO divided qid
Ticarcillin	Ticar (Smith-Kline Beecham)	1–3 gm q4–6h, maximum 16 gm/day
UREIDOPENICILLINS AND OTHER BROAD-SPECTRUM PCNS		
Azlocillin sodium	Azlin (Miles)	2–4 gm q4–6h, maximum 24 gm/24 hr
Mezlocillin sodium	Mezlin (Miles)	6–18 gm/day IM or OV divided q4–6h Uncomplicated *N. gonorrhoeae*: 1–2 gm IV or IM with 1 gm probenicid PO
Piperacillin sodium	Pipracil (Lederle)	12–24 gm/day IM or IV divided q4–8h Uncomplicated *N. gonorrhoeae*: 2 gm IM

37

enzymes, and this property may be transferred by plasmids (extrachromosomal DNA) that encode for its synthesis or may arise de novo from spontaneous mutation.

General Considerations

1. Discovered in 1928 by Alexander Fleming as a bactericidal mold.
2. Developed in 1940s.
3. Basic structure:
   a. Thiazolidine ring.
   b. ß-Lactam ring.
   c. Side chain.
4. Naturally occurring penicillins are derivatives of penicillin G (benzylpenicillin).
5. Changes in side chains result in semisynthetic PCNs and alter susceptibility to inactivating enzymes (ß-lactamases).
6. International unit of PCN is the specific PCN activity contained in 0.6 µg crystalline sodium salt of PCN-G.
7. Classification based on spectrum of antimicrobial activity (Table 3-4):
   a. PCN-G and PCN-V: effective against gram-positive cocci but hydrolyzed by penicillinase, so not active against most *S. aureus.*
   b. Penicillinase-resistant PCNs (e.g., methicillin, nafcillin, oxacillin, cloxacillin, dicloxacillin, floxacillin). Drugs of choice for infections because of *S. aureus;* less effective against organisms susceptible to PCN-G and PCN-V.
   c. Aminopenicillins (e.g., ampicillin, amoxicillin, hetacillin, cyclacillin, bacampicillin). Coverage extended to gram-negative microorganisms (e.g., *H. influenzae, E. coli, P. mirabilis*). Not penicillinase resistant.
   d. Carboxypenicillins (e.g., carbenicillin, ticarcillin). Coverage extended to *Pseudomonas, Enterobacter, Proteus.* Not penicillinase resistant.
   e. Ureidopenicillins and other extended-spectrum PCNs (e.g., azlocillin, mezlocillin, piperacillin); useful against *Pseudomonas, Klebsiella,* and other gram-negative bacteria. Aminocillin poor against gram-positive microorganisms but effective in treating *Enterobacteriaceae.* Not penicillinase resistant. May be used in combination with other ß-lactam antibiotics to achieve synergistic kill.

Table 3-4
ANTIBACTERIAL SPECTRUM PENICILLIN + β-LACTAM ANTIBIOTICS

Bacteria	PCN G and V	PCNase-resistant PCNs (Cloxacillin)*	Amino PCNs (Ampicillin)†	Carboxy PCNs (Ticarcillin)‡	Extended Spectrum PCNs (Piperacillin)§	Imipenem
GRAM-POSITIVE COCCI						
Peptococcus	+	–	+	+	+	+
Peptostreptococcus (anaerobic)	+	–	+	+	+	+
Staphylococcus	–	+	–	–	–	V
Streptococcus	+	–	+	+	+	+
faecalis (Enterococcus) other sp.	+	–	+	–	+	+
GRAM-POSITIVE BACILLI						
Actinomyces (anaerobic)	+	–	–	–	–	+
Clostridium difficile	–	–	+	+	+	+
Clostridium perfringens	+	–	+	+	+	+
Listeria	+	–	+	+	+	+

+, Sensitive; –, resistant; V, varied sensitivity.
*Penicillinase-resistant PCNs include nafcillin, oxacillin, dicloxacillin, methicillin, and floxacillin.
†Aminopenicillins include ampicillin, amoxicillin, cyclacillin, and bacampicillin.
‡Carboxypenicillins include carbenicillin and ticarcillin.
§Extended-spectrum penicillins include ureidopenicillins (azlocillin, mezlacillin, piperacillin).

Continued.

ANTIBIOTICS

Table 3-4
ANTIBACTERIAL SPECTRUM PENICILLIN + β-LACTAM ANTIBIOTICS—Cont'd

Bacteria	PCN G and V	PCNase-resistant PCNs Cloxacillin*	Amino PCNs (Ampicillin)†	Carboxy PCNs (Ticarcillin)‡	Extended Spectrum PCNs (Piperacillin)§	Imipenem
GRAM-NEGATIVE COCCI						
Neisseria	+	-	+	+	+	+
GRAM-NEGATIVE BACILLI						
Bacteroides (anaerobic)	>	-	-	>	+	+
Enterobacter	-	-	-	+	+	+
Escherichia coli	-	-	>	+	>	+
Haemophilus influenzae	>	-	>	+	+	+
Klebsiella	-	-	-	-	+	+
Proteus	-	-	>	+	+	>
Pseudomonas	-	-	-	>	+	+
Salmonella	-	-	>	>	>	+
Serratia	-	-	-	>	>	+
Shigella	-	-	>	-	>	+

8. After absorption:
   a. Achieve therapeutic levels in tissues and in certain secretions (e.g., joint, pleural, and pericardial fluid and bile).
   b. Low levels in prostatic secretions, brain tissue, intraocular fluid.
   c. Variable CSF levels: less than 1% of plasma levels unless inflammation present, then up to 5% plasma levels.
9. Rapidly eliminated by glomerular filtration and renal tubular secretion; thereby highly concentrated in urine.
   Contraindications: Known penicillin allergy or allergy to cephalosporins; significant asthma.

Adverse Reactions:

1. Hypersensitivity reactions are most common PCN side effect (0.7%–10%). PCNs are most common cause of drug allergy. Manifestations range from maculopapular or urticarial rash (common) and fever to bronchospasm, vasculitis, serum sickness, exfoliative dermatitis, Stevens-Johnson syndrome, and anaphylaxis (uncommon). Fatal episodes of anaphylaxis may occur even with very small doses of PCN, as used in skin testing. May also note eosinophilia and interstitial nephritis.
2. Minimal direct toxicity; thus other adverse reactions are rare:
   a. Pain and sterile inflammatory reaction at site of IM injection.
   b. Phlebitis or thrombophlebitis when given IV.
   c. Nausea, vomiting, diarrhea.
   d. Inadvertent injection of IM repository PCN intravascularly or immediately adjacent to an artery or sciatic nerve may result in severe neurovascular damage, with resultant paralysis, gangrene requiring amputation, or sloughing and necrosis at injection site.
3. Reactions unrelated to hypersensitivity or toxicity:
   a. Superinfection (e.g., candidiasis) secondary to changes in microflora.
   b. Pseudomembranous colitis because of *C. difficile* overgrowth and toxin production. Less frequent with parenteral than with oral administration.
   c. Jarisch-Herxheimer reaction seen in treatment of syphilis (fever, vascular collapse, sometimes fatal) because of hypersensitivity to antigens released during rapid lysis of spirochetes.

PENICILLIN G AND PENICILLIN V
■ Penicillin G Potassium (Pfizerpen; Roerig)

How Supplied:
Injection: 5 and 20 million U/vial.

Administration: IM, IV. Intrapleural, intrathecal, or other local infusion.

Dose: 5–30 million U/day in 4–6 divided doses, or continuous infusion.

Severe infections (e.g., meningitis): Dose every 2–3 hr or continuous infusion.

Elimination: Rapid renal excretion (elimination T½ 30 min). Half-life prolonged by renal failure, but toxic levels do not accumulate because of inactivation of 7%–10% of drug per hour by liver.

Spectrum (See Table 3-4):
1. Drug of choice for bacteremia, pneumonia, endocarditis, pericarditis, empyema, meningitis, and other severe infections because of susceptible strains of streptococci. Pneumococci and staphylococci: minimum 5 million U/day.
2. Syphilis: In adults, usually treated with penicillin G procaine (+probenicid) or penicillin G benzathine.
3. Gonorrheal endocarditis: 4–5 million U/day.
4. Meningococcic meningitis: 1–2 million U IM q2h, continuous IV drip 20–30 million U/day.
5. Actinomycosis: 1–20 million U/day, depending on site of infection.
6. Clostridial infections: 20 million U/day as adjunct to antitoxin.
7. *Listeria* monocytogenes: meningitis 15–20 million U/day × 2 wk; endocarditis 15–20 million U/day × 4 wk.
8. Gram-negative bacteremia because of *E. coli,* Enterobacter, *A. faecalis,* salmonella, shigella, and proteus; 20–80 million U/day.

Toxicity: Hypersensitivity reactions (see PCNs, p. 35). Large doses given parenterally (greater than 20 million U/day, or less in renal insufficiency) may be neurotoxic, with lethargy, confusion, myoclonus, or seizures. Hyperkalemia (1.7 mEq K or Na/L million U).

■ Penicillin G Benzathine (Bicillin L-A; Wyeth-Ayerst)

How Supplied:
IM injection: 300,000 U/ml in 10 ml multiple-dose vial.
    600,000 U/ml in 1, 2, 4 ml sterile cartridge-needle unit.

Dose: 0.6–2.4 million U × 1.

Elimination: See PCN-G, p. 35. Is slowly released from injection site to give uniform levels over 2–4 wk (longer with higher dose).

Spectrum   (see Table 3-4):

Indication:
1. Treatment/prophylaxis of group A ß-hemolytic streptococcal pharyngitis or pyoderma: PCN-G benzathine 1–2 million U single dose.
2. Treatment of primary, secondary, and latent syphilis of less than 1 year duration: PCN-G benzathine, single IM dose, 2.4 million U.
3. Latent syphilis of more than 1 year duration: PCN-G benzathine 2.4 million U/wk for 3–4 wk.
4. Neurosyphilis and cardiovascular syphilis: See PCN-G, p. 42.
5. Erysipeloid: PCN-G benzathine, 1.2 million U single dose.

Contraindications: Known PCN or cephalosporin allergy; significant asthma. Avoid intravenous or intraarterial administration or injection into or near major nerves or blood vessels to avoid neurovascular damage.

Toxicity: See PCN, p. 35. Ninety percent of patients with secondary syphilis (less frequently with other forms) experience Jarisch-Herxheimer reaction; chills, fever, headache, myalgias, arthralgias, and rash develop within a few hours of first PCN injection. Usually self-limited. Symptoms will not recur with subsequent PCN injections, and therapy should be continued.

■ Penicillin G Procaine (Wycillin; Wyeth-Ayerst)

How Supplied:
IM injection: 600,000 U/ml, 1, 2, 4 ml sterile cartridge-needle unit; 600,000 contains 120 mg procaine for anesthetic effects.

Dose: 0.3–1.2 million U/24 hr divided q12–24h; max 4.8 million U/day.

Elimination: See PCN-G, p. 42. Levels peak in 1–3 hr and are maintained for 2–4 days.

Spectrum   (See PCN-G, p. 42):
1. Indicated in treatment of moderately severe infections with PCN-G–sensitive strains that are sensitive to low but sustained serum levels common to this dosage form. Aqueous parenteral PCN-G in high doses preferable for acute infections, when bacteremia is present, and when high sustained serum levels are required.
2. In treatment of specific infections:
   a. Uncomplicated pneumococcal pneumonia, otitis media, or paranasal sinusitis: procaine PCN-G 300,000–600,000 U bid IM.
   b. Uncomplicated gonococcal urethritis or pharyngitis: PCN-G procaine, 4.8 million U injected into two sites with 1 gm probenecid PO.
   c. Syphilis: 600,000 U IM q day × 8 days or 10–15 days for late disease.
   d. Streptococcal pharyngitis secondary to *S. pyogenes* (group A ß-hemolytic *Streptococcus*): Procaine PCN-G, 600,000 U/day IM for 10 days.

Contraindications: See Penicillin G Benzathinen, p. 43.

Toxicity   (See PCN, p. 35):
1. Also, local sterile inflammatory reactions or sterile abscesses at injection site.
2. Contains 120 mg procaine/300,000 U; rapid liberation of procaine may cause an immediate reaction with CNS effects (tinnitus, headaches, hallucinations, and sometimes seizures), myocardial depression and conduction disturbances, or systemic vasodilatation.

Monitor: Renal and hematopoietic function with prolonged use.

Interactions: Potentiated by probenicid.

■ Penicillin G Benzathine, Penicillin G Procaine
(Bicillin C-R, Bicillin C-R 900/300; Wyeth-Ayerst)

How Supplied:
IM injection:
1. Bicillin C-R has equal amounts benzathine PCN-G and procaine PCN-G:
   a. 300,000 U/ml; 10 ml multiple-dose vial (150,000 U pro-
      caine + 150,000 U benzathine).
   b. 600,000 U/ml; 1, 2, and 4 ml sterile cartridge-needle
      unit, single dose.
2. Bicillin C-R 900/300 = 900,000 U benzathine PCN-G and
   300,000 U procaine PCN-G.
   a. 1.2 million U/2 ml; 2 ml sterile cartridge-needle, single-
      dose unit.

Dose:
Pneumococcal infections (except meningitis) 1:1.2 million
U/dose q2–3 days until afebrile for 48 hr.
Streptococcal infections (group A): 2.4 million U/dose × 1.

Elimination: See PCN-G, p. 42.

Spectrum:
1. Moderate to severe infection of upper respiratory tract, scar-
   let fever, erysipelas, and skin and soft tissue infections
   because of susceptible streptococci.
2. Group D strep enterococcus may be resistant.
3. PCN-G sodium or potassium recommended in presence of
   bacteremia.
4. Moderate to severe pneumonia or otitis media because of
   pneumococci.
5. PCN-G sodium or potassium preferred.
   a. In severe infections while acute.
   b. When high-sustained serum levels required.

Contraindication: See PCN-G Benzathine p. 43.

ANTIBIOTICS

Toxicity: See PCN-G procaine, p. 44.

Monitor: See PCN-G procaine p. 44.

■ **Penicillin V Potassium** (Betapen VK; Bristol-
Myers. Pen-Vee K; Wyeth-Ayerst. Veetids; Squibb)

How Supplied:
Tablet: 250 mg (400,000 U); 500 mg (800,000 U).
Solution: 125, 250 mg/5 ml in 100, 200 ml bottle.

Administration:
PO: Better absorbed from GI tract than PCN-G because resists
inactivation by gastric acid. Blood levels slightly higher when
taken on an empty stomach.
  250–500 mg/dose qid; continue for 10 days for streptococcal
infections of upper respiratory tract.

Elimination/Spectrum: See PCN-G, p. 42.

Contraindications: See PCN-G Benzathine p.43.

Toxicity: See PCN, p. 35. Contains 2.8 mEq K/gm.

Interactions: Potentiated by probenicid.

PENICILLINASE-RESISTANT PENICILLINS
■ **Cloxacillin Sodium** (Cloxapen; Smith-Kline
Beecham.)

How Supplied:
PO:
  Capsule: 250, 500 mg.
  Suspension: 125 mg/5 ml.

Administration:
PO: 1–2 hr before or 2 hr after meals. Rapidly absorbed; more
efficiently on an empty stomach.

Mechanism of Action: Isoxazolyl penicillin, resistant to cleav-
age by penicillinase.

Dose: 250–1000 mg qid.

Elimination: Rapidly excreted by kidney; half-life 30–60 min. No dose interval adjustment required with renal impairment.

Spectrum/Indications: (See Table 3-4.) Indicated for penicillinase-producing staphylococcus infections; particularly useful for *S. aureus*. Not a substitute for Penicillin G when susceptibility allows; oral route not a substitute for parenteral because of variability in intestinal absorption.

Contraindications: PCN, cephalosporin allergy.

Toxicity: Anaphylaxis, urticaria, GI upset, blood dyscrasias (mild reversible leukopenia), AST (SGOT) elevated.

Monitor: Blood, renal, and liver function with long-term use.

Interactions: Potentiated by probenicid.

■ Dicloxacillin Sodium (Pathocil; Wyeth-Ayerst)

How Supplied:
PO:
 Capsule: 250, 500 mg.
 Suspension: 62.5 mg/5 ml.

Administration:
PO: well absorbed.

Dose:
125–500 mg qid. Group A ß-hemolytic strep infections should be treated for 10 days to prevent development of acute rheumatic fever or glomerulonephritis.

Elimination: See Cloxacillin p. 46.

Spectrum: See Table 3-4 and Cloxacillin, p. 46.

Indications: Mild to moderate upper respiratory and localized skin and soft tissue infections because of susceptible organisms.

Contraindications: See Cloxacillin, p. 46.

Toxicity: See Cloxacillin, p. 46.

Monitor Interactions: See Cloxacillin, p. 46.

◼ Oxacillin Sodium (Bactocill; Smith-Kline Beecham)

How Supplied:
PO: 250, 500 mg capsules.

Administration:
PO: 1–2 hr before or 2 hr after meals; well absorbed.

Mechanism of action: See Cloxacillin, p. 46.

Dose: 2–4 gm/day divided qid × ≥ 5 days.

Elimination: See Cloxacillin, p. 46.

Spectrum: See Table 3–4 and Cloxacillin, p. 46.

Indications: See Cloxacillin, p. 46.

Contraindications: See Cloxacillin, p. 46.

Toxicity: See Cloxacillin, p. 46.

Monitor: See Cloxacillin, p. 46.

Interactions: See Cloxacillin, p. 46.

◼ Nafcillin Sodium (Unipen; Wyeth-Ayerst)

How Supplied:
PO: 250 mg capsules.
Parenteral: 1, 2 gm single-dose vial, buffered.
IV: 1, 2 gm single-dose piggyback, buffered.

Administration: Parenteral preferred to PO because of variable absorption.

Dose:
PO: 250–500 mg q4–6h; max 1 gm q4h.
IV: 500 mg to 1.5 gm q4h.

Elimination: See Cloxacillin, p. 46. Significant hepatic elimination in bile.

Spectrum: See Cloxacillin, p. 46. Adequate CSF levels obtainable for treatment of staphylococcal meningitis.

Indications/Contraindications/Toxicity: See Cloxacillin p. 46.

Monitor/Interactions: See Cloxacillin, p. 46.

AMINOPENCILLINS
■ **Ampicillin** (Omnipen, Omnipen-N; Wyeth-Ayerst. Principen; Squibb)

How Supplied:
PO:
    Capsule: 250, 500 mg.
    Suspension: 125 mg/5 ml; 250 mg/15 ml.
    Parenteral: 125, 250, 500 mg; 1, 2 gm single-dose vial;
    10 gm bulk vial.
    Administration: PO well absorbed, IV; IM.
    Mechanism of action: Bactericidal.

Dose:
PO: Preferably 1–2 hr before or 2 hr after meals. 250–1000 mg/dose q6h.
    Uncomplicated *N. gonorrhoeae:* 3.5 gm single dose with
    1 gm probenecid.
IM/IV:
    Meningitis and severe infections: 6–12 gm/day divided
    q4–6h.
    Other infections: 500–3000 mg/dose IV or 500–1500
    mg/dose IMq4–6h.

Elimination: Mostly renal, with half-life approximately 1 hr; dosage adjustment required in presence of renal dysfunction. Also appears in bile (unless common bile duct obstructed), undergoes enterohepatic circulation, and appears in feces.

Spectrum: (See Table 3-4). Bactericidal for gram-positive and gram-negative organisms. Not effective therapy for penicillinase-producing strains (e.g., *Staphylococcus, H. influenzae*).

Indications: GU and GI infections because of gonorrhea, *E. coli, P. mirabilis,* enterococci, shigella, salmonella; respiratory infections because of nonpenicillinase producing *H. influenza,* staphylococci, and streptococci (including *S. pneumoniae*); meningitis because of *N. meningitides.*

Contraindications: PCN or cephalosporin hypersensitivity; infection with penicillinase-producing organism.

Toxicity: Maculopapular rash (approximately 9% incidence, especially in patients with infectious mononucleosis or concurrently receiving allopurinol), pruritus, urticaria, GI distress including diarrhea (in more than 50% of patients taking more than 2 gm/day PO), eosinophilia, superinfection, bowel flora overgrowth, pseudomembranous colitis (more frequent after oral than parenteral administration). High doses sometimes result in seizures or CNS excitation. Contains approximately 3 mEq Na/gm.

Monitor: Phenotoin, hexobarbital levels when given concurrently.

Interactions: May potentiate carbamazepine, methylprednisolone, cyclosporine, digoxin, theophylline, warfarin, ergotamine, terfenadine, triazolam. Avoid use with lovastatin. Potentiated by probenicid.

■ **Amoxicillin** (Amoxil; Smith Kline Beecham. Wymox; Wyeth-Ayerst)

How Supplied:
PO:
   Capsule: 250, 500 mg.

Chewable tablet: 125, 250 mg.
Oral suspension: 125, 250 mg/5 ml.

Administration:
PO: Well absorbed (peak plasma concentration approximately twice that of ampicillin for same oral dose regardless of timing around meals).

Dose: Adults: 250–500 mg tid.
Uncomplicated *N. gonorrhoeae:* 3 gm with 1 gm probenecid as single dose.

Elimination: Eliminated by kidney; half-life 1 hr but prolonged with probenecid.

Spectrum/Indications/Contraindications: See Table 3-4 and Ampicillin, p. 49. Not as effective as ampicillin against shigellosis.

Toxicity: See Ampicillin, p. 49. Diarrhea less frequent than with ampicillin; superinfection usually involves *Enterobacter, Pseudomonas,* or *Candida* and warrants therapy discontinuation and change.

Monitor: Blood, renal, and liver function in long-term use.

Interaction: Antagonized by tetracycline; potentiated by probenicid.

■ Bacampicillin (Spectrobid; Roerig)

How Supplied:
PO:
Suspension: 125 mg/5 ml (70, 100, 140, 200 ml).
Tablet: 400 mg.

Administration:
PO: Well absorbed; peak levels three times that of equivalent dose of ampicillin. Rapidly hydrolyzed to ampicillin. Tablets may be given without regard to meals, but PO suspension should be taken on an empty stomach.

Dose: 400–800 mg bid; continue at least 10 days with infections because of hemolytic streptococci to prevent occurrence of acute rheumatic fever and glomerulonephritis.

Acute uncomplicated *N. gonorrhoeae:* 1.6 gm + 1 gm probenecid, single dose.

Elimination/Spectrum/Indications: See Table 3-4 and Ampicillin, p. 49.

Toxicity: See Ampicillin, p. 49. More likely to cause epigastric distress than ampicillin, but less frequently associated with diarrhea.

■ Carbenicillin Indanyl Sodium (Geocillin; Roerig)

How Supplied:
Tablet: 500 mg (equal to 382 mg carbenicillin).

Administration:
PO: Although only low serum levels obtained, is hydrolyzed rapidly to carbenicillin, which is rapidly excreted in urine; thus main indication is treatment of UTI and prostatitis.

Mechanism of Action: Bactericidal; interferes with final cell wall synthesis of susceptible bacteria.

Dose: 2–4 gm/day divided qid; higher dose range for chronic infections or those caused by *Pseudomonas.* Adjust dose if severe renal impairment (creatinine clearance <20 ml/min).

Elimination: Renal; primarily excreted in urine, 30% unchanged.

Spectrum: See Table 3-4. Especially useful for *P. aeroginosa; *ampicillin-resistant indole positive *Proteus; E. coli; Enterobacter.*

Indications: Clinical pharmacologic attributes (see Elimination above) make it particularly useful for upper and lower urinary tract infections, asymptomatic bacteriuria, and prostatitis.

Contraindications: PCN allergy.

Toxicity: Usual adverse reactions to PCNs in general (see p. 41); abnormal platelet aggregation.

Monitor: Sodium content may rarely precipitate congestive heart failure.

Interactions: Blood levels increased and prolonged with concurrent probenicid.

■ Ticarcillin Sodium (Ticar; Smith-Kline Beecham)

How Supplied:
  1, 3, 6 gm vial.
  20, 30 gm bulk pharmacy vial.
  3 gm piggyback bottle.

Administration:
IM, IV.

Dose: 150–300 mg/kg/day in divided doses q4–6h, depending on weight and severity of infection. Max 24 gm/day; max single IM dose 2 gm.

Elimination: Excreted unchanged by kidneys. Serum half-life approximately 70 min; prolonged with probenecid. Half-life in patients with renal failure approximately 13 hr.

Spectrum: See Carbenicillin, p. 52. More active (two to four times) than carbenicillin against *P. aeruginosa;* thus is carboxycillin of choice.

Indications: See Table 3-4. Particularly useful when anaerobic organisms are involved in infections of female genital tract including endometritis, PID, TOA, intraabdominal infection such as peritonitis and abscess; bacterial septicemia, lower respiratory tract infections such as emphysema, pneumonitis, and abscess; skin and soft tissue infections.

Contraindications: PCN allergy.

Toxicity: See Carbenicillin, p. 52. Contains 5.2–6.5 mEq Na/gm, but usually given in smaller doses than carbenicillin so that the incidence of electrolyte imbalance (e.g., hypernatremia) is lower.

Monitor: Electrolyte and cardiac status, including serum potassium, especially with long-term therapy.

UREIDOPENICILLINS AND OTHER BROAD-SPECTRUM PENICILLINS
■ Mezlocillin Sodium (Mezlin; Miles)

How Supplied:
Parenteral:
   1, 2, 3, 4 gm vial.
   2, 3, 4 gm infusion bottle.
   20 gm bulk package.

Administration:
IV, IM.

Dose: 100–300 mg/kg q4–6h; max 24 gm/24 hr. Usual dose 6–18 gm/day divided in 4–6 doses. Maximum single IM injection 2 gm. Usually given for 7–10 days. Treat group A ß-hemolytic streptococcal infections at least 10 days to decrease risk of rheumatic fever or glomerulonephritis.

   Acute uncomplicated gonococcal urethritis: 1–2 gm single dose IV or IM, usually with 1 gm probenecid PO.
   Prophylaxis:
      Vaginal hysterectomy: 4 gm IV 30–90 min before surgery and 4 gm at 6 hr and 12 hr.
      Cesarean section: 4 gm IV when cord is clamped and 4 gm at 4 hr and 8 hr.

Elimination: Renal excretion. Half-life approximately 1 hr; prolonged with probenecid or severe renal impairment.

Spectrum: See Table 3-2. More active than carbenicillin against *Klebsiella* and similar to ticarcillin.

Indications: See Table 3-4. For serious infections caused by susceptible microorganisms, especially gynecologic and intraabdominal infections such as PID, endometritis, and abscess resulting from *N. gonorrhoeae, Peptococcus, Peptostreptococcus, E. coli, Bacteroides, Proteus, Klebsiella,* and *Enterobacter.* Also useful for UTI, LRTI, septicemia, skin/skin structure infections because of above organisms.

Toxicity: (See PCNs p. 41.) Neuromuscular hyperirritability, seizures.

Monitor: Blood, renal, hepatic function; sodium levels.

■ Piperacillin Sodium (Pipracil; Lederle)

ANTIBIOTICS

How Supplied:
Parenteral:
   2, 3, 4 gm single use vial; 40 gm bulk vial.
   2, 3, 4 gm infusion bottle.

Administration:
IM, IV.

Dose: 12–24 gm/day, divided in 3–6 equal doses. Average duration of treatment is 7–10 days; in gynecologic infections treatment duration may be 3–10 days. Treat group A ß-hemolytic streptococcal infections at least 10 days to reduce risk of rheumatic fever or glomerulonephritis. Maximum single IM dose 2 gm per site (e.g., uncomplicated gonorrhea or UTI).
   Prophylaxis: 2 gm IV before surgery (or after the cord is clamped in case of cesarean section), 2 gm 2–6 hr later, then 2 gm 6 hr later.

Elimination: (See Mezlocillin, p. 54.)

Spectrum: (See Table 3-4). More active than carbenicillin against *Klebsiella* (see Mezlocillin p. 54), improved *Pseudomonas* coverage.

Indications: Also useful for bone and joint infections. If indicated, use as single-drug therapy or with an aminoglycoside in full therapeutic doses.

Toxicity: (See PCNs, p. 41.) Rarely, pseudomembranous colitis or interstitial nephritis. Approximately 1.85 mEq Na/gm.

Contraindications: PCN, cephalosporin allergy.

CEPHALOSPORINS

Mechanism of Action

Inhibits bacterial cell wall synthesis; therefore bactericidal.

General Considerations

1. Basic structure is 7-aminocephalosporanic acid (ß-lactam ring) nucleus with various semisynthetic side chains that confer different levels of antibacterial activity, changes in metabolism, and pharmacokinetics.
2. Classification by "generations" connotes features of antimicrobial activity (Table 3-5):
    a. First generation: e.g., cefazolin, cephalexin.
       Good against gram-positive bacteria, gram-positive cocci (except enterococci, *S. epidermidis,* and methicillin-resistant *S. aureus*); moderately active against gram-negative bacteria.
    b. Second generation: e.g., cefoxitin, cefamandole.
       Better against gram-negative microorganisms but not as good as third-generation cephalosporins.
    c. Third generation: e.g., ceftizoxime, ceftriaxone.
       Not as good against gram-positive cocci as first generation, but much more active against *Enterobacter* (even PCNase-producing strains).
       Subset (e.g., cefoperazone, ceftazidime, cefpiramide) also active against *Pseudomonas*.
3. Agents of choice for *Klebsiella* infections.
4. Certain second- and third-generation agents enter CNS/CSF in levels adequate for treatment of meningitis because of gram-negative enteric bacteria: cerfuroxime, moxalactam, cefotaxime, ceftizoxime, and ceftriaxone.
5. Primarily excreted by the kidney (except of cefoperazone); need to reduce dosage in patients with renal impairment. Probenecid lengthens half-life of all except moxalactam.
6. Widely used as prophylaxis during and after surgery.

7. Crosses the placenta.
8. Excreted into breast milk in low concentrations; however, potential adverse side effects for the nursing infant include modification of bowel flora, direct effects, and interference with culture results (e.g., fever workup).

Adverse Reactions

1. Hypersensitivity reactions are the most common side effects:
   a. Identical to those caused by PCNs, possibly because of shared ß-lactam ring.
   b. Immediate reactions: urticaria, bronchospasm, and anaphylaxis.
   c. Delayed reactions (after several days); maculopapular rash, with or without fever, and eosinophilia. More common than immediate reactions.
   d. May occur in 5%–20% of patients allergic to PCN.
   e. More likely in patients who report a recent, severe, immediate reaction to PCN; cephalosporins contraindicated in this group.
   f. Large doses may result in positive Coombs' test, usually without hemolysis.
   g. Rarely, bone marrow depression and granulocytopenia.
2. Nephrotoxicity:
   a. Not as common as with aminoglycosides or polymyxins.
   b. At higher risk:
      (1) If preexisting renal disease and no dosage adjustment.
      (2) Concurrent administration of gentamicin or tobramycin.
      (3) Older than 60 years of age.
3. GI effects: diarrhea, pseudomembranous colitis.
4. Intolerance to alcohol (disulfiram-like reaction) occasionally reported with cefamandole, moxalactam, and cefoperazone.
5. Vitamin K–reversible coagulopathy:
   a. Reported with cefamandole, moxalactam, and cefoperazone.
   b. Hypoprothrombinemia, thrombocytopenia, and/or platelet dysfunction.
   c. Patients who are elderly or malnourished or those with renal impairment at higher risk.

ANTIBIOTICS

FIRST-GENERATION CEPHALOSPORINS

■ **Cefazolin Sodium** (Ancef; Smith-Kline Beecham. Kefzol; Lilly)

How Supplied:
Parenteral:
    500 mg in 1 gm vial.
    500 mg in 1 gm dual-compartment vial.
    500 mg in 1 gm plastic bag for infusion.
    500 mg in 1 gm vial and diluent container.
    5, 10 gm multiple-dose vial.

Administration: *IM, IV.*

Dose: 500 mg to 1.5 gm tid–qid; max 12 gm/day. (Longer half-life allows less frequent dosing.) Adjust dose if renal impairment.

Elimination: Excreted by kidneys; half-life 1.8 hr.

Spectrum: (See Table 3-5.) Better against *E. coli* and *Klebsiella* than other first generation cephalosporins and not as resistant to degradation by staphylococcal ß-lactamase.

Indications: UTI, genital infections; biliary tract infections; septicemia; bone, joint, and skin infections; endocarditis; and perioperative prophylaxis for procedures classified as contaminated, potentially contaminated, or high risk if infection should occur.

Contraindication: Cephalosporin or PCN allergy.

Toxicity: See Cephalosporins, p. 57. Relatively less nephrotoxic. Contains 2.1 mEq NA/gm.

■ **Cephalexin** (Keflex, Keftab; Dista)

How Supplied:
PO:
    Pulvules: 250, 500 mg tablets,
    Suspension: 125 mg/5 ml and 250 mg/5 ml

Administration:
PO: Well absorbed without regard to meals.

Dose: 250–1000 mg qid. Use 500 bid for strep pharyngitis for 10 days, skin infections, uncomplicated cystitis.

Elimination: Renal excretion; half-life 0.9 hr.

Spectrum/Indications: (See Table 3-3, and Cefazolin, p. 58.)

Contraindications: (See Cefazolin p. 58.)

Toxicity: (See Cephalosporins, p. 57.) Not nephrotoxic.

■ **Cephradine** (Cephradine; Biocraft, Lederle, Warner Chilcott)

How Supplied:
PO:
   Capsule: 250, 500 mg.
   Suspension: 125 mg/5 ml and 250 mg/5 ml.

Administration:
PO: Well absorbed rapidly.

Dose: 250–1000 mg qid.

Elimination: Excreted unchanged by kidneys; half-life 0.8 hr.

Spectrum/Indications: (See Table 3-5 and Cefazolin, p. 58.)

Toxicity: (See Cephalosporins, p. 57.) Not nephrotoxic.

■ **Cefadroxil** (Duricef; Bristol-Myers, Squibb)

How Supplied:
PO:
   Capsules: 500 mg.
   Tablets: 1 gm.
   Suspension: 125, 250, and 500 mg/5 ml.

Table 3-5

ANTIBACTERIAL SPECTRUM: COMMONLY USED CEPHALOSPORINS

Bacteria	First-Generation*		Second-Generation†		Third-Generation‡	
	Cefazolin	Cephalexin	Cefoxitin	Cefotetan	Ceftriaxone§	Ceftazidime§
GRAM-POSITIVE COCCI						
Peptococcus	−	−	+	+	+	+
Peptostreptococcus (anaerobic)	−	−	+	+	+	+
Staphylococcus	+	+	+	+	+	+
Staphylococcus epidermidis	+	+	+	−	V	−
Streptococcus faecalis	−	−	−	−	−	−
Streptococcus enterococcus	−	−	−	−	−	−
Other sp.	+	+	+	+	+	+
GRAM-POSITIVE BACILLI						
Actinomyces (anaerobic)						
Clostridium difficile	−	−	−	−	−	−
Clostridium perfringens	−	−	+	+	+	−
Listeria	−	−	−	−	−	−
GRAM-NEGATIVE COCCI						
Neisseria	+	+	+	+	+	+

Table 3-5
ANTIBACTERIAL SPECTRUM: COMMONLY USED CEPHALOSPORINS—Cont'd

Bacteria	First-Generation*		Second-Generation†	Third-Generation‡		
	Cefazolin	Cephalexin	Cefoxitin	Cefotetan	Ceftriaxone§	Ceftazidime§
GRAM-NEGATIVE BACILLI						
Bacteroides fragilis (anaerobic)	-	-	+		-	-
Other sp.	-	-	+	>	-	>
Enterobacter	>	>	>	>	>	>
Escherichia coli	+	+	+	>	+	+
Haemophilus influenzae	-	>	+	+	+	+
Klebsiella	+	+	+	+	+	+
Proteus	>	>	+	-	+	+
Pseudomonas	>	-	-	-	-	+
Salmonella	>	>	+	+	+	+
Serratia	-	-	+	+	+	+
Shigella	-	+	+	+	+	+

-, Resistant; +, sensitive; V = varied sensitivity.
*First-generation cephalosporins include: cefazolin, cephalexin, cephradine, and cefadroxil.
†Second-generation cephalosporins include: cefoxitin, cefamandole, cefaclor, cefuroxime, cefmetazole, and cefonanide.
‡Third-generation cephalosporins include: cefotetan, ceftriaxone, ceftazidime, cefotaxime, moxalactam, cefprozil, ceftizoxime, cefoperazone, cefixime, and cefpodoxime.
§Sufficient CSF penetration for treatment of bacterial meningitis.

Administration: *PO:* Well absorbed rapidly, without regard to meals, but less GI distress if taken with food.

Dose: 1–2 gm/24 hr, single dose or divided every 12 hr.

Elimination: Renal excretion; half-life 1.5 hr.

Spectrum: (See Table 3-5, and Cefazolin, p. 58.)

Indications: Most often used for UTI because of *E. coli, P. mirabilis, Klebsiella;* skin infections because of staph and/or strep; URTI because of group A ß-hemolytic strep (although PCN is drug of choice here)

Toxicity: (See Cephalosporins.) Not nephrotoxic.

SECOND-GENERATION CEPHALOSPORINS
■ Cefamandole Nafate (Mandol; Lilly)

How Supplied:
Parenteral:
   1, 2, 100 gm (bulk) vial.
   1, 2 gm flexible plastic bag and diluent container.

Dose: 500 mg to 2 gm q4–8h; max 12 gm/day. Reduce dose with renal impairment.

Elimination: Excreted by kidneys; half-life 45 min.

Spectrum: (See Table 3-5.) More active than first-generation cephalosporins against certain gram-negative bacteria (e.g., *H. influenzae, Enterobacter,* indole-positive *Proteus, E. coli, Klebsiella*).

Indications: Most commonly used to treat lower respiratory tract infections, UTIs, peritonitis, septicemia, and skin and skin structure infections. Also used for preoperative prophylaxis in intraabdominal and gynecologic surgery.

Toxicity: (See Cephalosporins, p. 57.) Hypersensitivity reactions; GI distress, pseudomembranous colitis; thrombocytopenia, neutropenia, positive direct Coombs' test; elevation of liver function test values; nephrotoxicity, especially if used with aminoglycosides; vitamin K-reversible coagulopathy; disulfiram-like reaction with ingestion of alcohol (i.e., nausea, vomiting, hypotension). Contains 3.3 mEq Na/gm.

Monitor: Renal status in seriously ill patients receiving maximum doses.

■ Cefoxitin Sodium (Mefoxin; Merck)

How Supplied:
Parenteral:
  1, 2 gm vial.
  1, 2 gm infusion bottle.
  10 gm bulk bottle.
  1, 2 gm ADD-vantage vial and diluent container.
  1, 2 gm premixed IV solution, single dose.

Dose: 1–2 gm q6–8h; max 12 gm/24 hr; reduce with renal impairment.
  Uncomplicated gonorrhea: 2 gm IM with 1 gm probenecid PO.
  Prophylaxis: 2 gm IV or IM 30–60 min before surgery or when the cord is clamped during a cesarean section.

Elimination: Excreted by kidneys; half-life 40 min.

Spectrum: (See Table 3-5.) Advantages include high degree of resistance to gram-negative bacteria ß-lactamase and greater degree of activity against anaerobes (especially *B. fragilis*) than other first- or second-generation agents; thereby especially useful for treatment of certain anaerobic and mixed aerobic-anaerobic infections (e.g., pelvic inflammatory disease, lung abscess).

Indications: (See Cefamandole, p. 62.) Specific gynecologic indications include endometritis, pelvic cellulitis and PID because of *E. coli, N. gonorrhoeae* (both penicillinase and non-penicillianse producing), and *Bacteroides.*

Toxicity: (See Cephalosporins, p. 57 and Cefamandole, p. 62.) Most common adverse effect is local reactions at site of injection. Rarely, renal impairment in patients with preexisting dysfunction. Contains 23 mEq Na/gm.

■ Cefaclor (Ceclor; Lilly)

How Supplied:
PO:
　　Pulvules: 250, 500 mg.
　　Suspension: 125, 187, 250, 375 mg/5 ml.

Administration:
PO: Well absorbed.

Dose:　250–500 mg tid.

Elimination:　Renal excretion; half-life 0.8 hr.

Spectrum:　(See Table 3-3.) Some activity against certain ß-lactamase–producing strains of *H. influenzae.*

Toxicity:　(See Cephalosporins, p. 57.) Most common adverse side effects are gastrointestinal symptoms (2.5%), hypersensitivity reactions (1.5%), general pruritus or vaginitis (<1%), and rarely thrombocytopenia or reversible interstitial nephritis.

■ Cefuroxime Sodium (Ceftin; Glaxo. Kefurox; Lilly. Zinacef; Glaxo)

How Supplied:
PO:
　　Tablet: 125, 250, 500 mg.
　　Suspension: 125 mg/5 ml.
Parenteral:
　　0.75, 1.5, 7.5 gm vial.
　　750 mg, 1.5 gm flexible plastic bag.
　　750 mg, 1.5 gm vial and diluent container.

Administration:
PO, IM, IV.

Dose:　0.75–3 gm tid–qid; max 9 gm/24 hr.
　　Uncomplicated gonorrhea: 1.5 gm IM divided in two doses with 1 gm probenecid PO.

Elimination: Excreted by kidneys; half-life 1.7 hr.

Spectrum: (See Table 3-5.) Similar activity to cefamandole (see p. 62), but resistant to ß-lactamases. CSF penetration sufficient to treat meningitis secondary to *H. influenzae* (even some strains resistant to ampicillin), *N. meningitidis,* and *S. pneumoniae.*

Indications: (See Cefamandole, p. 62.)

Toxicity: (See Cephalosporins, p. 57 and Cefamandole on p. 62.) Most frequent adverse effects are thrombophlebitis after IV administration (1%–2%), GI symptoms (<1%), hypersensitivity reactions (<1%). Not considered nephrotoxic, but reduce dosage in patients with renal impairment. Contains 2.4 mEq Na/gm.

ANTIBIOTICS

■ **Cefonicid Sodium** (Monocid; Smith-Kline Beecham)

How Supplied:
Parenteral:
    500 mg, 1 gm vial.
    1 gm piggyback vial.
    10 gm bulk vial.

Administration:
IM, IV.

Dose: 1 gm q24h.
    Prophylaxis: Single 1 gm dose before surgery or when the cord is clamped during a cesarean section.
    Severe or life-threatening infection: 2 gm q24h divided between two sites if given IM.

Elimination: Excreted by kidneys; long half-life of 4.5 hr permits once-daily dosage.

Spectrum: (See Table 3-5 and Cefamandole, p. 62.)

Toxicity: (See Cephalosporins, p. 57.) Most frequent side effects are injection site phenomena (6%), eosinophilia (3%),

thrombocytosis (2%), elevated liver function test values
(1%–2%). Less frequent (<1%) side effects include hypersensitivity reactions, neutropenia, positive Coombs' test, renal impairment. Contains 3.7 mEq Na/gm.

■ **Cefmetazole Sodium** (Zefazone; Upjohn)

How Supplied:
Parenteral: 1, 2 gm/ vial or 50 ml container.

Administration: IV, IM.

Dose: 2 gm q6–12h 5–14 days, usually IV. Uncomplicated
gonorrhea: 1 gm IM plus probenicid 1 gm PO.

Elimination: 85% excreted uncharged in urine, resulting in
high urinary concentrations. Decreased clearance and prolonged
half-life in patients with reduced renal function.

Spectrum: (See Cephalosporins, p. 56 and Cefamandole,
p. 62.)

Indications: (See Cephalosporins, p. 56 and Cefamandole,
p. 62.) Also used to treat intraabdominal infections.

Toxicity: (See Cephalosporins, p. 57 and Cefamandole, p. 62.)

Interactions: Possible potentiation of aminoglycoside-induced
nephrotoxicity.

THIRD-GENERATION CEPHALOSPORINS
■ **Cefotaxime Sodium** (Claforan; Hoechst-
   Roussel)

How Supplied:
Parenteral:
   500 mg; 1, 2 gm vial.
   1, 2 gm infusion bottle.
   10 gm bottle.
   1, 2 gm vial and diluent container.

Dose: 1–2 gm q4–12h, max 12 gm/day.

Uncomplicated gonorrhea: 1 gm IM, single dose.

Prophylaxis: single 1 gm dose IM or IV 30–90 min before surgery; in case of cesarean section 1 gm IV when cord is clamped followed by 1 gm IM or IV 6 and 12 hr later. Decrease dose in presence of renal or hepatic impairment and in the elderly.

Elimination: Eliminated by kidneys; half-life 1.1 hr.

Spectrum: (See Table 3-5.) Advantages include high degree of resistance to ß-lactamases and penetration into CSF adequate for treatment of gram-negative bacterial meningitis. (Not as good in treatment of *B. fragilis* as clindamycin and metronidazole.)

Indications: Lower respiratory tract infections, GU and gynecologic infections, bacteremia, and skin and intraabdominal infections because of susceptible organisms.

Toxicity: (See Cephalosporins, p. 57.) Most frequently, local reactions at site of injection (4%), hypersensitivity reactions (2%), and GI symptoms (1%) including pseudomembranous colitis. Contains 2.2 mEq Na/gm.

■ Cefixime (Suprax; Lederle)

How Supplied:
PO:
    Tablet: 200, 400 mg.
    Suspension: 100 mg/5 ml.

Administration: PO

Dose: 400 mg/day, in one or 2 doses.

Uncomplicated gonorrhea: 400 mg single dose.

Adjust dose with renal impairment or the elderly.

Elimination: 50% excreted unchanged in urine.

Spectrum: UTI, otitis media, bronchitis, gonorrheal cervicitis, and urethritis.

ANTIBIOTICS

Toxicity: (See Cephalosporins, p. 57 and Cefotaxime, p. 67.) Gastrointestinal events most commonly reported (up to 20%–30%) such as diarrhea or nausea; rarely, pseudomembranous enterocolitis. Overdosage may trigger seizures, especially in patients with renal impairment if dosage not reduced.

■ CeFZIL (Cefprozil; Bristol-Myers, Squibb)

How Supplied:
PO:
  Tablets: 250, 500 mg.
  Suspension: 125 mg/5 ml, 500 mg/5 ml.

Administration: PO; well absorbed.

Dose: 500 mg q12–24h. Reduce dose with renal impairment.

Elimination: 60% of administered dose recoverable in urine.

Spectrum/Indications: (See Table 3-5 and Cefotaxime, p. 67.) Most strains of *B. fragilis* resistant.

Contraindications: Cephalosporin allergy; prior history of colitis.

Toxicity: (See Cephalosporins, p. 57 and Cefotaxime, p. 67.)

Interactions: Aminoglycosides, potent diuretics given concurrently increase the risk for nephrotoxicity.

■ Ceftizoxime Sodium (Cefizox; Fujisawa)

How Supplied:
Parenteral:
  500 mg; 1, 2 gm vial and single dose container.
  10 gm bulk vial.
  1, 2 gm piggyback vial.

Administration:
IM, IV.

Dose: 1–2 gm bid–tid; max 2 gm/4 hr in life-threatening infections. Uncomplicated gonorrhea: 1 gm IM, single dose. Reduce dose with renal impairment.

Elimination: Excreted by kidneys; half-life 1.8 hr.

Spectrum: (See Table 3-5; Cefotaxime, p. 67.)

Indications: PID; uncomplicated gonorrhea; intraabdominal infections; septicemia; UTI; lower respiratory infections; meningitis; skin, bone, and joint infections.

Toxicity: (See Cephalosporins, p. 57.) Most frequent (1%–5%) adverse reactions are mild hypersensitivity reactions; transient rise in liver function test values; eosinophilia, thrombocytosis, and positive Coombs' test; local injection site symptoms. Rarely, pseudomembranous colitis. Not considered nephrotoxic. Contains 2.6 mEq Na/gm.

Interactions: Avoid concurrent furosemide, ethacrynic acid, aminoglycosides, and other nephrotoxic drugs.

■ Ceftriaxone Sodium (Rocephin; Roche)

How Supplied:
Parenteral:
  250, 500 mg; 1, 2 gm vial.
  1, 2 gm piggyback bottle.
  10 gm bulk container.
  1, 2 gm vial and diluent container.

Administration:
IM, IV.

Dose: 1–2 gm q12–24h.
  Uncomplicated gonorrhea: 250 mg IM single dose.

Elimination:
60% eliminated by kidneys, 40% by biliary secretion; half-life 8 hr.

Spectrum: (See Table 3-5; Cefotaxime, p. 67.) Advantages include long half-life (bid dosage feasible), good CSF penetration for treatment of bacterial meningitis, and good activity against *N. gonorrhoeae,* including penicillinase-producing strains.

Indications: (See Cefotaxime, p. 67.) Specific gynecologic indications include uncomplicated gonorrhea (i.e., cervical, urethral, rectal, pharyngeal infections, and PID [both penicillinase and nonpenicillinase producing organisms]).

Toxicity: (See Cephalosporins, p. 57.) Most commonly mild local or hypersensitivity reactions, eosinophilia, thrombocytosis or leukopenia, diarrhea, elevated liver function test, or BUN values. Contains 2.6 mEq Na/gm.

■ Cefotetan Disodium (Cefotan; Stuart)

How Supplied:
Parenteral:
    1, 2 gm vial; vial and diluent container.
    10 gm/100 ml bulk vial.

Administration:
IV, IM.

Dose: 1–2 gm bid; max 6 gm/day in life-threatening infections.

Elimination: Excreted by kidneys; half-life 3–0.5 hr.

Spectrum: (See Table 3-5.)

Toxicity: (See Cephalosporins, p. 57.) Most frequently nausea or diarrhea; eosinophilia, positive direct Coombs' test, thrombocytosis; elevated liver enzymes; mild hypersensitivity reactions. Contains 2.3 mEq Na/gm.

■ Cefoperazone Sodium (Cefobid; Roerig)

How Supplied:
Parenteral:
    1, 2 gm vial.
    1, 2 gm piggyback unit.

Administration:
IM, IV.

Dose: 1–2 gm q12h; max 12 gm/day.

Elimination: Mostly excreted in bile, only 25% in urine. Half-life 2.1 hr; can be prolonged in hepatic dysfunction or biliary obstruction. (No dose alteration in renal impairment.)

Spectrum: (See Table 3-5.) Main advantage is greater activity against *P. aeruginosa;* less active than cefotaxime and other third-generation agents against gram-positive microorganisms and some gram-negative bacteria.

Indications: (See Cefotaxime, p. 67.) Specific gynecologic infections include PID, endometritis, and other female genital tract infections resulting from *N. gonorrhoeae, E. coli, Clostridium,* and *Bacteroides.*

Toxicity: (See Cephalosporins, p. 57.) Most commonly mild allergic reactions; diarrhea; mild neutropenia, anemia, and eosinophilia; transient elevation of liver enzymes, BUN, and creatinine. Suppression of gut flora that synthesize vitamin K may lead to coagulopathy. Disulfiram-like reaction with flushing, headache, and tachycardia if ethanol ingested within 72 hr. Contains 1.5 mEq Na/gm.

Monitor: Liver function; prothrombin time if poor nutritional status, alcoholic, malabsorption state, or recent hyperalimentation.

Interactions: Avoid alcohol for at least 72 hr after dosing; aminoglycosides may potentiate nepthrotoxicity.

ANTIBIOTICS

■ **Ceftazidime** (Ceptaz, Fortaz; Glaxo. Tazicef; Smith-Kline Beecham. Tazidime; Lilly)

How Supplied:
Parenteral:
  500 mg; 1, 2 gm vial.
  1, 2 gm flexible plastic bag.
  1, 2 gm vial and diluent container.
  6, 10 gm bulk package.

Dose: 1–2 gm q8–12h; max 6 gm/day in treatment of meningitis.

Elimination: Mainly excreted by kidneys (glomerular filtration); half-life 1.5–2 hr.

Spectrum: (See Table 3-5.) Main advantage is good activity against *Pseudomonas*. Use maximum dosage to treat meningitis.

Indications: (See Cefotaxime, p. 67; Cefoperazone on p. 71.)

Toxicity: (See Cephalosporins, p. 57.) Most commonly mild local effects, hypersensitivity reactions, and GI symptoms.

Monitor: Contains 2.3 mEq Na/gm.

Interactions: Increased risk of nephrotoxicity with aminoglycosides or potent diuretics (e.g., furosemide).

■ **Cefpodoxime Proxetil** (Vantin; Upjohn)

How Supplied:
PO:
  Tablets: 100, 200 mg.
  Oral suspension: 50, 100 mg/ml.

Administration: PO: tablets should be taken with food.

Dose: 100–400 mg q12h × 7–14 days.
  Uncomplicated gonorrhea: 200 mg single dose.
  Increase dosing interval to 24 hr with severe renal impairment.

Elimination: One-third excreted unchanged in urine.

Spectrum: (See Table 3-5.)

Toxicity: (See Cephalosporins, p. 57.)

Interaction: Concomitant administrations of high doses of antacids or H_2-blockers reduce peak plasmas levels by 24%–42%. Monitor renal function closely when given with potentially nephrotoxic drugs.

AMINOGLYCOSIDES

Mechanism of Action

Bind irreversibly to bacterial ribosomes, thereby inhibiting protein synthesis.

General Considerations

1. Basic structure is amino sugar in glycosidic linkage.
2. Highly polar cations; poorly absorbed from the GI tract and penetrate poorly into most cells, including eye and CSF, thus inadequate for treatment of gram-negative bacterial meningitis.
3. Rapidly excreted in normal kidney by glomerular filtration but can accumulate if this is impaired; dosage reduction necessary in patients with renal dysfunction.
4. Bactericidal.
5. Primarily used to treat infections caused by aerobic, gram-negative bacteria.
6. Little activity against anaerobes, facultative anaerobes, or gram-positive bacteria.
7. Demonstrates synergism when given with PCN.
8. Crosses placenta.

Adverse Reactions

1. Ototoxicity:
   a. Drug accumulates in perilymph and endolymph of inner ear with progressive destruction of vestibular or cochlear sensory cells, which do not regenerate.
   b. Degree of permanent dysfunction correlates with the number of damaged cells; thus increased with sustained exposure to drug.

c. Older patients may be more susceptible because the number of cells decreases with age; patients with preexisting impairment are also at a higher risk.

d. Cochlear damage:

   (1) Since high-frequency sensory cells are lost first, the patient may not have symptoms or complain of high-pitched tinnitus, which may persist several days after the drug is discontinued.

   (2) Early changes may be reversible with calcium.

   (3) Retrograde degeneration of auditory nerve results in irreversible hearing loss; may occur several weeks after the drug is discontinued.

   (4) Seen more frequently with amikacin, kanamycin, neomycin, and tobramycin.

e. Vestibular damage:

   (1) First warning of labyrinthine dysfunction may be intense headache lasting 1–2 days.

   (2) Acute labyrinthitis characterized by nausea, vomiting, difficulty with balance; may last 1–2 wk. May be associated with vertigo while upright, especially with eyes closed; difficulty with reading as eyes drift at the end of a movement; positive Romberg's sign; spontaneous nystagmus.

   (3) Chronic labyrinthitis manifested by lack of symptoms while lying down but difficulty with walking or making sudden movements and ataxia; chronic phase may persist 1–2 mo.

   (4) Compensatory phase may last 12–18 mo, during which symptoms are latent and become manifest only with the eyes closed. Some residual permanent damage in most cases.

   (5) Most common with streptomycin; also with gentamicin and tobramycin to some extent.

2. Nephrotoxicity:

   a. Toxicity results from accumulation and retention of drug in renal cortex by proximal tubular cells.

   b. Usually reversible because these cells can regenerate (but reduced drug excretion may lead to ototoxicity).

   c. Commonly occurs to a mild degree in 8%–26% of patients on aminoglycoside therapy for more than several days.

   d. Signs:
      (1) Initially, mild proteinuria with hyaline and granular casts.
      (2) After several days, decrease in GFR.
      (3) Mild rise in serum creatinine (0.5–2.0 mg/dl).
      (4) Rarely, hypokalemia, hypocalcemia, hypophosphatemia, and severe acute tubular necrosis.
   e. Toxicity correlates with total amount of drug administered and constant drug concentrations above a critical level.
   f. Greatest risk with neomycin (therefore never given parenterally), gentamicin, and tobramycin.
   g. Other drugs given concurrently can potentiate toxicity: amphotericin B, vancomycin, cisplatin, cyclosporine, and cephalothin.
   h. Furosemide therapy and advanced age may increase risk, although all data is inconclusive.
3. Miscellaneous nervous system toxic effects:
   a. Neuromuscular blockade:
      (1) Can result in acute muscular paralysis and apnea.
      (2) Most likely with neomycin followed by kanamycin, amikacin, gentamicin, and tobramycin.
      (3) More likely after intrapleural or intraperitoneal instillation but also reported with IV, IM, and even PO therapy.
      (4) Most reports associated with concomitant anesthesia or use of neuromuscular blocking agents.
      (5) Patients with myasthenia gravis or chronic obstructive pulmonary disease (COPD) are at highest risk.
      (6) Reverse with IV calcium salt.
   b. Optic nerve dysfunction:
      (1) Presents as scotomas or enlargement of blind spot.
      (2) Streptomycin most often implicated.
   c. Peripheral neuritis:
      (1) Especially if nerve accidentally injected.
      (2) May see paresthesias, especially circumoral, within 30–60 min of injection; these may persist for hours.
4. Hypersensitivity reactions (rare):
   a. Skin rashes, eosinophilia, fever, blood dyscrasias, angioedema, exfoliative dermatitis, stomatitis, and anaphylactic shock.
5. Overgrowth of nonsusceptible organisms, including fungi.

ANTIBIOTICS

■ Streptomycin Sulfate (Roerig)

How Supplied:
Parenteral: 1 gm/2.5 ml ampule.

Administration: Intermittent, deep IM injection. (No longer used IV, intrathecally, or intraperitoneally.)

Dose: 1–2 gm/day (15–25 mg/kg/day) divided bid; max 2 gm/day. Usual therapy not more than 7–10 days, except for TB or bacterial endocarditis.

Therapeutic Levels:
Peak: 20–30 µg/ml.
Trough: Less than 5 µg/ml.

Spectrum: Aerobic gram-negative bacteria. Most commonly:
1. TB: Usually as a 4th drug in a regimen of INH, rifampin, and pyrazinamide for initial treatment, or when one or more of the drugs listed above contraindicated because of toxicity or intolerance.
3. Tularemia (*F. tularensis*).
4. Plague (*P. pestis*).
5. Brucellosis: Add to usual tetracycline therapy in severe cases and in those secondary to *Brucella suis* or *melitensis*.

Contraindications: Pregnancy (risk of congenital ototoxicity); history of hypersensitivity to streptomycin.

Toxicity: (See Aminoglycosides, p. 73.) More commonly associated with permanent ototoxicity and vestibular damage than with nephrotoxicity. Vestibular dysfunction related to cumulative daily dose; more frequent in the elderly or in patients with renal impairment, especially with large doses for prolonged periods. May also see myocarditis, serum sickness–like reaction, hot tender mass at site of injection, optic nerve dysfunction, and peripheral neuritis.

Monitor: Baseline and periodic caloric stimulation and audiometric testing.

Interaction: Avoid concommitant use of other nephrotoxic or ototoxic agents (see Aminoglycosides, p. 73.); nephrotoxicity may also be potentiated by concommitant ethacrynic acid, furosemide, mannitol, and other diuretics.

■ Gentamicin Sulfate (Garamycin; Schering)

How Supplied:
Parenteral:
    10 mg/ml as 2 ml vial.
    40 mg/ml as 2 ml vial.
    1.5, 2 ml disposable syringe.
Intrathecal: 2 mg/ml as 2 ml vial.
Ophthalmic ointment: 3 mg/gm in 3.5 gm tube.
Ophthalmic solution: 3 mg/ml in 5 ml plastic dropper bottle.
Dermatologic cream: 0.1% in 15 gm tube.
Dermatologic ointment: 0.1% in 15 gm tube.

Administration:
Parenteral:
IM, IV, intrathecal: Absorption and plasma concentrations variable so must follow levels (see below) to avoid toxicity, especially if given for several days because it may accumulate.
Opthalmic: Ointment or solution is placed in conjunctival sac; ointment may slow corneal healing.
Topical: Absorption better with cream than ointment, especially when applied to large denuded areas such as extensive burns.

Dose:
IM/IV:
    3–4 mg/kg/day divided q8h; max 300 mg/day.
    Life-threatening infections: Begin with 5 mg/kg/day divided q8h; reduce to 3 mg/kg/day as soon as clinically indicated.
Opthalmic:
    Solution: 1–2 drops q4h; 2 drops qh if severe infection.
    Ointment: Apply small amount to conjunctival sac bid or tid.
Topical: Gently apply small amount to lesion tid or qid.

Therapeutic Levels:
Peak: 6–10 μg/ml.
Trough: 2 μg/ml.

ANTIBIOTICS

Elimination: Renal excretion by glomerular filtration; reduce dose in patients with renal impairment. Half-life approximately 2 hr.

Spectrum: Aerobic gram-negative bacteria. Usually interchangeable with tobramycin, amikacin, and netilmicin. (See Table 3-2.)

Indication:
1. Complicated UTI (e.g., pyelonephritis): Begin therapy with aminoglycoside (with ampicillin, if desired), but discontinue aminoglycoside treatment if sensitivity reports nonsusceptible organism. (Not indicated for uncomplicated UTI.)
2. Pneumonias:
    a. *Pseudomonas:* With an antipseudomonal PCN.
    b. *Klebsiella:* With cephalosporin, mezlocillin, or piperacillin.
    c. *E. coli, Proteus mirabilis:* With ampicillin.
3. Meningitis: Infrequently used since only effective when injected intrathecally or intraventricularly and because 3rd-generation cephalosporins are superior, especially moxalactam and cefotaxime.
4. Peritonitis secondary to peritoneal dialysis: Add to dialysate.
5. Enterococcal endocarditis: Superior to streptomycin when used with a PCN.
6. *Pseudomonas* sepsis in granulocytopenic patient: Combine with antipseudomonal PCN.

Toxicity: (See Aminoglycosides, p. 73.) Most importantly, irreversible ototoxicity, and nephrotoxicity.

Interactions: (See Aminoglycosides, p. 75.) Reduced bactericidal activity when used with chloramphenicol.

■ **Tobramycin Sulfate** (Nebcin; Lilly)

How Supplied:
Parenteral:
   20 mg or 80 mg/2 ml multiple-dose vial.
   1.2 gm/30 ml bulk vial.
   60 mg/1.5 ml, 80 mg/2 ml disposable syringe.
   60 mg/6 ml, 80 mg/8 ml vial and diluent container pack.

Administration:
Parenteral: (See Gentamicin, p. 77.)

Dose: (See Gentamicin, p. 77.)

Therapeutic Levels:
Peak: 4–10 µg/ml.
Trough: <2 µg/ml. Rising trough implies accumulation because of renal impairment and requires dose adjustment.

Elimination: (See Gentamicin, p. 78.)

Spectrum: (See Gentamicin, p. 78; Table 3-2.) Superior to gentamicin for *Pseudomonas* bacteremia, osteomyelitis, and pneumonia (use with appropriate PCN); less effective against enterococci or mycobacteria.

Toxicity: (See Aminoglycosides, p. 73.) May be slightly less nephrotoxic or ototoxic than gentamicin.

Interactions: (See Aminoglycosides, p. 75; Gentamicin, p. 78.)

■ **Amikacin Sulfate** (Amikacin Sulfate; Elkins-Sinn. Amikin; Apothecon)

How Supplied:
Parenteral:
    100, 500 mg/2 ml vial.
    1 gm/4 ml bulk vial.
    500 mg/2 ml disposable syringe.

Administration:
IM/IV.

Dose: 15 mg/kg/day divided bid or tid; max 1.5 gm/day. Limit treatment to 7–10 days.

Therapeutic Levels:
Peak: 20–30 µg/ml.
Trough: 5–10 µg/ml.

Elimination: Excreted by kidney via glomerular filtration; half-life 2–3 hr.

Spectrum: (See Gentamicin, p. 78; Table 3-2.) Resistant to aminoglycoside-inactivating enzymes; thus has broadest spectrum of group. Particularly useful in hospitals with a high incidence of gentamicin-resistant or tobramycin-resistant gram-negative organisms (e.g., *P. rettgeri, P. stuartii, S. marcescens,* and *P. aeruginosa*). Also effective against *M. tuberculosis* and some atypical mycobacteria.

Toxicity: (See Aminoglycosides, p. 73.) Ototoxicity more common than nephrotoxicity. May provoke anaphylactic-like asthma symptoms in individuals sensitive to sodium bisulfite.

Interaction: (See Aminoglycosides, p. 75.)

■ Netilmicin Sulfate (Netromycin; Schering)

How Supplied:
Parenteral: 150 mg/1.5 ml vial.

Administration:
IM, IV

Dose: 3–4 mg/kg/day divided bid or tid, 7–14 days.
Life-threatening infection: 4.0–6.5 mg/kg/day.
Decrease dose in presence of renal impairment.

Therapeutic Levels:
Peak: 6–10 μg/ml.
Trough: 0.5–2 μg/ml.

Elimination: Excreted by kidney via glomerular filtration. Half-life, 2–2.5 hr; increases as dosage increases.

Spectrum: (See Gentamicin, p. 78; Table 3-2.) Resistant to most aminoglycoside-inactivating enzymes like amikacin.

Toxicity: (See Aminoglycosides, p. 73, Amikacin, p. 73.) Neuromuscular blockage more common than with other aminoglycosides, but not more nephrotoxic or ototoxic than aminoglycisodes.

Interactions: (See Aminoglycosides, p. 75.)

■ Neomycin Sulfate (Biocraft. Roxane)

How Supplied:
500 mg tablet.
100,000 U/ml suspension.

Administration:
PO: Poorly absorbed. (Not for parenteral use because of high incidence of nephrotoxicity and ototoxicity.)

Dose: 50–100 mg/kg/day divided qid or tid; max 12 gm/day.

Elimination: 97% of oral dose excreted unchanged in feces.

Spectrum: Susceptible organisms include *E. coli, Enterobacter aerogenes, Klebsiella pneumoniae, Proteus vulgaris, S. aureus, S. faecalis, M. tuberculosis.*

Indications: Preoperative bowel preparation, usually with erythromycin base; treatment of hepatic coma to decrease blood ammonia levels.

Toxicity: Spruelike malabsorption syndrome with diarrhea, steatorrhea, and azotorrhea; superinfection with intestinal yeast overgrowth.

TETRACYCLINES
Common tetracyclines (TCNs) are listed in Table 3-6.

Mechanism of Action
Bind to bacterial 30S ribosome and inhibit protein synthesis. Primarily bacteriostatic; only affect multiplying organisms.

ANTIBIOTICS

Table 3-6
TETRACYCLINES

Chemical Name	Brand Name (Manufacturer)	How Supplied	Usual Dose
INCOMPLETELY ABSORBED			
Tetracycline HCl	Achromycin (Lederle)	PO: 250, 500 mg	250–500 qid
Oxytetracycline HCl	Terramycin (Pfizer, Roerig)	IM: 100, 250 mg (with 40 mg procaine HCl)	250–300 mg/day
		PO: 250, 500 mg	
		IM: 100 mg/2 ml, 250 mg/2 ml, 500 mg/10 ml	
INTERMEDIATE ABSORPTION			
Demeclocycline HCl	Declomycin (Lederle)	PO: 150, 300 mg	150 mg qid to 300 mg bid
Methacycline HCl	Rondomycin (Wallace)	PO: 150, 300 mg	150 mg qid to 300 mg bid
WELL ABSORBED			
Doxycycline hyclate	Doryx (Parke-Davis)	PO: 50, 100 mg	100–200 mg/day, divided
	Vibramycin, IV, Vibra-Tabs (Pfizer, Roerig)	IV: 100, 200 mg	100–200 mg/day
Minocycline HCl	Dynacin (Medicis); Minocin (Lederle)	PO: 50, 100 mg	200 mg, then 100 bid
		IV: 100 mg	200 mg, then 100 bid

Absorption

Incompletely but adequately absorbed from GI tract. Absorption decreased by milk products and antacids containing aluminum, magnesium, or calcium in addition to iron (because of chelation and an increase in gastric pH).

Classification

Based on dosage and frequency of oral administration required:

1. Oxytetracycline and tetracycline: Incompletely absorbed, short half-life; qid dosage.
2. Demeclocycline and methacycline: Intermediate absorption, longer half-life.
3. Doxycycline and minocycline: Well absorbed (even on full stomach), long half-life; bid dosage.

Elimination

Concentrated in liver, excreted via bile into intestine, and partially reabsorbed (enterohepatic circulation); thus longer half-life in presence of hepatic dysfunction or common bile duct obstruction. Remainder of drug cleared by kidney via glomerular filtration.

Penetration

Passes into CSF (even without meningeal inflammation) and synovial fluid, across placenta, and into breast milk.

Spectrum and Indications (see Table 3-2):

1. Rickettsial infections: Rocky Mountain spotted fever; epidemic, murine, and scrub typhus; rickettsialpox; Q fever.
2. *Mycoplasma pneumoniae* pneumonia.
3. *Chlamydia,* lymphogranuloma venereum (treatment of choice), psittacosis, inclusion conjunctivitis, trachoma, nonspecific urethritis, and epididymitis.
4. Sexually transmitted diseases (in patients unable to tolerate PCN): Gonorrhea, including gonococcal salpingitis; syphilis; chancroid; and granuloma inguinale.
5. Bacillary infections: Brucellosis, tularemia, and cholera.
6. Acute urethral syndrome.
7. Miscellaneous: Actinomycosis, nocardiosis (with a sulfonamide), yaws and relapsing fever (with PCN), and Lyme disease.
8. Acne.

ANTIBIOTICS

Contraindications

Pregnancy, lactation, and children younger than 12 years (see below).

Adverse Effects

1. Toxicity:
   a. GI: Irritation of GI tract with pyrosis, nausea, vomiting, diarrhea; decreased incidence if taken with food or antacids not containing aluminum, magnesium, or calcium. (Separate entity from pseudomembranous colitis; see below.)
   b. Phototoxicity: Sunburnlike reaction, sometimes with onycholysis and nail pigmentation. More common with demeclocycline and doxycycline.
   c. Hepatic toxicity: Acute fatty liver type of syndrome; more frequent with large parenteral doses. Jaundice followed by azotemia, acidosis, and possibly irreversible shock; pregnant women particularly susceptible. Less likely with oxytetracycline and tetracycline.
   d. Nephrotoxicity:
      (1) TCNs may inhibit protein synthesis; in patients with renal disease the net catabolic effect results in increased metabolism of amino acids and worsening azotemia. Less likely with doxycycline.
      (2) Rarely, diabetes insipidus in patients receiving demeclocycline.
      (3) Ingestion of outdated and degraded TCN may result in a Fanconi-type syndrome:
         Nausea, vomiting, polydipsia, polyuria, glycosuria, proteinuria, acidosis, and aminoaciduria. Usually reversible after discontinuation of therapy.
   e. Calcified tissue effects:
      (1) Permanent brown discoloration of teeth in children because of the formation of a tetracycline-calcium orthophosphate complex. Risk is highest in neonates but still exists until 5 years of age when the teeth are being calcified.
      (2) Permanent discoloration of teeth in offspring of pregnant women treated with TCNs. May still see effects in children as old as 7 years of age.
      (3) Depressed bone growth is seen in fetuses and young

children treated with TCN; effects reversible with short-term therapy.

f. Miscellaneous toxic effects:

(1) Thrombophlebitis after IV administration, especially if repeated infusion at same site; severe pain if given IM without local anesthetic.

(2) Blood dyscrasias: Leukocytosis, atypical lymphocytes, toxic neutrophilic granulation, and purpura.

(3) Pseudotumor cerebri-like syndrome with increased intracranial pressure and normal CSF. More common in young infants.

(4) Vestibular toxicity with nausea, vomiting, vertigo, and ataxia beginning soon after first dose of minocycline and ending 1–2 days after therapy is stopped. Seen more frequently in women than men and with higher doses.

2. Hypersensitivity reactions (cross-sensitization common):

a. Skin reactions (rare): Urticaria, morbilliform rash, fixed drug eruptions, and exfoliative dermatitis.

b. Allergic reactions: Angioedema and anaphylaxis. May even follow oral administration.

c. Miscellaneous: Burning eyes, cheilosis, glossitis, or vaginitis; fever; eosinophilia; and asthma.

3. Miscellaneous biologic effects:

a. Superinfections, usually results from resistant bacterial strains or fungi; may be oropharyngeal, vaginal, or systemic.

b. Pseudomembranous colitis: Fever, severe diarrhea containing mucous membrane shreds and many neutrophils. Occurs secondary to overgrowth of *Clostridium difficile;* clostridial toxin damages mucosal cells and causes shallow ulcerations. Symptoms usually subside after discontinuation of TCN but sometimes require oral vancomycin, too.

Interactions

May depress plasma prothrombin activity; dosage adjustment may be necessary in patients receiving anticoagulants. Antacids containing aluminum, calcium, or magnesium impair PO form of absorption.

ANTIBIOTICS

■ Tetracycline HCl (Achromycin, Achromycin V; Lederle)

How Supplied:
PO:
250, 500 mg capsules.
Ophthalmic:
1%, 5 ml unit dose dropper suspension.
3%, 1/8 oz tube ointment.
Topical: 3%, 1 oz tube ointment.

Administration:
PO: Give 1 hr before or 2 hr after meals; not to be taken with milk or dairy products or aluminum, calcium, iron, or magnesium preparations.

Dose (Adults):
PO: 1–2 gm/day divided bid–qid.
Uncomplicated gonorrheal urethritis or pharyngitis (in patients sensitive to PCN): 1.5 gm PO, then 500 mg q6h × 4 days for total dose of 9 gm. (Not indicated in treatment of anorectal gonorrhea in men because of high relapse rate.)
Gonococcal salpingitis: Continue treatment 10 days.
Syphilis (patient sensitive to PCN):
Early (less than 1 year's duration) 500 mg qid × 15 days.
Late (more than 1 year's duration) 500 mg qid × 30 days.
Uncomplicated chlamydial cervicitis: 500 mg qid × 7–10 days.

Elimination: Primarily renal excretion via glomerular filtration; half-life 6–9 hr. With severe renal impairment, may need to reduce individual dosage or extend dosing interval.

Spectrum: (See Table 3-2.)

Indications: (See Tetracyclines, p. 83.)

Toxicity: (See Tetracyclines, p. 84.)

■ Oxytetracycline (Terramycin; Roerig)

How Supplied:
PO: 500 mg/10 ml multiple-dose vial.

Administration:
IM: (See Table 3-6.) Lower blood levels with IM than with PO therapy (thus reserve IM form for patients unable to tolerate PO).

Dose:
IM: 250 mg q24h or 300 mg divided bid–tid; change to PO therapy as soon as possible.

Elimination/Spectrum/Toxicity: (See Tetracyclines, p. 83–84.)

■ Demeclocycline HCl (Declomyicn; Lederle)

How Supplied:
PO: 150, 300 mg tablets.

Administration:
PO: (See Tetracyclines, p. 84.)

Dose: 150 mg qid or 300 mg bid.
Uncomplicated gonorrhea (in patients sensitive to PCN): 600 mg stat, then 300 mg bid × 4 days (total, 3 gm).

Elimination: Primarily glomerular filtration.

Spectrum/Indications: (See Table 3-2.)

Toxicity: (See Tetracyclines, p. 84.) Photosensitivity more common than with other TCNs.

■ Doxycycline Hyclate (Doryx; Parke-Davis. Monodox-Oclassen, Vibramycin; Pfizer, Roerig. Vibra-Tabs; Pfizer)

How Supplied:
PO:
Capsules: 50, 100 mg.
Tablets: 100 mg.
Suspension: 25 or 50 mg/5ml
Parenteral: Injection—100 mg vial.

Administration:
PO: (See Table 3-6.) May be taken with food or milk to lessen GI distress.
IV: Avoid too rapid administration.

Dose:
PO: 100 mg bid × 2 doses, then 100 mg/day (given as single dose or 50 mg bid).
    Uncomplicated gonorrhea: 100 mg bid × 7–10 days.
    Uncomplicated chlamydial urethritis, cervicitis, or proctitis: 100 mg bid × 7–10 days.
IV: 100–200 mg/24 hr given in 1 or 2 divided doses.
    Primary and secondary syphilis: 300 mg/day × 10 days.
    Acute pelvic inflammatory disease: 100 mg bid until oral therapy clinically indicated, followed by 100 mg bid PO for 10–14 days. Usually given with cefoxitin or other broad-spectrum cephalosporin to cover doxycycline-resistant organisms (anaerobes, facultative aerobes, and certain penicillinase-producing strains of *N. gonorrhoeae*).

Elimination: Enterohepatic circulation in bile and excreted in feces, mostly as inactive conjugate. No dose adjustment with renal impairment. Half-life 16 hr.

Spectrum: (See Table 3-2.)

Toxicity: (See Tetracyclines, p. 84.) Slightly higher incidence of phytotoxicity than other TCNs.

Interaction: (See Tetracyclines, p. 84.) Half-life shortened in patients receiving long-term barbiturate or phenytoin therapy.

■ **Minocycline HCl** (Minocin; Lederle. Dynacin; Medicis)

How Supplied:
PO:
    Capsules: 50, 100 mg.
    Suspension: 50 mg/5ml.
    Parenteral: 100 mg vial.

Administration:
PO: (See Table 3-6.)
IV: (See Table 3-6.)

Dose:
PO: 200 mg loading dose, then 100 mg bid.
   Syphilis: Usual dosage, extended to 10–15 days.
   Gonorrhea (patient sensitive to PCN): Usual dosage × 4 days min; cure culture 2–3 days posttherapy.
   Meningococcal carrier state: 100 mg bid × 5 days.
   Mycobacterium marinum: 100 mg bid × 6–8 wk.
   Uncomplicated urethritis, cervicitis, and proctitis because of *Chlamydia trachomatis* or *Ureaplasma urealyticum:* 100 mg bid × 7 days min.
   Uncomplicated gonococcal urethritis in men: 100 mg bid × 5 days.
IV: 200 mg loading dose, then 100 mg bid; max 400 mg/24 hr.

Elimination: Metabolized in liver, excreted by glomerular filtration. Half-life 18 hr; not prolonged in patients with hepatic failure. Dosage in renal impairment may need to be decreased or interval between doses extended to avoid toxicity.

Spectrum/Toxicity/Interaction: (See Tetracycline, p. 83–84)

Indications: (See Tetracycline, p. 83.) Useful in treatment of *N. gonorrhoeae* in men when PCN contraindicated; also as adjunctive treatment of severe acne.

ERYTHROMYCIN

■ **Erythromycin** (Erythromycin: Abbott. E-mycin; Boots. Ery-Tab, PCE Dispertab; Abbott. Ilotycin; Dista. ERY-C; Parke-Davis)

How Supplied:
PO:
   Tablets: 250, 333, 500 mg.
   Capsules: 250 mg.
   Parenteral: 1 gm/30 ml vial.

Administration:
PO: Fairly well absorbed, more rapidly on an empty stomach.
IV.

Mechanism of Action: Macrolide structure; binds reversibly to 50S ribosome and inhibits protein synthesis.

Penetration: Diffuses into most intracellular fluids except brain and CSF, crosses placenta, and appears in breast milk.

Dose: 1–2 gm/day divided qid–bid (individual dose not to exceed 1 gm).
Specific infections in adults:
1. Streptococcal infections (in patients sensitive to PCN): Continue treatment of active infections for minimum of 10 days to avoid potential sequelae such as glomerulonephritis; continuous prophylaxis in patient with history of rheumatic heart disease is 250 mg bid.
2. Prophylaxis against bacterial endocarditis in patients with valvular heart disease: 1 gm PO 1.5–2 hr before procedure, then 500 mg qid × 8 doses; or 1 gm 1 hr before and 500 mg 6 hr after procedure.
3. *Chlamydia* urogenital infection in pregnancy: 500 mg qid × 7 days or 250 mg qid × 14 days.
4. Uncomplicated chlamydial urethritis, cervicitis, or proctitis in nonpregnant patients unable to tolerate TCN: 500 mg qid × 7 days min.
5. Primary syphilis: 30–40 gm in doses divided over 10–15 days.
6. Acute *N. gonorrhoeae* pelvic inflammatory (PID): After initial dose of 500 mg erythromycin lactobionate IV qid × 3 days, 250 mg PO qid × 7 days.
7. Legionnaire's disease: 1–4 gm/day in divided doses.
8. *Mycoplasma* pneumonia: 500 mg tid or qid.

Elimination: Concentrated in liver; active form excreted in bile. Half-life 1.6 hr.

Spectrum: (See Table 3-2.) Considered an acceptable substitute for PCN (e.g., in hypersensitive patients) in treatment of group A ß-hemolytic *Streptococcus*, α–hemolytic *Streptococcus,* and *Treponema pallidum* and as acceptable alternative to TCN (e.g., in pregnancy) for treatment of *Chlamydia, Mycoplasma,* and *Rickettsia.* Also active against *Actinomyces israelii, Corynebacterium diphtheriae,* and *Bordetella pertussis.*

Toxicity: Allergic reactions including fever, eosinophilia, and rash. Epigastric distress, especially with large oral doses.

Interaction: Can prolong serum levels and potentiate effects of theophylline, carbamazepine, corticosteroids, cyclosporine, digoxin, hexobarbital, phenytoin, lovastatin, bromocriptine, and warfarin. When given with (dihydro) ergotamine, may precipitate acute ergot toxicity with severe peripheral vasospasm and dysesthesia.

■ Erythromycin Estolate (Ilosone; Dista)

How Supplied:
PO:
>   *Pulvules:* 250 mg.
>   *Tablets:* 500 mg.

Administration:
PO: Well absorbed without regard to meals.

Dose: 250 mg qid; max 4 gm/day.
>   Specific infections: (See Erythromycin, p. 90.)

Elimination: (See Erythromycin, p. 90.)

Spectrum: (See Erythromycin, p. 90.)

Toxicity: (See Erythromycin, p. 91.) Also may see cholestatic hepatitis with symptoms of GI distress, jaundice, elevated liver enzymes, and cholestasis on biopsy; usually resolves several days after discontinuation of therapy. Pregnant women may demonstrate reversible asymptomatic elevation of SGOT. Rarely, reversible hearing impairment may follow treatment with large doses.

Interaction: (See Erythromycin, p. 91.)

■ **Erythromycin Ethylsuccinate** (EES, EryPed; Abbott)

How Supplied:
PO:
  Tablets: 250, 333, 400, 500 mg.
  Suspension: 200 mg/ml.

Administration:
PO: without regard to meals.

Dose: 400 mg every 6 hr; 4 gm/day max in severe infections.

Elimination/Spectrum/Interaction: (See Erythromycin, p. 90–91.)

Toxicity: (See Erythromycin, p. 91.) Cholestatic hepatitis rare (see Erythromycin Estolate, p. 91).

■ **Erythromycin Gluceptate** (Ilotycin Gluceptate; Dista)

How Supplied:
Parenteral: 1 gm in 30 ml vial.

Administration:
IV.

Dose: 15–20 mg/kg/day divided bid–qid; max 4 gm/day.
  Switch to PO therapy as soon as possible.
  Specific infections: (See Erythromycin, p. 90.)

Spectrum: (See Erythromycin, p. 90.)

Toxicity: (See Erythromycin, p. 91.) Minimize risk of thrombophlebitis by using slow infusion rates. Rarely, transient auditory impairment at higher doses.

Interaction: (See Erythromycin, p. 91.)

■ Erythromycin Lactobionate (Elkins-Sinn; Lederle)

How Supplied:
Parenteral: 500 mg, 1 gm vial.

Administration:
IV.

Dose: (See Erythromycin Glucepate, p. 92.)

Elimination/Spectrum/Interaction: (See Erythromycin, p. 90–91.)

Toxicity: (See Erythromycin glucepate, p. 92.)

■ Clarithromycin (Biaxin; Abbott)

Mechanism of Action: Semisynthetic macrolide antibiotic. Binds to 50S ribosomal bacterial subunit inhibiting protein synthesis.

How Supplied:
PO:
   250, 500 mg tablets.
   125, 250 mg/5 ml oral suspension.

Administration: PO without regard to meals. Rapidly absorbed.

Dose: 250–500 mg q12h × 7–14 days. Decrease dose or prolong dosing intervals in presence of severe renal impairment.

Spectrum: Indicated for mild-to-moderate infections because of *S. pyogenes* and pneumoniae, *H. influenzae,* mycobacteriae, mycoplasma pneumoniae, and *S. aureus* (e.g., upper and lower respiratory tract infections and skin infections).

Toxicity: Mostly mild and transient: diarrhea, nausea, or headache.

Interactions: Temporary increase in concomitantly administered theophylline or carbamezapine levels; decrease in concomitantly administered zidovudine levels.

■ Clindamycin HCl (Cleocin HCl; Upjohn)

■ Clindamycin Phosphate (Cleocin Phosphate; Upjohn)

How Supplied:
PO: 75, 150, 300 mg capsule.
Parenteral:
    150 mg/ml vial.
    300, 600, and 900 mg/50 ml container.

Administration:
PO: Well absorbed and not affected by presence of food in stomach.
IM/IV.

Mechanism: Binds to 50S subunit of bacterial ribosome and inhibits protein synthesis.

Dose:
PO: 150–300 mg qid; max 450 mg qid in more severe infections.
IM/IV: 600–1200 mg/day divided bid–qid. More severe infections, especially if resulting from *Bacteroides fragilis, Peptococcus,* or *Clostridium* (other than *C. perfringens*): 1200–2700 mg/day divided q6–12h.

Elimination: Metabolized in liver; excreted in urine and bile. Half-life, 2.5–3 hr; slightly prolonged in severe renal or hepatic dysfunction.

Spectrum: (See Table 3-2.) Particularly useful in treating anaerobic infections, especially *B. fragilis;* recommended in combination therapy with an aminoglycoside for intraabdominal and pelvic abscesses and peritonitis. Not effective against aerobic gram-negative microorganisms and certain *Clostridium* species.

Toxicity:
GI: Diarrhea (2%–20% incidence); pseudomembranous colitis with bloody mucoid diarrhea, pain, and fever; stools test positive for *Clostridium difficile* toxin (0.01%–10%).
Skin: Rash (10%).
Miscellaneous (rare): Stevens-Johnson syndrome (exudative erythema multiforme); transient ALT or AST (SGOT or SGPT) elevation; granulocytopenia, thrombocytopenia; anaphylaxis; local thrombophlebitis after IV administration.

Interaction: May potentiate effects of neuromuscular blocking agents given simultaneously.

■ Colistin (Colistimethate Sodium, Coly-Mycin M; Parke-Davis)

How Supplied:
Parenteral: 150 mg vial.

Administration:
IM/IV.

Mechanism: Surface-active agent that penetrates and disrupts integrity of bacterial cell membranes.

Dose: *Adults/children:* 2.5–5 mg/kg/day divided bid–qid; reduce dose with renal impairment.

Elimination: Excreted by kidneys; adjust dosage and exercise extreme caution in patients with renal impairment.

Spectrum: Restricted to gram-negative bacteria, particularly *P. aeruginosa, E. aerogenes, E. coli, Klebsiella pneumoniae;* also *Salmonella, Bordetella, Pasturella,* and *Shigella.*

Toxicity:
Major: Extreme nephrotoxicity now limits usefulness parenterally (topical forms also available; see *PDR*); also may see respiratory arrest secondary to concurrent use of agents (e.g., guccibylcholine with neuromuscular blocking potential).
Minor: Paresthesias, urticaria, drug fever, GI distress, and vertigo.

■ Spectinomycin HCl (Trobicin; Upjohn)

How Supplied:
Parenteral: 2, 4 gm vial.

Administration:
IM: rapidly absorbed.

Mechanism: Bacteriostatic. Inhibits protein synthesis in gram-negative bacteria selectively by binding to 30S ribosomal subunit.

Dose:
1. Acute genital and rectal gonorrhea in patients allergic to PCN or infected with PCN-resistant organism: 2 gm × 1 dose (cure rate, 95%).
2. In localities in which antibiotic resistance is prevalent: 4 gm × 1 dose.
3. Gonococcal pharyngitis: 2 gm bid × 3 days.

Elimination: Excreted in urine.

Spectrum: Sole indication: Uncomplicated gonococcal infections in patients with known PCN hypersensitivity or with PCNase-producing microorganisms.

Toxicity: Rarely, urticaria, chills, fever, vertigo, or nausea.

■ Vancomycin HCl (Vancocin; Lilly. Vancoled; Lederle).

How Supplied:
PO: 125, 250 mg pulvules.
Parenteral: 500 mg; 1, 5, and 10 gm vial.

Administration:
PO: Poorly absorbed; therefore only indicated in treatment of colitis secondary to toxin-producing bacteria (see below).
IV.

Mechanism: Rapidly bactericidal; inhibits cell wall synthesis.

Penetration: CSF (when meninges is inflamed), bile, pleural and pericardial cavities, synovial fluid, and ascitic fluid.

Dose:
PO: 500 mg qid × 7–10 days.
IV: 2 gm/day divided qid or bid.

Elimination:
PO: Excreted in stool.
Parenteral: Excreted by glomerular filtration; half-life 6 hr. Dosage adjustment important in renal impairment.

Spectrum: (See Table 3-2.) Most useful for serious infections resulting from gram-positive bacteria:
1. Staphylococcal infections: Those resistant to ß-lactamase antibiotics or occurring in PCN-sensitive patients, including pneumonia, empyema, endocarditis, osteomyelitis, and soft-tissue abscesses.
2. *Streptococcus viridans* endocarditis: In patients allergic to PCN.
3. *Streptococcus faecalis* endocarditis: In combination with aminoglycoside (monitor carefully for potential ototoxicity; see below).
4. *Staphylococcus aureus* ileocolitis.
5. *Clostridium difficile* pseudomembranous colitis.

Toxicity:
1. Auditory: Possibly permanent ototoxicity, especially with preexisting renal or auditory impairment, with concurrent treatment with a potentially ototoxic drug, or at sustained plasma levels greater than 30 µg/ml.
2. Renal: Unusual, unless dosage not adjusted for decreased renal function or aminoglycosides given concomitantly.
3. Infusion related: "Red neck syndrome" if given too rapidly with upper body flushing and sudden severe hypotension or pain and muscle spasm; phlebitis.

Interaction: Avoid simultaneous therapy with possibly nephrotoxic and neurotoxic agents (e.g., amphotericin B, amino-glycosides, bacitracin, colistin, cisplatin).

ANTIBIOTICS

■ Troleandomycin (Tao; Roerig)

How Supplied:
PO: 250 mg capsules (equivalent to 250 mg oleandomycin).

Administration: PO.

Dose: 250–500 mg qid; continue for 10 days with streptococcal infections.

Elimination: Primarily excreted by the liver.

Spectrum: Streptococcus pyogenes; Diplococcus pneumoniae; Group A ß-hemolytic strep.

Indications: Pneumococcal pneumonia; URTI.

Contraindications: Pregnancy; hepatic dysfunction.

Adverse Effects: GI distress, diarrhea, urticaria, and rash.

Toxicity: Allergic cholestatic hepatitis.

Monitor: Liver function tests; theophylline levels.

Interaction: Concurrent use of ergotamine containing drugs may induce ischemic reactions; possible elevated serum levels of theophylline.

■ Chloramphenicol (Chloromycetin; Parke-Davis)

How Supplied:
PO: 250 mg capsule.
Parenteral: 100 mg/ml vial.

Administration:
PO: IV only in severe, life-threatening infection; switch to PO as soon as clinically feasible.

Dose: 50 mg/kg/day divided qid; max 100 mg/kg/day or 4 gm/day; decrease dose to 50 mg/kg/day as soon as possible.

Mechanism of Action: Binds reversibly to 50S ribosomal subunit, inhibits protein synthesis.

Therapeutic Levels: 15–25 µg/ml. Levels >50 µg/ml associated with a high incidence of toxicity.

Spectrum/Indications: See Table 3-2. Primarily bacteriostatic (bactericidal for *H. influenzae*). Indicated only for serious infections in which other antimicrobials are not effective (e.g., *Salmonella* species, including *S. typhi; H. influenzae,* particularly meningitis; *Rickettsia* (tetracyclines preferable in most cases); serious anaerobic or mixed aerobic-anaerobic infections with foci in the bowel or pelvis (clindamycin or metronidazole usually preferable).

Elimination: Metabolized in liver to the inactive glucuronide; then excreted in urine by glomerular filtration and tubular secretion. Adjust dose in presence of hepatic cirrhosis; adjustment not necessary in patients with renal impairment. Half-life 4 hr.

Toxicity:
1. Hematologic:
   a. Aplastic anemia: Most common cause of drug-induced pancytopenia, leukopenia, thrombocytopenia, marrow aplasia, and fatal pancytopenia. More common with prolonged or repeated therapy; possible genetic or idiosyncratic susceptibility. Incidence 1/30,000; high mortality rate; high incidence of acute leukemia in survivors.
   b. Reversible erythroid precursor suppression: With reticulocytopenia. Incidence and severity dose related, especially with plasma level >25 µg/ml over prolonged period.
   c. Depression of erythropoiesis: Frequent in presence of hepatic disease (especially if with ascites and jaundice) or renal insufficiency.
2. Gray baby syndrome: In neonates, especially premature infants, when exposed to higher doses. Initial manifestations of vomiting and irregular respiration; progress to diarrhea, cyanosis, and refractory lactic acidosis; death in 40% of patients. Occurs secondary to inadequate glucuronidation and drug excretion.

ANTIBIOTICS

3. Hypersensitivity reaction (rare): Vesicular/macular skin rashes, fever, and angioedema; Herxheimer reaction when used to treat syphilis, brucellosis, or typhoid fever.
4. Miscellaneous: Nausea or vomiting, diarrhea, blurred vision, optic neuritis, digital parethesias, and encephalopathic changes; cardiomyopathy.

Precautions: Monitor baseline and serial hematologic studies; avoid concurrent therapy with other potential bone marrow depressants (e.g., phenylbutazone, glutethimide). Avoid repeated or prolonged courses of therapy or excessively high doses.

Contraindications: Pregnancy at or near term, lactation; known hypersensitivity to drug.

Interaction: May prolong half-life of dicumarol, phenytoin, chlorpropamide, and tolbutamide because of effects on hepatic microsomal enzymes. Long-term phenobarbital therapy may shorten half-life.

AGENTS TO TREAT URINARY TRACT INFECTIONS

Agents that do not achieve therapeutic levels in plasma but are concentrated in the renal tubules; effective concentrations reach only renal pelves and bladder.

■ **Methenamine** (Urised; Webcon. Uro-Phosphate; ECR)

■ **Methenamine Hippurate** (Urex; 3M)

■ **Methenamine Mandelate** (Uroqid-Acid No. 2; Beach)

Mechanism of Action: Hexamethylenamine structure converts to formaldehyde, the active antibacterial agent. Acidification of urine speeds conversion (low pH by itself also bacteriostatic); acidify by adding hippurate or mandelate.

Administration:
PO: Well absorbed. Acidify urine to promote antibacterial action with high-protein diet, cranberry juice, ascorbic acid, prunes, plums, and methionine.

Spectrum: Almost all bacteria is sensitive to free formaldehyde; certain organisms with urea-splitting activity (e.g., *Proteus,* some *Pseudomonas*) will raise pH and thereby inhibit formaldehyde release. Particularly useful in suppressing *E. coli,* common gram-negative bacteria, *S. aureus,* and *S. epidermidis. Enterobacter* is usually resistant.

Indication: Not a primary drug for acute urinary tract infection (UTI), but indicated for long-term suppression.

Contraindications: Conversion to active ingredient produces ammonia as a byproduct, so contraindicated in hepatic dysfunction; acids may be detrimental in renal insufficiency.

Toxicity: GI distress at larger doses; dysuria, frequency, and rashes on high-dose prolonged therapy.

Specific Agents:
Urised (Webcon): 1 tablet = 40.8 mg methenamine.
    Dose: 2 tablets qid.
Uro-Phosphate (ECR): 1 tablet = 300 mg methenamine.
    Dose: 2 tablets qid.
Urex (3M): 1 tablet = 1 gm methenamine hippurate.
    Dose: 1 tablet bid.
Uroquid-Acid No. 2 (Beach): 1 tablet = 500 mg methenamine mandelate.
    Dose: 2 tablets qid, then 2–4 per day in divided doses.

ANTIBIOTICS

QUINOLONES AND CONGENERS

■ Cinoxacin (Cinobac; Oclassen)

How Supplied:
Tablet: 250, 500 mg.

Administration:
PO: Well absorbed without regard to meals.

Mechanism of Action: (See Nalidixic Acid, p. 103.)

Dose: 1 gm/day, divided bid or qid, × 7–14 days.

Elimination: Renal excretion; half-life 1.5 hr. Reduce dosage in renal dysfunction.

Spectrum/Toxicity: (See Nalidixic Acid, p. 103–104.)

Contraindications: Hepatic insufficiency, anuria, prepubertal children, pregnancy, and lactation (may cause arthropathy in neonates).

■ Ciprofloxacin (Cipro; Miles)

How Supplied:
PO: 250, 500, 750 mg.
Parenteral:
    200 mg/20 ml vial or 100 ml D5W.
    400 mg/40 ml vial or 200 ml D5W.

Administration:
PO: Well absorbed; not substantially affected by presence of food; IV.

Mechanism of Action: (See Nalidixic Acid, p. 103.)

Dose: 250–500 mg bid.

Elimination: Partially metabolized and partially excreted by kidney via glomerular filtration and tubular secretion, as well as in bile. Half-life 4 hr. Adjust dosage in patients with renal dysfunction.

Spectrum: Broader activity and more potent than others in this class (see Nalidixic Acid, p. 103).

Indication (with susceptible organisms): UTI; lower respiratory infections; infections of skin, soft tissue, bones, and joints; infectious diarrhea.

Contraindications: (See Nalidixic Acid, p. 104.)

Toxicity: (See Nalidixic Acid, p. 104.)

Interaction: Concurrent therapy with antacids containing magnesium or aluminum interferes with drug bioavailability.

■ Nalidixic Acid (NegGram; Winthrop)

How Supplied:
PO:
    250, 500, 1000 mg capsules.
    250 mg/ml suspension.

Administration:
PO: Well absorbed.

Mechanism of Action: Bactericidal; inhibits DNA gyrase and thus proper DNA synthesis during bacterial replication.

Dose: 1 gm qid × 1–2 wk, then 2 gm/day in divided doses.

Elimination: Conjugated in liver, excreted by kidney (both as conjugated form and as parent drug).

Spectrum: Most common gram-negative bacteria, especially *E. coli, Enterobacter, Klebsiella,* and most *Proteus. Pseudomonas* and *S. faecalis* usually insensitive.

Indication: UTI.

Contraindications: Neonates; prepubertal children (theoretical potential to erode cartilage in weight-bearing joints); first-trimester pregnancy; pregnancy near term.

Toxicity: GI distress; allergic reactions such as urticaria, rash, fever, eosinophilia, and photosensitivity; rarely, cholestasis, blood dyscrasias, or hemolytic anemia. Potential CNS effects include headache, vertigo, convulsions, and pseudotumor cerebri (seen more in extremely young or extremely old patients or with inappropriately high doses).

Interaction: Therapeutic activity inhibited by nitrofurantoin.

■ Nitrofurantoin (Macrodantin, Macrobid; Proctor & Gamble)

How Supplied:
PO: 25, 50, 100 mg capsules.

Administration:
PO: Rapidly and well absorbed; slower with macrocrystalline form. Take with meals to improve absorption and decrease GI side effects.

Mechanism of Action: Bacteriostatic; inhibits several bacterial enzymes.

Dose:
Treatment of acute infection: 50–100 mg bid–qid.

Prophylaxis: 50–100 mg nightly (qhs).

Elimination: Excreted by kidney mostly via glomerular filtration; half-life 0.3–1 hr.

Spectrum/Indication: UTI secondary to *E. coli,* enterococci, *S. aureus,* and susceptible strains of *Klebsiella, Enterobacter,* and *Proteus.* However, many strains of *Enterobacter, Klebsiella,* and most *Proteus* and *Pseudomonas* are resistant.

Contraindications: Significant renal impairment, G-6-PD deficiency, pregnancy at term, lactation, and infants younger than 1 month of age.

Toxicity:
1. GI distress: Decreased if given with food or split dosage.
2. Hypersensitivity reactions:
   a. Chills, fever, leukopenia, granulocytopenia, and hemolytic anemia (if G-6-PD deficiency).
   b. Cholestatic jaundice, hepatocellular damage, and chronic active hepatitis.
   c. Acute pneumonitis, which may progress to interstitial pulmonary fibrosis (geriatric age group more susceptible).
3. Neurologic: Headache and vertigo; rarely, severe polyneuropathies with demyelination and nerve degeneration; more common in patients with renal impairment or receiving prolonged therapy.

ANTIBIOTICS

■ **Norfloxacin** (Noroxin; Merck)

How Supplied:
Tablet: 400 mg.

Administration:
PO: Well absorbed; best taken 1 hr before or 2 hr after meals.

Mechanism of Action: (See Nalidixic Acid, p. 103.)

Dose:
Uncomplicated UTI: 400 mg bid × 7–10 days.
Complicated UTI: 400 mg bid × 10–21 days.

Elimination: Metabolized and excreted in bile and in kidney by glomerular filtration and tubular secretion. Half-life, 3–4.5 hr. Dosage adjustment required with significant renal impairment.

Spectrum: (See Table 3-2.) Fairly broad spectrum against gram-positive and gram-negative aerobic bacteria, including *E. coli, Klebsiella pneumoniae, Proteus mirabilis, Pseudomonas aeruginosa, Staphylococcus saprophyticus,* and enterococci.

Indication: UTI; uncomplicated urethral and cervical gonorrhea (including penicillinase-resistant).

Contraindications: Prepubertal children; pregnancy, lactation.

Toxicity: (See Nalidixic Acid, p. 104.)

Monitor: Theophylline levels if given concurrently.

Interaction: Probenecid given concurrently can delay drug excretion; nitrofurantoin may antagonize antibacterial effect; antacids also interfere with effectiveness. Possible increased plasma levels of theophylline and theophylline side effects. May enhance oral anticoagulant effects (e.g., warfarin).

■ **Ofloxacin** (Floxin; McNeil)

How Supplied:
PO: 200, 300, 400 mg tablets.
IV:
    200 mg in 50 ml flexible container (4 mg/ml).
    400 mg in 10 ml vial (40 mg/ml).
        20 ml vial (20 mg/ml).
        100 ml D5W bottle or flexible container (4 mg/ml).

Administration:
PO: Well absorbed.
Parenteral: IV only.

Dose:
200–400 mg bid. Decrease dose in presence of severe renal or hepatic impairment (max 400 mg/day).
Acute uncomplicated gonorrhea: 400 mg PO single dose.
Cervicitis/urethritis because of *Chlamydia, N. gonorrhoeae:* 300 mg bid × 7 days.

Elimination: Mainly renal excretion.

Spectrum: (See Table 3-2.)

Indications: Cervicitis and urethritis because of *C. trachomatis* or gonorrhea; UTI because of *Citrobacter, Enterobacter, E. coli, Klebsiella,* and *P. mirabillis;* skin and skin structure infections resulting from *S. aureus,* strep pyogenes, or *P. mirabillis;* bacterial exacerbation of chronic bronchitis and community-acquired pneumonia because of *H. influenza* or strep pneumoniae.

Contraindications: Pregnancy and lactation; history of hypersensitivity to quinolones; younger than 18 years of age.

Toxicity: CNS stimulation, phytotoxicity, GI upset, insomnia, headaches, dizziness, local reactions, or IV site.

Monitor: Maintain adequate hydration; monitor serum creatinine in patients with severe renal impairment.

Interactions: If taken less than 2 hr before, antacids containing calcium, magnesium, or aluminum interfere with absorption. Concommitant use of NSAIDs may increase risk of CNS stimulation and seizures. Drug may also potentiate theophylline warfarin.

ß-LACTAM ANTIBIOTICS
■ Aztreonam (Azactam; Briston-Myers Squibb)

How Supplied:
Parenteral:
    500 mg; 1, 2 gm single-dose vial.
    500 mg; 1, 2 gm IV infusion bottle.

Administration:
IM/IV.

Mechanism of Action: Monobactam (monocyclic ß-lactam) structure; bactericidal. Interacts with bacterial penicillin-binding proteins to induce aberrant bacterial structure formations.

Dose:
1. UTI or uncomplicated localized infection: 500 mg to 1 gm bid–tid.
2. Moderate to severe systemic infection: 1–2 gm bid–qid.
3. *P. aeruginosa* infection: 2 gm tid–qid.

Elimination: Cleared by kidney via glomerular filtration and tubular secretion; half-life, 1.5–2 hr.

Spectrum: Best against gram-negative aerobic organisms, especially *P. aeruginosa.* Enterobacteriaceae, and *N. gonorrhoeae.* Useful in treatment of UTI; lower respiratory tract infections; septicemia; skin and soft-tissue infections; and intraabdominal and gynecologic infections including endometritis, pelvic cellulitis, peritonitis, and abscesses.

Contraindications: Use extreme caution in patients with known hypersensitivity with rash and eosinophilia, GI distress, and transient AST (SGOT) elevation.

■ Imipenem-Cilastatin Sodium (Primaxin; Merck)

How Supplied:
Parenteral: 250 mg imipenem + 250 mg cilastatin, 500 mg imipenem + 500 mg cilastatin as vial, infusion bottle, and diluent container.

Administration:
IV.

Mechanism of Action:
Imipenem: Bactericidal by inhibition of bacterial cell wall synthesis; if given alone, it is quickly metabolized in kidneys by dehydropeptidase I.
Cilastatin: Inhibitor of renal dehydropeptidase I; thus prevents full metabolism of imipenem, so that adequate antibacterial levels achieved in urine.

Dose: 250–1000 mg qid–tid, depending on severity of infection; max 4 gm/day or 50 mg/kg/day, whichever is achieved first. Higher dosages for *Pseudomonas* infections; decrease dosage proportionately in patients weighing less than 70 kg.

Elimination: Excreted by kidneys; half-life of both imipenem and cilastatin is 1 hr.

Spectrum: (See Table 3-4.) Highly resistant to ß-lactamases synthesized by both gram-positive and gram-negative bacteria. Excellent activity against streptococci, enterococci, staphylococci, *Listeria;* most strains of *Pseudomonas* and *Acinetobacter;* and anaerobes such as *B. fragilis* and *Clostridium difficile. Pseudomonas maltophilia* and some methicillin-resistant staphylococci are resistant.

Indications: Gynecologic infections, including postpartum endomyometritis; intraabdominal infections, such as complications of appendicitis; lower respiratory tract infections; and skin and skin structure infections.

Contraindications: Patients with history of anaphylaxis to PCN may exhibit cross-reactivity. No adequate data on usage in pregnancy, lactation, and children younger than 12 years of age.

Toxicity: GI distress; rash, fever, and hypotension. Most serious side effects rare (fewer than 1%) but related to CNS: confusion, myoclonic activity, and seizures; higher incidence in patients with preexisting CNS disorders and renal impairment. Contains 3.2 mEq Na/gm.

COMBINATION ANTIBIOTIC ß-LACTAMASE INHIBITORS
■ Amoxicillin/Clavulanate Potassium
(Augmentin, Smith-Kline Beecham)

How Supplied:
PO:
    250 mg amoxicillin + 125 mg clavulanate tablet.
    500 mg amoxicillin + 125 mg clavulanate.
    125 mg amoxicillin + 31.25 mg clavulanate chewable tablet.
    250 mg amoxicillin + 62.5 mg clavulanate.

Administration:
PO: Well absorbed without regard to meals.

Mechanism of Action: Bactericidal; clavulanate binds to and inactivates bacterial ß-lactamases, thus preventing amoxicillin degradation and thereby extending spectrum.

Dose: 1 tablet, 250–500 mg, tid.

Elimination: Both constituents excreted by kidneys. Half-life, 1–1.3 hr.

Spectrum: Amoxicillin's usual spectrum extended to ß-lactamase–producing strains of staphylococci, *H. influenzae,* gonococci, and *E. coli.*
    Indicated in treatment of lower respiratory tract infections, otitis media, sinusitis, skin and soft-tissue infections, and UTI.

Contraindications: History of allergic reaction to PCNs; mononucleosis (high incidence of skin rash). No adequate data on usage in pregnancy and lactation.

Toxicity: Most mild and transient (e.g., GI distress and hypersensitivity reactions with skin rash and urticaria). (See Amoxicillin, p. 51.)

■ Ampicillin Sodium/Sulbactam (Unasyn; Roerig)

Mechanism of Action: (See Ampicillin, p. 50.) Sulbactam confers ß-lactamase resistance.

How Supplied:
Parenteral:
    1.5 gm vial bottle (1 gm ampicillin + 0.5 gm sulbactam as sodium salt).
    3 gm vial, bottle (2 gm ampicillin + 1 gm sulbactam as sodium salt).

Administration: IV, IM.

Dose: 1.5–3 gm q6h; lengthen dosing interval in presence of impaired renal function.

Elimination: 75%–85% excreted unchanged in urine. Usual serum half-life 1 hr; longer with concomitant probenicid.

Spectrum: Indicated for gynecologic, intraabdominal, and skin infections because of ß-lactamase producing strains of *E. coli,* bacteroides species including *B. fragilis, Klebsiella, Enterobacter,* staph aureus, *Proteus mirabilis,* and *A. cinetobacter.* Broad spectrum activity allows administration before organism isolation.

Toxicity: Pain at injection site (16% with IM), thrombophlebitis (3%); diarrhea (2%); rash; hypersensitivity reactions (especially with history of penicillin allergy).

Interactions: Concomitant probenicid results in increased and prolonged blood levels.

■ Piperacillin Sodium/Tazobactam (Zosyn; Lederle)

Mechanism of Action: Bactericidal (see Piperacillin, p. 55); tazobactam is a ß-lactamase inhibitor.

How Supplied:
Parenteral: 40.5 gm bulk vial (36 gm piperacillin + 4.5 gm tazobactam sodium)

Administration: IV infusion over 30 mins.

Dose: 3.375 gm (12 gm/1.5gm) q6h.

Elimination: Excreted via kidney; 68%/80% as unchanged drug. Adjust dose in presence of severe renal impairment.

Spectrum: See Piperacillin p. 55. Indicated for moderate to severe infections caused by ß-lactamase producing susceptible strains of E. coli, *Bacteroides, H. influenza,* such as pelvic inflammatory disease, endometritis, appendicitis, peritonitis, intraabdominal abscess, community-acquired pneumonia, and skin infections. Useful as presumptive therapy before organism isolation because of broad spectrum bactericidal activity against gram-positive and gram-negative aerobic and anerobic organisms.

Toxicity: Diarrhea, nausea, vomiting, constipation (1%–10%), rash (4%); headaches (7%).

Interactions: Concomitant administration can result in aminoglycoside inactivation.

■ Ticarcillin Disodium/Clavulanate Potassium
(Ticar, Timentin; Smith-Kline Beecham)

How Supplied:
Parenteral:
   3 gm ticarcillin +0.1 gm clavulinic acid as 3.1 gm vial,
   3.1 gm piggyback bottle, 3.1 gm vial and diluent container.
   3 gm ticarcillin +0.2 gm clavulinic acid as 3.2 gm vial,
   3.2 gm piggyback bottle.
   30 gm ticarcillin +1 gm clavulinic acid as 31 gm bulk vial.

Administration: *IV.*

Mechanism of Action: Bactericidal, clavulinic acid binds to and inactivates bacterial b-lactamases, preventing ticarcillin degradation and extending antibiotic spectrum.

Dose: 3.1 gm q4–6h.
   UTI: 3.2 gm tid.

Elimination: Cleared by kidneys; half-life 1.1 hr. Adjust dosage only in severe renal impairment.

Spectrum: See Amoxicillin/Clavulanate Potassium, p. 110. Clavulanate component extends spectrum to many ß-lactamase–synthesizing microorganisms.

Contraindications: Known history of penicillin hypersensitivity reaction.

Toxicity: Hypersensitivity reactions with rash, urticaria, drug fever, and possible anaphylaxis; CNS hyperirritability or seizures; GI distress; blood dyscrasias including prolongation of prothrombin time and bleeding time; elevation of liver enzymes or BUN and/or creatinine; thrombophlebitis; hypokalemia. Contains 4.75 mEq Na/gm. See also Ticarcillin, p. 53–54.

ANTIMICROBIAL AGENTS TO TREAT TUBERCULOSIS

First-line Drugs:

- Isoniazid.
- Rifampin.
- Ethambutol HCl.
- Streptomycin.
- Pyrazinamide.

1. Best efficacy with acceptable level of side effects.
2. Treatment of active disease with combination therapy to avoid emergence of resistant strains:
   a. Nine–month regimen: Isoniazid and rifampin
   b. Six–month regimen: Isoniazid, rifampin, and pyrazinamide × 2 mo followed by isoniazid and rifampin × 4 mo.
   c. Initial therapy should involve four drugs in area where primary resistance to isonizid is high: rifampin, isoniazid, pyrazinamide, and ethambutol (or streptomycin) until sensitivity tests completed.

Second-line Drugs:

- Ethionamide.
- Aminosalicylic acid.
- Cycloserine.
- Amikacin.
- Kanamycin.
- Capreomycin.

May be needed in case of resistant organisms to suit individual patient tolerance.

Treatment Guidelines

I. Patients with active infections:

Outpatient treatment with visits at frequent intervals.

Notify local health department; seek out contacts (see Prophylaxis below).

To prevent development of resistance during course of therapy, treatment must include at lest two drugs to which organism is sensitive.

Standard 6-month treatment usually preferred: isoniazid, rifampin, and pyrazinamide × 2 months, then isoniazid and rifampin equally effective.

ANTIBIOTICS

Use three drugs initially in life-threatening disease, large cavitary disease, or renal TB.

Use four drugs initially in patients exposed to drug-resistant strains; Asians and Hispanics, especially if recent immigrants; miliary, or other extra pulmonary TB; meningitis, extensive pulmonary disease. Fourth agent either ethambutol 1 gm/day, or streptomycin 1 gm daily × 2 months, then 1 gm 2 × /wk.

II. Patients infected with HIV:

CDC (1989) advises minimum 9-month treatment: 2 months isoniazid, rifampin, and pyrazinamide, then at least 7 months isoniazid and rifampin.

Add ethambutol to initial regimen if CNS or disseminated TB or if suspect isoniazid-resistant strain.

Continue treatment at least 3 months after three negative cultures.

If unable to use isoniazid or rifampin, continue therapy 12–18 months after negative cultures.

III. Chemoprophylaxis:

Goal is to prevent development of active TB in patients at risk.

Isoniazid usually given 300 mg/day.

For household and close contacts with negative skin tests, continue therapy × 6 months after contact has been broken (12 months if skin test turns positive).

Skin test converts from negative to positive within last 2 years without evidence of active disease; 12-month regimen.

Positive skin test at any time and high-risk status are patients younger than 35 years old with HIV, leukemia, lymphoma, silicosis, or on immunosuppressive therapy; 12-month regimen. (In patients older than 35 years old, the risk of isoniazid toxicity may outweigh the potential benefit of therapy.)

Patients with old, "inactive" TB who never received adequate therapy should be treated for 1 year.

In pregnant women, delay prophylaxis until after delivery.

IV. Chemotherapy failure:

Most frequently because of poor patient compliance and irregular/inadequate therapy resulting in persistant/resistant mycobacteria, misuse of a single drug with interruption necessitated by toxicity or hypersensitivity, or primary resistant strain.

■ **Ethionamide** (Trecator-SC; Wyeth-Ayerst)

How Supplied:
Tablet: 250 mg.

Administration:
PO: Adequately absorbed. Distributes itself throughout blood and various organs including CSF.

Mechanism: Bacteriostatic.

Dose: Initially 250 mg bid, then increase by 125 mg every 5 days to max 1 gm/day. Avoid GI upset by taking with meals; concurrent pyridoxine recommended.

Elimination: Metabolized in liver; half-life approximately 2 hr.

Spectrum: *Mycobacterium tuberculosis.*

Indication: Considered a secondary agent to be used as part of multidrug therapy only when adequate treatment with primary agents fail.

Contraindications: Pregnancy, lactation, significant hepatic dysfunction, and known hypersensitivity.

Toxicity: GI distress (common), reversible hepatitis (more common in diabetic patients), postural hypotension, peripheral neuritis, optic neuritis, psychic disturbances, rash, and menorrhagia.

Monitor: AST and ALT (SGOT and SGPT) as baseline and every 2–4 wk.
NOTE: Diabetic patients may need insulin/hypoglycemic agent dosage adjustment; adverse effects of other antituberculous agents may intensify (e.g., convulsions more common when taken with cycloserine).

■ **Aminosalicylic Acid**

How Supplied:
PO: 500, 1000 mg tablets.

ANTIBIOTICS

Administration:
PO; well absorbed.

Mechanism of Action: Bacteriostatic structural analog of paraminobenzoic acid; mechanism of action similar to sulfonamides.

Dose: 14–16 gm/day, divided tid–qid; after meals to minimize GI irritation.

Elimination: Largely renal excretion; half-life 1 hr. Excretion greatly retarded with renal dysfunction and probenicid.

Spectrum: *M. tuberculosis.*

Indications: Second-line agent in combination treatment of TB.

Contraindications: Renal dysfunction; history of peptic ulcer.

Adverse reactions: Seen in 10%–30% patients; GI distress symptoms predominate. Hypersensitivity reactions 5%–10% with fever, rash, malaise, joint pains, and blood dyscrasias.

■ Cycloserine (Seromycin; Lilly)

How Supplied:
250 mg pulvules.

Administration:
PO: Rapidly absorbed. Penetrates all body fluids and tissues, including CSF.

Mechanism of Action: Bacteriostatic; inhibits cell wall synthesis.

Dose: 500 mg to 1 gm/day divided bid; given with 200–300 mg pyridoxine per day to reduce neurotoxicity.

Elimination: One third metabolized in liver, two thirds excreted unchanged in urine. Half-life 15–25 hr. Adjust dose in renal insufficiency.

Spectrum: *M. tuberculosis:* certain gram-positive and gram-negative bacteria, including *Enterobacter* species and *E. coli.*

Indication: As second-line agent; usefulness in anti-TB therapy limited to retreatment or when organisms are resistant to other drugs. Must be used as part of combination therapy.

Contraindications: Known hypersensitivity to cycloserine; seizure disorder; depression, severe anxiety, or psychosis; severe renal impairment; excessive alcohol intake; and lactation. Used in pregnancy only if absolutely necessary.

Toxicity: CNS effects predominate (more common at doses in excess of 500 mg/day or plasma level >30 μg/ml) such as somnolence, vertigo, headache, mental disorientation, psychosis, and seizures (increased risk of convulsions with ingestion of ethanol). Symptoms usually appear within first 2 wk, disappear when therapy is discontinued. Rarely, megaloblastic anemia.

Interaction: Concurrent administration of isoniazid or ethionamide may potentiate CNS and neurotoxic effects.

■ Capreomycin Sulfate (Capastat Sulfate; Lilly)

How Supplied:
Parenteral: 1 gm/10 ml vial.

Administration: Deep IM injection only (superficial injection may be associated with pain or sterile abscess development).

Mechanism: Bactericidal; inhibits protein synthesis.

Dose: 1 gm/day (max 20 mg/kg/day) for 60–120 days, then 1 gm 2–3 times/wk.

Elimination: Excreted via kidneys.

Spectrum: *M. tuberuclosis* only.

Indication: Pulmonary infections susceptible strains when primary agents have been ineffective because of resistance or toxicity. Usually given as part of continuing combination therapy.

Contraindications: Infancy, childhood, pregnancy, lactation, and known hypersensitivity. Use only with great caution in patients with preexisting renal or auditory impairment.

Toxicity:
Renal: Proteinuria, abnormal urinary sediment, and rise in BUN; hypokalemia; rarely, tubular necrosis and severe renal failure.
Auditory: Subclinical auditory loss, usually reversible; tinnitus; vertigo.
Blood: Eosinophilia (common), leukocytosis, leukopenia, thrombocytopenia.
Miscellaneous: Rash; fever; abnormal liver function tests; pain, induration, or sterile abscess at injection site.

Monitor: Baseline and serial audiometric and vestibular evaluation, baseline and weekly renal function studies, periodic serum potassium. In presence of renal impairment, maintain serum drug levels at 10 µg/ml.

Interaction: Streptomycin or other potentially nephrotoxic or ototoxic agents (e.g., gentamicin, tobramycin, vancomycin) given concurrently may potentiate nephrotoxicity or ototoxicity.

■ Isoniazid (Isoniazid; Duramed. Nydrazid; Apothecon)

How Supplied:
PO: 300 mg tablets.
Parenteral: 100 mg/10 ml vial.

Administration:
PO: Well absorbed (unless taken with aluminum-containing antacids). Penetrates well into all body fluids and cells, including CSF and caseous material; crosses placenta and passes into breast milk.
IM administration only indicated when PO route is not possible.

Mechanism of Action: Bactericidal for rapidly dividing microorganisms by inhibition of synthesis of mycobacterial mycolic acid cell wall constituents.

Dose:
Prophylaxis:
Children: 10 mg/kg/day as single dose; max 300 mg.
Adults: 300 mg/day, single dose.
Treatment:
Children: 10–20 mg/kg/day as single dose; max 500 mg/day
in very severe infections.
Adults: 5 mg/kg/day as single dose; max 300 mg/day.
Give with pyridoxine (15–20 mg/day) to avoid neuropathy
(see Toxicity below).

Elimination: Renal and hepatic metabolization by acetylation
and dehydralization. Half-life varies from 1–4 hr; prolonged in
"slow acetylators" (50% of Caucasians and African-Americans)
and hepatic insufficiency.

Spectrum: *M. tuberculosis* and *M. kansasii.*

Contraindications: Acute or chronic liver disease; known
hypersensitivity to isoniazid. Prophylaxis contraindicated in
patients with heavy alcohol intake and during pregnancy (delay
start of therapy until after delivery). Breast-fed neonates should
be observed carefully for adverse effects.

Toxicity: Overall incidence 5.4%.
Hepatic: Symptoms usually begin 4–8 wk after starting therapy; may progress to severe, possibly fatal hepatitis with jaundice, elevated liver enzymes, and multilobular necrosis.
Increased risk with increasing age or preexisting liver disease.
Neurologic: Peripheral neuritis (if not receiving pyridoxine
concurrently); convulsions (more common in patients with
seizure disorders); optic neuritis; paresthesias, vertigo, stu-
por, mental disorientation, hallucinations, or coma (may also
be seen with overdosage).
Hypersensitivity: Fever, rash, blood dyscrasias, and vasculitis.
Miscellaneous: Systemic lupus erythematosus (SLE)-like
syndrome; rheumatic syndrome.

Monitor: Liver enzymes and ophthalmologic exam as baseline
and periodically thereafter (liver enzymes monthly); phenytoin
levels if receiving concurrent therapy; renal function if attempt-
ing to rule out drug toxicity vs. hypersensitivity reaction.

ANTIBIOTICS

Interaction: May need to lower dosage of phenytoin, carbamazepine, diazepam, or prednisone because of isoniazid inhibition of liver microsomal enzymes. Daily alcohol users may have a higher incidence of isoniazid hepatitis.

■ Ethambutol HCI (Myambutol; Lederle)

How Supplied:
PO: 100, 400 mg tablets.

Administration:
PO: Well absorbed without regard to meals.

Mechanism of Action: Tuberculostatic by means of impairment of cell metabolism and arrest of multiplication.

Dose (as part of combination therapy):
Initial treatment: 15 mg/kg, single daily dose.
Retreatment (i.e., history of previous antituberculous therapy): 25 mg/kg as single dose; decrease to 15 mg/kg single dose after 60 days.

Elimination: Renal excretion by tubular secretion and glomerular filtration. Half-life 3–4 hr. Adjust dose in renal insufficiency.

Spectrum: *M. tuberculosis* and *M. kansasii.* Used only in treatment of pulmonary TB, most commonly in combination with isoniazid or isoniazid and streptomycin.

Contraindications: Children younger than 13 years of age (usual visual acuity assessment may be difficult), optic neuritis, and known hypersensitivity to ethambutol. Pregnancy not a contraindication.

Toxicity: Overall incidence less than 2%.
Optic neuritis with decreased visual activity and loss of red-green differentiation; dose and duration related, unilateral or bilateral; usually reversible.
Hypersensitivity: Reactions such as rash, fever, and joint pain.
Miscellaneous: Peripheral neuritis (rare), GI distress, mental state changes and elevation of serum uric acid.

Monitor: Ophthalmologic exam baseline and monthly, including visual acuity and red-green color discrimination, if receiving >15 mg/kg/day. Also, periodic liver enzymes, renal function tests, CBC.

■ Pyrazinamide (Lederle)

How Supplied:
PO: 500 mg tablets.

Administration:
PO: Well absorbed.

Mechanism of Action: Bactericidal; exact mechanism unknown.

Dose: 20–35 mg/kg/day divided tid or qid; max 2 gm/day.

Elimination: Hepatic metabolism and renal excretion via glomerular filtration.

Spectrum: *M. tuberculosis.* Used mainly as initial part of (6 months or longer regimen of) combination therapy, particularly in underdeveloped areas with high degree of primary resistance.

Contraindication: Hepatic dysfunction.

Toxicity: Elevated liver enzyme values with jaundice, and rarely, fatal hepatic necrosis (more common at doses of 40–50 mg/kg/day), elevated uric acid levels with symptoms of acute gout, arthralgias, GI distress, and fever.

Monitor: Baseline and serial liver function tests.

COMBINATION FIRST-LINE AGENTS
■ Rifampin and Isoniazid (Rifamate; Marion Merrell Dow)

■ Rifampin, Isoniazid, and Pyrazinamide (Rifater; Marion Merrell Dow)

How Supplied:
PO: 120 mg rifampin/50 mg isoniazide/300 mg pyrazinamide per tablet.

Administration: *PO.*

Dose: 4–6 tablets (depending on body weight) single dose q day 1 hr before or 2 hr after a meal with a full glass of water.

Elimination/Spectrum: (See individual agents Isoniazid, p. 119, Rifampin, p. 123, and Pyrazinamide, p. 121.)

Indications: Is daily part of initial 2 months phase of short course TB therapy.

Contraindications/Toxicity/Interactions: (See individual drugs.)

■ **Rifampin** (Rifadin; Marion Merrell Dow. Rimactane; CIBA)

How Supplied:
PO: 150, 300 mg.
Parenteral: 600 mg vial.

Administration:
PO: Well absorbed. Give 1 hr before or 2 hr after meals. PAS may delay absorption (give at least 4 hr apart). Adequate levels reached in most body fluids, including CSF. Do not give intermittently (less than 2 times/wk).
Parenterally: give IV only; avoid extravasation.

Mechanism of Action: Bactericidal; inhibits DNA-dependent RNA polymerase and thus protein synthesis in bacterial, but not mammalian cells.

Dose:
Tuberculosis: As part of long-term (e.g., 9 mo) combination therapy, usually with isoniazid: 600 mg/day, single dose.

M. carriers (N. meningitidis and *H. influenzae):* 600 mg/day given once daily × 4 days.

Elimination: Metabolized in liver by deacetylation; eliminated via enterohepatic circulation in bile and by kidney. Half-life 1.5–5 hr, longer in patients with liver dysfunction. Body fluids (i.e., urine, feces, saliva, sputum, tears, sweat) become orange-red.

Spectrum: *Mycobacterium, N. meningitidis, H. influenzae.* Also active against most gram-positive bacteria, *S. aureus,* and *L. pneumophila.*

Contraindications: Pregnancy <16 weeks gestation (high incidence of fetal malformations); may be used after 16 weeks gestation, but only if microorganisms and not sensitive to isoniazid or ethambutol (preferred agents for treatment of active tuberculosis in pregnancy). Also contraindicated in patients with known hypersensitivity to the drug. Use with great caution in patients with chronic liver disease or alcoholism or in older patients (increased risk of hepatotoxicity, see below).

Toxicity: Overall incidence, 3%–4%.
   Hepatic: Jaundice and possible fatal hepatitis. Increased risk in patients with liver disease or alcoholism, or in older patients.
   Hypersensitivity: Rash, fever, GI distress, and blood dyscrasias.
   Miscellaneous: Flulike syndrome when given intermittently (less than twice weekly), with fever, myalgias, interstitial nephritis, acute tubular necrosis, hemolytic anemia, and shock.

Interaction: Induces liver microsomal enzymes, thereby decreasing the half-life of concurrently administered coumarin, digitoxin, quinidine, propranolol, metoprolol, prednisone, keto-conazole, verapamil, phenytoin, theophylline, methadone, barbiturates, or oral hypoglycemics. Possible decreased efficacy of oral contraceptives if receiving combination TB therapy with at least one other drug.

ANTIBIOTICS

CHAPTER 4

ANTIINFECTIVES

ANTIFUNGAL AGENTS

■ **Amphotericin B** (Fungizone; Apothecon)
(Common antifungals and indications are listed in Table 4-1.)

How Supplied:
Parenteral: 50 mg vial.

Administration: *IV:* Crosses inflamed pleura, peritoneum, synovium, and aqueous humor. Does not penetrate CSF (requires direct intrathecal injection to treat meningitis). Therapy usually lasts 6–10 wk but possibly up to 4 mo, except for some candidal infections.

Dose:
IV:
1. Test dose: 1 mg in 20 ml D5W infused over 20–30 min; monitor vital signs every 30 min for 4 hr.
2. Initial daily dose:
    a. If no or mild reaction to test dose and good cardiorenal status: 0.25 mg/kg over 2–6 hr.
    b. If severe, rapidly progressive infection: 0.3 mg/kg.
    c. With severe reaction to test dose or cardiorenal impairment: 5–10 mg/day over 2–6 hr.
3. Increment dosage: Gradually increase dose by 5–10 mg/day to final dose of 0.5–0.7 mg/kg.
4. Usual daily dose: 0.5–1.0 mg/kg.
5. Maximum dose: 1.0 mg/kg/day or 1.5 mg/kg every other day (qod).
    Alternate day dosage may decrease anorexia and phlebitis.

Mechanism: Increases cell membrane permeability; fungistatic or fungicidal, depending on drug concentration and organism sensitivity.

Elimination: Biliary excretion; half-life 1–15 days.

TABLE 4-1
ANTIFUNGAL AGENTS

Organism	First-Line Treatment	Second-Line Treatment
ASPERGILLUS	*AMPHOTERICIN B*	
BLASTOMYCES DERMATITIDIS	*AMPHOTERICIN B*	*KETOCONAZOLE*
Nonmeningeal	1.5 gm total dose over 6–10 wk	400–800 mg/day
CANDIDA SPECIES	*AMPHOTERICIN B*	*KETOCONAZOLE*
Disseminated disease	40 mg qod, total of 600–1000 mg	
Esophagitis	20 mg/day × 10 days	200–400 mg/day × several wk
Endocarditis	With or without flucytosine	
Chronic mucocutaneous		600 mg/day
Oral thrush		*KETOCONAZOLE*
COCCIDIOIDES IMMITIS	*AMPHOTERICIN B*	
Disseminated disease	1 mg/kg qod, long term	
Meningitis	0.5–1 mg, intrathecal, 3 times/wk, until CSF sterile × 3 mo or no positive complement-fixation antibody test	
Relapse or resistant cases	Add immunotherapy with transfer factor	
Nonmeningeal		400–800 mg/day

Continued.

125

TABLE 4-1
ANTIFUNGAL AGENTS—Cont'd

Organism	First-Line Treatment	Second-Line Treatment
CRYPTOCOCCUS NEOFORMANS		
Meningitis	*AMPHOTERICIN B*	
	0.4–1 mg/kg/day × 6–10 wk	
	0.3 mg/kg/day with flucytosine,	
	150 mg/kg/day × 6 wk	
Nonmeningeal disease		*KETOCONAZOLE*
HISTOPLASMA CAPSULATUM		*KETOCONAZOLE*
Severe/prolonged pulmonary infection	*AMPHOTERICIN B*	400–800 mg/day × 6–12 mo
	0.4–0.7 mg/kg/day,	
	total of 800–1000 mg	
Chronic cavitary	Total, 1.5–2 gm over 10 wk	
Progressive disseminated	Total, 2 gm over 10 wk	
PARACOCCIDIOIDES BRASILIENSIS	*KETOCONAZOLE*	*SULFONAMIDES*
Nonmeningeal	200–400 mg/day	
Meningeal	*AMPHOTERICIN B*	
SPOROTHRIX SCHENKII	*AMPHOTERICIN B*	*KETOCONAZOLE*
Systemic, especially if bone and	1.5–2 gm × 6–10 wk	
joint involvement		
Cutaneous-lymphatic	*IODIDE*	
TINEA VERSICOLOR	*KETOCONAZOLE*	
ZYGOMYCETES	*AMPHOTERICIN B*	

Spectrum: *Aspergillus, Blastomyces dermatitidis, Candida, Coccidioides immitis, Cryptococcus neoformans, Histoplasma capsulatum, Paracoccidioides brasiliensis, Rhodotorula, Sporothrix schenckii.*

Indications: See Table 4-1. Progressive, potentially fatal fungal infections only. May be used in pregnancy; no evidence of fetal toxicity has been reported, but long-term studies have yet to be performed; thus, breastfeeding not advised.

Toxicity: Fever, chills, vomiting; common after initial IV dose but usually less severe with each subsequent dose. Also, decreased renal function in 80% of patients (minimize with adequate hydration); largely reversible, but some residual decrease in GFR to be expected. Mild renal tubular acidosis and hypokalemia frequent; hypomagnesemia. May also see normochromic and normocytic anemia, leukopenia, thrombocytopenia; anaphylaxis, convulsions; phlebitis; anorexia. Intrathecal injection may be followed by pain along lumbar nerve distribution, headache, nerve palsies, paresthesias, and visual impairment. Immediate reactions (fever, etc.) may be lessened with concurrent corticosteroid administration. Rarely, may see cardiac dysrhythmias, ventricular fibrillation, cardiac arrest; acute liver failure; agranulocytosis.

Monitor: CBC, UA, potassium, magnesium, BUN, bilirubin, AST (SGOT); creatinine, 2–3 times per week initially (as dosage is increased), then weekly. Discontinue therapy if BUN exceeds 40, creatinine exceeds 3, or liver function tests become abnormal.

Interactions: Corticosteroids, ACTH, or nonreabsorbable anions (e.g., carbenicillin) may potentiate hypokalemia, which itself may result in digitalis toxicity or enhanced curariform effect of certain skeletal muscle relaxants. Other nephrotoxic agents (aminoglycosides, cyclosporine, nitrogen mustards) given concurrently may enhance potential for renal damage. Synergism with flucytosine may allow decrease in dosage but may also delay excretion and thus increase toxicity.

■ **Fluconazole** (Diflucan; Roerig)

How Supplied:
PO: Tablet: 50, 100, 150, 200 mg.
  Oral Suspension: 350 mg, 1400 mg/35 ml.
Parenteral: 200 mg/100 ml, 400 mg/200 ml glass bottle or flexible plastic container.

Administration: *PO,* rapidly and almost completely absorbed; *IV.*

Mechanism of Action: Fungistatic; selective inhibitor of fungal cytochrome P-450 sterol C-14 alpha-demethylation.

Dose:
General principles: PO absorption rapid and almost as complete as IV, so daily dose same. Give twice the usual dose on the first day as loading dose to achieve steady state plasma concentration by day two. Inadequate period of treatment may lead to recurrence. Patients with AIDS, cryptococcal meningitis, or recurrent oropharyngeal candidiasis usually need maintenance therapy to prevent relapse.

  Vaginal candidiasis: 150 mg PO single dose.

  Oropharyngeal candidiasis: 200 mg on day one, then 100 mg/day, for at least two weeks.

  Esophageal candidiasis: Same as for oropharyngeal; maximum dose 400 mg/day, for at least 2–3 weeks and at least two weeks after symptoms resolve.

  Candidal UTI and peritonitis: 50–200 mg/day.

  Systemic candidal infections (e.g., candidemia, pneumonia): up to 400 mg/day.

  Cryptococcal meningitis: 400 mg on day one, then 200 mg/day, up to 400 mg/day for 10–12 weeks after CSF culture negative; continue at 200/mg/day in AIDS patients to prevent relapse.

  Prevention of candidiasis in patients undergoing bone marrow transplant: 400 mg/day, single dose, beginning several days before transplant if neutropenic.

Elimination: Excreted by the kidney unchanged; reduce dose by 50% if creatinine clearance less than 50 ml/min.

Spectrum: *Cryptococcus neoformans; Candida.*

Indications: Candidal infections of the oropharynx, esophagus, genitourinary tract and peritonitis; and systemic infection, including candidemia and pneumonia; cryptococcal meningitis; prophylaxis against candidiasis in patients about to undergo bone marrow transplant or chemotherapy or radiation.

Contraindications: Hypersensitivity to fluconazole or other azoles.

Adverse effects: GI distress; headache; exfoliative dermatitis; liver reactions (see below), leukopenia; thrombocytopenia.

Toxicity: Potentially fatal liver failure, more common in patients with AIDS, malignancy, or on multiple other medications.

Monitor: Liver function tests; CBC; platelets; theophylline phenytoin levels if taken concurrently; serum creatinine if on cyclosporine; prothrombin time if on coumadin.

Interactions: Clinically significant hypoglycemia if on oral hypoglycemic agents; prothrombin time may increase if on coumadin-type anticoagulants; increased theophylline and phenytoin levels; increased cyclosporine levels in renal transplant patients; rifampin speeds diflucan metabolism and dose increase should be considered.

■ Flucytosine (Ancobon; Roche)

How Supplied:
Capsule: 250, 500 mg.

Administration: *PO:* rapidly and well absorbed; widely distributed in body tissues including in CSF and aqueous humor.

Dose: 50–150 mg/kg/day divided qid; decrease in patients with renal dysfunction.

Mechanism of Action: Competitively inhibits purine and pyrimidine uptake; also, is metabolized in cells to 5-fluorouracil (5-FU) with subsequent incorporation into fungal RNA and inhibition of DNA and RNA synthesis.

Elimination: Renal excretion via glomerular filtration. Half-life 3–6 hr in presence of normal renal function; up to 200 hr with renal failure.

Spectrum: *Cryptococcus neoformans,* certain strains of *Candida.*

Indications: See Table 4-1. Yeast and fungal infections; usually used with amphotericin B because of rapid emergence of drug-resistant strains when given as a single agent. Treatment of choice (administered with amphotericin B) for cryptococcal meningitis.

Contraindications: Exercise caution in patients with renal impairment or bone marrow depression. Potential teratogenicity of 5-FU metabolites limits use in pregnancy to life-threatening situations; breastfeeding discouraged.

Toxicity:
1. More common in patients with azotemia or when serum drug concentrations exceed 100 µg/ml.
2. Bone marrow depression: Anemia, leukopenia, and thrombocytopenia; more common in patients with underlying hematologic disorder, undergoing radiation treatment, or receiving other bone marrow depressant drugs.
3. GI: Nausea, vomiting (minimize by administering dose over 15 min), diarrhea, enterocolitis.
4. Hepatotoxicity: Liver enzyme elevation and hepatomegaly (5% patients), usually reversible.
5. Renal: Increased BUN or creatinine.

Monitor: CBC, BUN, creatinine, electrolytes, LFTs. If used in renal impairment, watch serum drug levels and maintain peak at 50–100 µg/ml.

Drug Interactions: Synergistic with polyene antibiotics including amphotericin B; cytosine arabinoside may inactivate antifungal activity.

■ **Griseofulvin** (Fulvicin P/G, P/G 165, P/G 330, Schering. Grifulvin V; Ortho. Grisactin, Grisactin Ultra; Wyeth-Ayerst. Gris-PEG; Allergan Herbert)

How Supplied:
PO: 125, 165, 250, 330, 500 mg tablet.
Suspension: 125 mg/5 ml in 4 oz bottle.

Administration: PO. Absorption variable; increased in ultra-microsized form or if taken with meals, especially fatty; decreased if taken with barbiturates. Deposited in keratin precursor cells (hair, nails, skin). Half-life approximately 24 hr.

Dose: 500 mg/day as single dose or divided qid; maximum starting dose 1 gm/day if lesions widespread.

Mechanism of Action: Fungistatic; inhibits fungal mitosis.

Spectrum: *Microsporum, Epidermophyton, Trichophyton.*

Indication: Mycotic diseases of the skin (tinea cruris, tinea corporis, ringworm, and "athlete's foot"), hair (tinea capitis), beard, and nails.

Contraindications: Embryotoxic and teratogenic, with at least two reported cases of conjoined twins after use in first trimester of pregnancy. Should also not be used in patients with porphyria, hepatocellular failure, or a history of hypersensitivity to the drug.

Toxicity:
1. Hypersensitivity (common): Rash, urticaria, photosensitivity, angioneurotic edema (rare).
2. Nervous system: Headache (15% patients), peripheral neuritis, fatigue, confusion, vertigo.
3. GI: Nausea, vomiting, diarrhea.
4. Hematologic (rare): Leukopenia, granulocytopenia.
5. Miscellaneous: Hepatotoxicity, proteinuria.

Monitor: CBC, BUN, and creatinine; liver function tests.

Interaction: May induce hepatic microsomal enzymes and necessitate increase in warfarin-type anticoagulant dosage. Barbiturates may decrease efficacy. In theory, may reduce oral contraceptive efficacy or result in increased incidence of breakthrough bleeding.

ANTIINFECTIVES

■ Itraconazole (Sporanox; Janssen)

How Supplied:
PO: 100 mg capsule.

Administration: *PO;* best absorbed with food.

Mechanism of Action: Inhibits cytochrome P-450 dependent synthesis of ergosterol, vital component of fungal cell membranes.

Dose:
Usual: 200 mg/day, single dose.
    If no improvement: Increase by 100 mg up to 400 mg/day maximum in two divided doses.
    In life-threatening situations: 200 mg tid for first 3 days, then continue at 200–400 mg/day.

Elimination: Metabolized by liver; 40% excreted as inactive metabolites in urine. No need to decrease dose with renal impairment.

Spectrum: *Blastomyces dermatitis, Histoplasma* species, *Aspergillus* species, *Cryptococcus neoformans.*

Indications: Pulmonary and extrapulmonary blastomycosis; histoplasmosis including chronic cavitary pulmonic and disseminated nonmeningeal infections; pulmonary and extrapulmonary aspergillosis refractory to amphotericin B.

Contraindications: Known itraconazole hypersensitivity; coadministration of terfenadine or astemizole.

Adverse effects/Toxicity: GI distress, vomiting; edema, skin rash; headache; rarely, potentially fatal reversible idiosyncratic hepatitis.

Monitor: Liver function tests; prothrombin time if on coumadin-type anticoagulant; itraconazole serum levels when given with isoniazid; digoxin and phenytoin levels.

Drug Interactions: May elevate terfenadine plasma levels leading to potentially fatal cardiac dysrhythmias; increased plasma levels of cyclosporine and digoxin; potentiates coumadin-type anticoagulants and oral hypoglycemics; reduced drug levels when given with isoniazid.

■ Ketoconazole (Nizoral; Janssen)

How Supplied:
PO: 200 mg tablet.
Topical: 2% cream in 25, 30, 60 gm tube.

Administration:
PO: Fairly well absorbed unless given with agents that decrease gastric acidity such as antacids and H_2 blocking agents (these should be taken 2 hours after ketoconazole). GI upset minimized by administration with meals, but this may also diminish absorption. Penetrates CSF poorly, but appears in breast milk.
Topical: No systemic absorption.

Mechanism of Action: Fungicidal imidazole. Inhibits synthesis of ergosterol, the main fungal cell sterol, and thus alters cell membrane permeability.

Dose:
PO: 200 mg/day as single dose; 400 mg/day in severe infections. Continue therapy 1–2 weeks for candidiasis; 6 months or longer for other systemic mycoses.
Topical: Apply to affected area and immediate surrounding area every day × 2 wk; bid in cases of seborrheic dermatitis.

Elimination: Hepatic metabolism; half-life approximately 90 min (longer with larger doses).

Spectrum: *Candida* species, *Histoplasma capsulatum, Coccidioides immitis, Blastomyces dermatitidis, Paracoccidioides brasiliensis, Phialophora* species, *Trichophyton, Epidermophyton* and *Microsporum* species.

Indication: See Table 4-1. Particularly useful for systemic fungal infections: candidiasis, chronic mucocutaneous candidiasis, oral thrush, histoplasmosis, paracoccidiomycosis, blastomycosis, coccidioimycoses, and chromomycosis. Also used for severe recalcitrant cutaneous dermatophyte infections not responding to topical therapy or oral griseofulvin. Insufficient CSF penetration to treat fungal meningitis.

Contraindications: Pregnancy, lactation (teratogenic in rats); concurrent INH, rifampin, terfenadine, astemizole; known hypersensitivity to the drug.

Adverse effects: Nausea and vomiting (common), anorexia, headache, photophobia, paresthesias; rash; thrombocytopenia; gynecomastia, reversible lowering of serum testosterone; transient asymptomatic elevation of plasma transaminase in 5%–10%.

Toxicity: Serious hepatic toxicity, rarely fatal, in 1/15,000 patients, especially if on other potentially hepatotoxic drugs or with history of liver disease; cardiac dysrhythmias if taken with astemizole or terfenadine.

Monitor: Baseline and monthly alkaline phosphatase, bilirubin, SGGT, AST (SGOT), ALT (SGPT); PT if on coumadin-type anticoagulant; ketoconazole and phenytoin levels if taken concurrently.

Interactions:
1. Decreases phenytoin blood levels.
2. Potentiates effects of oral anticoagulants and oral hypoglycemic agents.
3. Increases blood levels of cyclosporin A (leading to possible resultant renal toxicity) and methylprednisolone.
4. Concurrent administration with isoniazid or rifampin reduces ketoconazole levels.
5. Administration with terfenadine or astemizole increases the levels of the two latter drugs, with possible resultant cardiac dysrhythmia.

■ **Miconazole** (Monistat IV; Janssen)

How Supplied:
Parenteral: 10 mg/ml in 20 ml ampule.

Administration:
Intravenous. Initial test dose of 200 mg should be given under closely monitored conditions with physician in attendance, because of risk of anaphylaxis. Penetrates joints but not CSF.
Intrathecal: Needed for treatment of fungal meningitis.
Bladder instillation: For UTI.

Dose:
IV: 200–3,600 mg/day, depending on infection, divided tid; continue for 1–20 weeks, depending on severity of infection. Maximum 15 mg/kg per infusion.
Intrathecal: 20 mg/dose q3–7 days.
Bladder instillation: 200 mg in diluent.

Mechanism of Action: See Ketoconazole, p. 000.

Elimination: Metabolized in liver; half-life 24 hr. Pharmacokinetics not altered in renal insufficiency.

Spectrum: *Candida albicans, Coccidioides immitis, Cryptococcus neoformans, Pseudoallescheria boydii (Petriellidium boydii, Allescheria boydii)* and *Paracoccidioides brasiliensis.*

Indications: See Table 4-1, Severe systemic fungal infections, and chronic mucocutaneous candidiasis.

Contraindications: Known hypersensitivity to drug.

Adverse effects:
1. Common (10%–30% patients): Nausea, vomiting; (lessen by giving antiemetics prior or by slowing infusion rate), diarrhea; pruritus and/or rash, phlebitis; fever.
2. Rarely, thrombocytopenia, hyperlipidemia.

Toxicity: Anaphylaxis; cardiopulmonary arrest, cardiac dysrhythmia (more common with too rapid infusion of undiluted drug); hyperlipidemia (secondary to cremophor el vehicle); hyponatremia.

Monitor: Hemoglobin, hematocrit, electrolytes, lipid profile.

ANTIINFECTIVES

Interactions: Given concurrently, augments systemic concentrations/effects of anticoagulants, oral hypoglycemic agents, phenytoin, cyclosporine and carbamezapine.

■ **Miconazole Nitrate** (Monistat; Janssen. Monistat-Derm; Ortho)

How Supplied:
Topical: (Monistat-Derm)
    2% cream in 15 gm; 1, 3 oz tube.
Vaginal: (Monistat)
    Cream: 45 gm (1.59 oz) tube and applicator.
    Suppository: 100 mg (7–day therapy).
        200 mg (3–day therapy).

Administration:
Topical: Apply bid × 2–4 wk (apply sparingly in intertriginous areas to avoid maceration)
Vaginal:
    One full applicator cream: qh × 7 days.
    Suppository: 100 mg qh × 7 days.
    200 mg suppository qh × 3 days.

Mechanism of Action: Fungicidal.

Elimination: Less than 1% absorbed from skin, 1.3% from vagina.

Spectrum: *Candida* species; common dermatophytes (trichophyton, epidermophyton)

Indication: Vulvovaginal and cutaneous candidiasis; tinea pedis, tinea cruris, tinea corporis, and tinea versicolor.

Contraindications: Known hypersensitivity to drug (vaginal preparation only). Since small amounts can be absorbed from the vagina, not recommended for use during first trimester of pregnancy or with ruptured membranes.

Adverse reactions: Vulvovaginal burning, itching, irritation (2%).

■ Nystatin (Mycostatin; Westwood-Squibb; Bristol-Myers Squibb. Nilstat; Lederle)

How Supplied: *Oral:* Suspension 100,000 U/ml; powder for suspension; 50, 150, 500 million and 5 billion U per vial; 200,000 unit pastille.
Topical:

    Cream: 15, 30 gm tube.
    Ointment: 25 gm tube.
    Ointment with triamcinolone acetonide: 15, 30 gm tube.
    100,000 U per gm topical powder; 15 gm plastic squeeze bottle.
    500,000 U vaginal tablets.

Administration: *PO:* Absorption negligible. Thoroughly rinse mouth and retain as long as possible before swallowing. Topical and vaginal as directed.

Dose:
Topical: Apply bid–tid.
Vaginal: Every night (qh) or bid × 14 days.

Mechanism of Action: Increases cell membrane permeability; fungistatic and fungicidal.

Elimination: Excreted unchanged in feces.

Spectrum: *Candida, Cryptococcus, Histoplasma, Blastomyces.*

Indications: See Table 4-1. *Candida* infections of skin, mucous membranes (including vaginitis and stomatitis), and GI tract.

Toxicity: Nausea, vomiting and diarrhea observed rarely after oral administration.

■ Clotrimazole (Lotrimin; Schering. Mycelex, Mycelex-G; Miles)

How Supplied:
PO: 10 mg troche.

Topical:
> 1% cream in 15, 30, 45, 90 gm tube.
> 1% lotion in 30 ml bottle.
> 1% solution in 10, 30 ml bottle.

Vaginal:
> 1% cream in 45, 90 gm tube with applicator.
> 100 mg tablet (7–day therapy) with applicator.
> 500 mg tablet (1–day therapy) with applicator.

Administration/Dose:
PO: Dissolve 1 lozenge slowly in mouth 5 times a day × 14 days.
Topical: Gently massage into affected and surrounding skin bid × 1–4 wk. Systemic absorption less than 0.5%.
Vaginal:
> One full applicator cream qh × 7.
> One 100 mg tablet qh × 7.
>> 500 mg tablet hs as single dose.

Mechanism of Action: Fungicidal: Causes leakage of intracellular phosphorus compounds with concomitant breakdown of cellular nucleic acids and accelerated potassium efflux.

Elimination: Metabolized in liver and excreted in bile.

Spectrum: *Candida,* most common dermatophytes (*Trichophyton, Microsporum, Epidermophyton*), *Malassezia furfur.*

Indications:
Troche: Oropharyngeal candidiasis.
Topical: Tinea pedis, tinea cruris, tinea corporis, tinea versicolor and candidiasis.
Vaginal: Candida vulvovaginitis.

Contraindications: Known drug hypersensitivity; first trimester of pregnancy or with ruptured membranes.

Adverse effects:
PO: Mild (15%) elevation of AST (SGOT); nausea and vomiting.
Topical/vaginal: Local irritation or burning.

■ **Econazole Nitrate** (Spectazole; Ortho)

How Supplied:
Topical: 1% cream in 15, 30, 85 gm tube.

Administration/Dose: Cover affected areas once (tinea) or twice daily (candidiasis) 2–4 wk. Less than 1% absorbed systemically.

Mechanism of Action: See Ketoconazole, p. 133.

Spectrum: Broad activity against many species of *Trichophyton, Microsporum, Epidermophyton,* and yeasts, including *Candida.*

Indication: Tinea pedis, tinea cruris, tinea corporis, tinea versicolor, and cutaneous candidiasis.

Contraindications: Known hypersensitivity. Use only with caution in pregnancy and lactation.

Adverse effects: Local erythema, burning, and itching (3% of patients).

■ **Terconazole** (Terazol 3, Terazol 7; Ortho)

How Supplied:
Vaginal:
    0.4% cream in 45 gm tube with applicator.
    0.8% cream in 20 gm tube with applicator.
    80 mg suppository in package of 3 with applicator.

Administration/Dose:
1 full applicator (5 gm) 0.4% cream intravaginally hr × 1 wk.
1 full applicator (5 gm) 0.8% cream intravaginally hr × 3 nights.
1 suppository intravaginally qh × 3 nights.
    5%–16% systemic absorption.

Mechanism of Action: Triazole fungicide.

Elimination: Renal and hepatic.

Spectrum: *Candida albicans.*

Indication: Vulvovaginal candidiasis.

Contraindications: Known drug hypersensitivity; first trimester of pregnancy.

Adverse effects: Headache; dysmenorrhea; vaginal irritation (rare).

■ Butoconazole Nitrate (Femstat; Syntex)

How Supplied:
Vaginal: 2% cream as single 28 gm tube or as set of 3 prefilled applicators (5 gm each).

Administration/Dose: 1 applicatorful qh × 3 (or × 6 if pregnant second and third trimester).

Mechanism of Action: See Ketoconazole, p. 133.

Spectrum: Fungicidal activity against Candida species; in vitro also against *Trichophyton, Microsporum,* and *Epidermophyton.*

Indication: Vulvovaginal candidiasis.

Contraindications: Known drug hypersensitivity; first trimester pregnancy and lactation.

Adverse effects: Rarely, local irritation.

■ Tioconazole (Vagistat-1; Bristol-Myers)

How Supplied:
Vaginal: 6.5% ointment in 4.6 gm prefilled applicator.

Administration/Dose:
One full applicator intravaginally at bedtime as single dose. Systemic absorption in nonpregnant patient negligible.

Mechanism of Action: See Ketoconazole, p. 133.

Spectrum: In vitro activity against *Candida* species and *Torulopsis glabrata.*

Indication: Vulvovaginal candidiasis.

Contraindications: Known hypersensitivity to imidazole antifungal agents; pregnancy, lactation.

Adverse effects: Local burning and itching (5%); rarely, vulvar edema, pain, dysuria, dyspareunia.

■ **Tolnaftate** (Tinactin; Schering)

How Supplied:
Topical: 1% cream, solution, aerosol liquid, and powder.

Administration/Dose: Apply locally bid × 2–4 wk.

Spectrum: Many species of *Trichophyton, Epidermophyton, Microsporum,* and *Pityrosporum orbiculare.*

Indications: Cutaneous mycoses caused by susceptible organisms.

Contraindications: Pregnancy, lactation.

Adverse effects: Mild irritation and sensitivity.

ANTIBACTERIAL/ANTIPARASITIC AGENTS

■ **Metronidazole** (Flagyl; Searle. Metronidazole; Lederle. Protostat; Ortho)

How Supplied:
PO: 250, 500 mg tablet.
Parenteral: 500 mg single-dose vial.

Administration:
IV, PO.

Dose:
IV:

Loading or preoperative prophylaxis: 15 mg/kg over 1 hr (1 gm for 70 kg adult).
Maintenance: 7.5 mg/kg infused over 1 hr q6h; max 4 gm/24 hr.

PO:

Trichomoniasis: 250 mg tid × 7 days or 2 gm PO at once.
Gardnerella vaginalis: 250 mg qid or 500 mg bid × 7 days.

Mechanism of Action: Selectively toxic to certain protozoal organisms and anaerobic-microaerophilic microorganisms via impairment of proper DNA synthesis.

Elimination: Hepatic metabolism; 60%–80% excreted in urine. Normal half-life 8 hr, prolonged with liver impairment.

Spectrum: Anaerobic gram-negative bacilli (including *Bacteroides* sp. and *Fusobacterium*), gram-positive bacilli (including *Clostridium* sp.), anaerobic gram-positive cocci, *Trichomonas, Entamoeba histolytica; Giardia lamblia.*

Indications:
IV: Serious anaerobic infections: intraabdominal, pelvic, skin, bone, joint, CNS, and endocarditis.
PO: Trichomoniasis, amebiasis, bacterial vaginosis; or as continuation of IV therapy.

Contraindications: Known drug hypersensitivity, first trimester of pregnancy, lactation, active CNS disease.

Toxicity: Convulsive seizures, peripheral neuropathy, GI upset, Antabuse-like reaction if taken with ethanol.

Interactions: Elimination accelerated by phenobarbital and phenytoin, slowed with cimetidine; may potentiate oral anticoagulants; increased risk of lithium toxicity.

ANTIVIRAL AGENTS

■ Acyclovir (Zovirax; Burroughs Wellcome)

How Supplied:
PO: 200 mg capsule.
   400, 800 mg tablets.
   200 mg/5 ml suspension.
Parenteral: 50 mg/ml; 10, 20 ml vial.
Topical: 5% ointment in 3, 15 gm tubes.

Administration:
PO: Bioavailability 20%.
IV: Infuse over 1 hr.
Topical: Apply to affected skin with finger cot or rubber glove to prevent autoinoculation.

Dose for herpes simplex:
   Genitalis, severe initial infection: 5 mg/kg IV q8h × 5 days.
   Genitalis, mild-moderate initial infection: 200 mg PO q4h, 5 × per day × 10 days. (or ointment q3h, 6 times per day × 7 days).
   Genitalis, recurrent: 200 mg PO q4h, 5 × per day × 5 days.
   Genitalis, chronic suppressive therapy: 400 mg bid for up to 12 hrs; then reevaluate.
   Encephalitis: 10 mg/kg IV q8h × 10 days.
   Mucosal and cutaneous infections in immunocompromised patients: 5 mg/kg IV q8h × 7 days.

Dose for varicella-zoster:
   Chicken pox (initial infection): 20 mg/kg (800 mg maximum) PO qid × 5 days.
   Zoster (shingles), acute: 800 mg PO q4h, 5 times per day × 7–10 days.
   Zoster in immunocompromised patients: 10 mg/kg (maximum 500 mg/ml) IV q8h × 7 days.
   Renal impairment: Lengthen dosing interval and decrease dose by one-third to one-half.

Mechanism of Action: Infected cells convert acyclovir into nucleotide analog, which interferes with viral DNA polymerase and inhibits viral DNA replication. If incorporated into growing viral DNA chain, DNA chain terminated.

Elimination: Excreted in kidney by glomerular filtration and tubular secretion; dosage adjustment required in presence of renal impairment. Half-life 2.5 hr in normal patients. Penetrates most tissues including brain, CSF, kidney, lung, liver, uterus and vaginal mucosa and secretions.

Spectrum: Herpes simplex type I and II, varicella-zoster virus, Epstein-Barr virus, cytomegalovirus.

Indications: Oral: Initial and recurrent genital herpes; herpes zoster (shingles); chickenpox (varicella).

    Ointment: Initial herpes genitalis; limited non-life threatening mucocutaneous herpes simplex in immunocompromised patients.

    IV: Severe initial genital herpes; initial and recurrent mucosal and recurrent mucocutaneous herpes simplex and varicella. Zoster (shingles) in immunocompromised patients; herpes simplex encephalitis.

Contraindications: Known hypersensitivity to the drug; pregnancy, lactation. Exercise caution and adjust dose in patients with renal dysfunction.

Adverse effects:
Topical: Transient local burning, pain, rash, vulvitis (rare).
Oral: GI distress, headache, rash.
IV: Local phlebitis, rash, nausea, hypotension, diaphoresis.
Toxicity: Transient rise in serum creatinine in 10% of patients; more often in those who are dehydrated, have preexisting renal impairment, or are receiving concurrent therapy with other nephrotoxic agents. Very rarely, signs of neurotoxicity (e.g., lethargy, disorientation, hallucinations, seizures, coma).

Interactions: Half-life increased by probenecid. Exercise caution when administering to patients with prior history of neurologic reactions to cytotoxic drugs or those receiving concomitant intrathecal methotrexate or interferon.

■ **Amantadine** (Amantadine Hydrochloride; Barre-National. Duramed; Warner Chilcott)

How Supplied:
PO: Capsule: 100 mg.
Syrup: 50 mg/5 ml.

Administration: PO; very well absorbed.

Mechanism of Action: Blocks a late stage in assembly of influenza A virus. Does not inhibit development of specific antiviral antibody or interfere with immunogenicity of inactivated influenza A virus vaccine. As an antiParkinsons agent, amantadine causes release of dopamine from central neurons and facilitates its release by nerve impulses.

Dose: 200 mg/day (100 mg/day if person over 65 yr.) Begin prophylaxis as soon as possible after exposure; continue for a minimum of 10 days, and up to 90 days in case of possible repeated and unknown exposures (i.e., community epidemic). If prophylactic therapy is begun in conjunction with inactivated influenza A virus vaccine, continue until protective antibody responses develop (i.e., 2–3 wk).

Elimination: Excreted unchanged by kidney via glomerular filtration and tubular secretion. Half-life 15 hr; prolonged in patients with kidney dysfunction.

Spectrum: Most strains of influenza A virus.

Indications: Prevention or chemoprophylaxis of influenza A virus illness, especially for unimmunized patients at high risk for development of complications from influenza, such as those with chronic cardiopulmonary disease and persons over 65. Also useful as single agent in treatment of mild Parkinson's disease or to maximize improvement when combined with levodopa.

Contraindications: Known drug hypersensitivity, pregnancy, and lactation. Use with caution in patients with a history of epilepsy, congestive heart failure, cerebral atherosclerosis, renal impairment, liver disease, recurrent eczematoid rash, or psychiatric disorders.

ANTIINFECTIVES

Adverse effects:
1. Most frequently (5%–10%): Nausea, dizziness, insomnia.
2. Less frequently (1%–5%): Depression, anxiety, hallucinations, ataxia, cutis marmorata, orthostatic hypotension.

Toxicity: Rare (<1%): Congestive heart failure, psychosis, ataxia, convulsions, edema. CNS toxicity associated with plasma levels of 1–5 µg/ml.

Monitor: Watch for emergence of resistant viral strains.

Interaction: Hallucinations, confusion and nightmares are more common when given with CNS stimulants and anticholinergics and may require reduction in dosage of one or both drugs.

■ Famciclovir (Famvir; Smith-Kline Beecham)

How Supplied:
PO: 500 mg tablets.

Administration: *PO:* Fairly well absorbed without regard to meals.

Mechanism of Action: Undergoes rapid biotransformation to active agent penciclovir, which, in infected cells, inhibits HSV 2 polymerase and therefore viral DNA synthesis and replication.

Dose: 500 mg q8h × 7 days; most useful when begun within 48 hr of rash onset. Lengthen dosing interval in presence of renal impairment (creatinine clearance <60 ml/min).

Elimination: Renal excretion.

Spectrum: Herpes simplex virus I & II; varicella-zoster virus.

Indications: Acute herpes zoster (shingles).

Contraindications: Known hypersensitivity to famciclovir; pregnancy; lactation.

Adverse effects: GI distress, headache, paresthesias; rash.

Monitor: Creatinine clearance (with renal dysfunction).

Interactions: Drug levels increased with concurrent administration of probenecid.

■ Foscarnet Sodium (Foscavir; Astra)

How Supplied:
Parenteral:
24 mg/ml; 250, 500 ml bottle.

Administration:
IV: Diluted to 12 mg/ml with D5W or 0.9 NS and given over at least 1 hour in a large vein to avoid local phlebitis. Maintain adequate hydration to establish diuresis and thus minimize renal toxicity.

Mechanism of Action: Organic analog of inorganic pyrophosphate; selectively inhibits virus-specific DNA polymerases and reverse transcriptases at pyrophosphate binding site.

Dose: Induction therapy: 60 mg/kg over 1 hr q8h × 2–3 wk. Maintenance: 90–120 mg/kg/day as single infusion over 2 hr. Decrease dose in presence of renal impairment.

Elimination: Renal excretion by tubular secretion and glomerular filtration.

Spectrum: Cytomegalovirus (CMV), herpes simplex I & II, human herpesvirus 6, Epstein-Barr virus, varicella-zoster virus.

Indications: CMV retinitis in AIDS patients.

Contraindications: Known sensitivity to foscarnet; pregnancy; lactation. Use with caution if there is history of renal impairment or concurrent use of drugs known to influence minerals (especially calcium, phosphate and magnesium).

Adverse effects: Electrolyte changes (8%–16%): decrease in serum calcium, magnesium and potassium; hypo/hyperphosphatemia.

Anemia (33%): Granulocytopenia (17%), marrow suppression (10%).

Misc: fever (65%); phlebitis at injection site, skin ulceration; GI distress (30%–47%); headache; rash.

Toxicity: Renal impairment (33%); increased serum creatinine, acute renal failure, potentially fatal, usually but not uniformly reversible with dose adjustment or discontinuation; may occur even with normal baseline renal function.

Neurotoxicity: Seizures (10%), especially if patient has active or past CNS condition (e.g., toxoplasmosis, HIV encephalopathy), receives excessive dose or has associated renal/electrolyte disturbance.

Monitor: Baseline and periodic 24-hour creatinine clearance. Baseline and 2–3 times/wk while on induction therapy and q 1–2 wk during maintenance: serum creatinine, calcium, magnesium, potassium and phosphorus; CBC.

Interactions: Concomitant IV netamidine may increase risk of serious hypocalcemia or nephrotoxicity. Avoid use with other potentially nephrotoxic drugs such as aminoglycosides and amphotericin B. Concurrent zidovudine may increase risk of anemia. Use caution when giving with other drugs that can affect calcium or electrolyte levels.

■ Ganciclovir Sodium (Cytovene; Syntex)

How Supplied:
Parenteral: 50 mg/ml, 10 ml vials.

Administration: IV only, by reconstituting with 10 ml sterile water (not bacteriostatic containing parabens), then adding to 100 ml 0.9 NS, D5W, Ringer's Injection or LR and infusing into large vein more than 1 hour. Maintain adequate hydration to ensure normal clearance.

Mechanism of Action: Inhibits viral DNA synthesis by competitive inhibition of viral DNA polymerases and direct incorporation into viral DNA, resulting in termination of viral DNA elongation.

Dose: Induction: 5 mg/kg q12h × 14–21 days (7–14 days if for CMV prevention).

Maintenance: 5 mg/kg q day, single dose, or 6 mg/kg q day, single dose, 5 days per week. Decrease dose amount and lengthen dosing interval with renal impairment (creatinine clearance less than 80 ml/min).

Elimination: Renal excretion by glomerular filtration.

Spectrum: Cytomegalovirus (CMV), herpes simplex virus I & II, Epstein-Barr virus, varicella-zoster virus.

Indications: CMV retinitis in immunocompromised patients (e.g., AIDS); prevention of CMV disease in at risk transplant recipients.

Contraindications: Hypersensitivity to ganciclovir or acyclovir; pregnancy; lactation; absolute neutrophil count <500 cells/ mm₃ or platelets <25,000. Use with caution if preexisting or history of cytopenia or cytopenic drug reaction.

Adverse effects: Anemia, fever, rash, abnormal LFTs. Retinal detachment also reported; exact relationship to drug unknown. Theoretically inhibits spermatogenesis and is teratogenic; advise reproductive-age patients to use effective contraception.

Toxicity:
Hematologic (up to 45%): Usually reversible, rarely fatal granulocytopenia; neutropenia (especially if given with zidovudine); thrombocytopenia.
Renal (up to 58%): Usually transient/intermittent increased serum creatinine (especially if given with cyclosporine or amphotericin B); increased BUN.
CNS: Seizures (if given with imipenem-cilastin); headache; confusion.
Misc: Phlebitis at injection site; sepsis.

Monitor: Neutrophil and platelet counts q 2 days during bid dosing and q wk after; check neutrophils daily if there is history of prior leukopenic drug reaction or if baseline count is <1000 cells/mm₃. Serum creatinine or creatinine clearance > q 2 wks.

Interactions: Renal clearance reduced with probenecid and similarly acting agents. Potential for additional inhibited replication of rapidly dividing cell populations (e.g., marrow, GI mucosa) when used with dapsone, pentamidine, flucytosine, vincristine, vinblastine, doxorubizin HCl, amphotericin B, trimethoprim/sulfamethoxazole; avoid concomitant use if possible. Increased risk of granulocytopenia when given with zidovudine; increased risk seizures with imipenem/cilastin; increased risk elevated serum creatinine with cyclosporine, amphotericin B.

■ Interferon alfa-n 3 (Alferon N; Purdue Frederick)

How Supplied:
Injectable solution: 5 million IU/1 ml vial.

Administration: Intralesional injection.

Mechanism of Action: Single subtype recombinant interferon, human leukocyte derived. Binds to specific membrane receptors and induces protein synthesis, resulting in inhibition of virus replication, suppression of cell proliferation and immunomodulation (enhancement of phagocytosis by macrophages, augmentation of lymphocyte cytotoxicity and enhanced human leukocyte antigen expression).

Dose: 0.05 ml per wart, twice weekly, for up to 8 weeks; maximum 0.5 ml (2.5 million IU) per session. Wait 3 months before retreatment unless warts enlarge or new warts develop.

Spectrum: Human papilloma virus.

Indications: Refractory/recurrent external condyloma acuminata.

Contraindications: Hypersensitivity to human interferon alpha, mouse immunoglobulin (IgG), egg protein, or neomycin; pregnancy; lactation; age younger than 18 years. Use with caution in patients with debilitating medical conditions such as cardiopulmonary disease (e.g., unstable angina, uncontrolled CHF, COPD) or DM with ketoacidosis; coagulation or seizure disorders; severe myelosuppression.

Adverse effects: Flu-like symptoms (fever, myalgias, headaches) in up to 30%, mostly after first treatment. Because of theoretical mutagenicity in nonhuman data, reproductive-age patients should use effective contraception.

■ Ribavirin (Virazole; ICN Pharmaceuticals)

How Supplied:
6 gm/100 ml vial for inhalation solution.

Administration: Continuous aerosol via small particle aerosol generator.

Mechanism of Action: Purine nucleoside analog; inhibits viral replication.

Dose: 20 mg/ml for 12–18 hr/day × 3–7 days; specialized equipment necessary in patients on mechanical ventilation to avoid drug precipitation.

Spectrum: Respiratory syncytial virus (RSV); influenza A & B viruses; herpes simplex virus.

Indications: Now approved for severe lower respiratory tract infections in children because of RSV. Encouraging data also for treating young adults with influenza A or B viral infection, and to delay progression from ARC to AIDS.

Elimination: Plasma half-life 9.5 hr; concentrated and persists in RBCs for their entire life span.

Contraindications: Hypersensitivity to ribavirin; women who are or may become pregnant during drug exposure.

Adverse effects: Anemia caused by extravascular hemolysis and marrow suppression, with elevated bilirubin, iron and uric acid; GI distress; conjunctival irritation; reversible deterioration in pulmonary function. Teratogenic, mutagenic in small animals.

■ Rimantidine Hydrochloride (Flumadine; Forest)

How Supplied:
PO: 100 mg tablets.
50 mg/5 ml syrup.

Administration: Oral; slowly but efficiently absorbed with good concentrations achieved in respiratory secretions.

Mechanism of Action: Structural analog of amantadine. Exerts inhibitory effect early in viral replicative cycle, possible by inhibiting viral uncoating.

Dose: 100 mg bid × 7 days; 100 mg/day if severe hepatic dysfunction, renal failure or elderly. Continue therapy for 2–4 weeks for prophylaxis.

Elimination: Extensively metabolized in liver.

Spectrum: Influenza A.

Indications: Prophylaxis and treatment of influenza A.

Contraindications: Hypersensitivity to adamantine-type drugs; pregnancy; lactation. Use caution in patients with epilepsy or severe renal/hepatic dysfunction.

Adverse effects: Rare: GI distress, insomnia, dizziness, seizure-like activity.

Monitor: Renal/hepatic functions; watch for emergence of resistant virus strain.

Interactions: Clearance reduced by cimetidine; plasma levels decreased by acetaminophen and aspirin.

■ **DIDANOSINE** (Videx; Bristol-Myers Squibb Oncology)

How Supplied:
PO: 25, 50, 100, 150 mg chewable/dispersible buffered tablets; each contains 264.5 mg sodium.
Oral solution: 100, 167, 250, 375 mg single dose buffered powder; each packet contains 1380 mg sodium.

Administration: *PO,* on empty stomach; 2 tablets at each dose so that adequate buffering is provided to prevent gastric acid drug degradation. Tablets may be dissolved in 1 oz water; powder may be dissolved in 4 oz water (not fruit juice or other acid-containing liquid).

Mechanism of Action: Nucleoside analog of deoxyadenosine, that, when incorporated into viral DNA, leads to chain termination and thus inhibition of viral replication. Also interferes with HIV-RNA-dependent DNA polymerase (reverse transcriptase).

Dose:
Patients >60 kg weight: 200 mg tablets bid, or 250 mg powder bid.
Patients <60 kg weight: 125 mg tablets bid, or 167 mg powder bid.
 Consider dose reduction with liver dysfunction or serum creatinine <1.5 mg/dl or creatinine clearance <60 ml/min.

Elimination: Renal clearance by active tubular secretion and glomerular filtration.

Spectrum: HIV-infected cells.

Indications: Patients with HIV infections who have received prolonged prior zidovudine therapy, or who have demonstrated intolerance or clinical/immunologic deterioration on zidovudine (zidovudine should still be considered first-line initial therapy).

Contraindications: Hypersensitivity to didanosine. Use with caution in patients with hepatic/renal impairment; avoid use with other drugs that may increase risk of neurotoxicity or pancreatic toxicity (e.g., IV pentamidine) (see p.154). Use in pregnancy only if clearly needed.

Adverse Effects: Diarrhea; neuropathy; rash/pruritus; headache.

Toxicity:

Pancreatitis: Occasionally fatal; increased amylase; abdominal pain. Possible increased risk if past history of pancreatitis, advanced HIV stage, or renal impairment not on reduced dose.

Peripheral neuropathy: Possibly dose related; more frequent in patients with history of neuropathy or neurotoxic drug therapy.

Liver failure: Rarely fatal.

Retinal depigmentation (reported in pediatric patients).

Monitor: Avoid use with potentially neurotoxic or pancreatic toxicity (e.g., IV pentamidine). Coadministration will lessen tetracycline absorption. Quinolone levels decreased if taken within 2 hr of didanosine. Concomitant administration of magnesium or aluminum containing antacid may potentiate the antacid's adverse effects.

■ **Interferon alfa-2a, recombinant** (Roferon-a; Roche)

How Supplied:

Parenteral: 3 million IU/ 1 ml vial, solution.

9 million IU/ 0.9 ml vial, solution.

18 million IU/ 1 ml vial, solution and sterile powder.

Administration: Injection IM; subcutaneous (particularly useful for thrombocytopenic patients).

Mechanism of Action: Recombinant interferon with direct antiproliferative action against tumor cells; also modulates host immune response.

Dose: Hairy cell leukemia and AIDS-related Kaposi's sarcoma.

Contraindications: Hypersensitivity to alfa interferon, mouse immunoglobulin; visceral AIDS-related Kaposi's sarcoma in rapidly progressing/life-threatening disease. Use with caution if there is significant preexisting cardiac, renal, or hepatic disease or myelosuppression. No data on use in pregnancy; advise discontinuation of nursing; must use effective contraception.

Adverse effects/Toxicity: Decrease in WBC, platelets, Hb (Kaposi's sarcoma patients); elevated LFTs; flu-like symptoms, GI distress, dizziness, decreased mental status.

Monitor: CBC; platelets; LFTs.

Interactions: Synergistic marrow toxicity if given with myelo-suppressive drugs such as zidovudine.

■ Interferon alfa-2b (Intron-a; Schering)

How Supplied:
Parenteral:
As recombinant powder:
   3, 5 million IU/ 1 ml vial or syringe.
   10 million IU/ 2 ml vial.
   18 million IU/ 3.8 ml vial.
   25 million IU/ 1 ml vial.
As recombinant solution:
   10 million IU/ 2 ml vial.
   25 million IU/ 5 ml vial.

Administration:
Systemic: IM
Subcutaneous (preferred for patients with thrombocytopenia)
Intralesional.

Mechanism of Action: See Interferon alfa-2a, p.154.

Dose:
Condyloma acuminatum: Reconstitute 10 million IU vial with 1 ml diluent (bacteriostatic water); inject 0.1 ml into base of each wart with 23–30-gauge needle, 3 times/week (qod) × 3 weeks. Repeat course after 12–16 weeks if there is inadequate improvement.

Hairy cell leukemia: 2 million IU/m² IM or subcutaneous, 3 times a week.

AIDS-related Kaposi's sarcoma: 30 million IU/m² 3 times/week, subcutaneous or IM.

Chronic hepatitis non-A, non-B/C: 3 million IU 3 times/week × 6 months, subcutaneous or IM.

Chronic hepatitis B: 30–35 million IU/week in divided doses × 16 weeks, subcutaneous or IM.

Spectrum/Indications: External genital condyloma acuminatum; refractory to other therapy; hairy cell leukemia; AIDS–related Kaposi's sarcoma; chronic hepatitis non–A, non–B/C with compensated liver disease; history of blood product exposure and/or HCV Ab positive; chronic hepatitis B in patients with compensated liver disease and HBeAg positive.

Contraindications: Hypersensitivity to interferon alfa or its components; preexisting psychiatric condition, especially depression. Use cautiously in debilitated patients, patients with history of thromboembolism, severe myelosuppression, unstable angina, CHF, or recent MI.

Adverse effects: Common: flu–like symptoms; GI distress; mild alopecia; leukopenia, elevated LFTs.

Toxicity: Rare with systemic therapy. Cardiac dysrhythmia, cardiomyopathy; severe/suicidal depression; thyroid abnormalities; potentially fatal liver failure; potentially fatal pneumonitis and pneumonia; retinal hemorrhages and artery/vein obstruction; anaphylaxis; exacerbation of psoriasis.

Monitor:
All patients: baseline and periodic CBC, LFTs.
Patients receiving systemic therapy: CBC, platelets, LFTs, bilirubin, albumin, creatinine, TSH.

Interactions: Possible potentiation of myelosuppressive effect of other drugs such as zidovudine.

■ Rifabutin (Mycobutin; Pharmacia Adria)

How Supplied: *PO:* 150 mg capsules.

Administration: *PO:* 53% absorbed from GI tract.

Mechanism of Action: Semisynthetic ansamycin antibiotic derived from rifamycin. Inhibits DNA-dependent RNA polymerase in certain organisms, but not mammalian cells.

Dose: 300 mg/day, single dose; 150 bid with food if having GI upset.

Elimination: Mixed hepatic/renal clearance.

Spectrum: *Mycobacterium avium* complex (MAC) organisms including *M. avium* and *M. intracellulare*.

Indications: Prevention of disseminated MAC disease in advanced HIV-infected patients.

Contraindications: Known hypersensitivity to any rifamycin-type drug. Not to be used alone in patients with active TB, as this would be inadequate therapy (see Antitubercular drugs, p. 113). HIV–positive patient may need special testing to rule out false negative PPD (see Monitor below).

Adverse effects: Rash, GI distress; neutropenia; thrombocytopenia; myositis; uveitis; discolored urine and tears (may permanently stain contact lenses).

Monitor: CBC, platelets; LFTs.

Interactions: Liver-inducing properties may reduce activity of concomitant dapsone, narcotics, anticoagulants, corticosteroids, cyclosporine, cardiac glycosides, quinidine, oral contraceptives, oral hypoglycemics, analgesics, ketoconazole, barbiturates, diazepam, verapamil, beta-adrenergic blockers, clofibrate, progestins, disopyramide, mexiletine, theophylline, chloramphenicol and anticonvulsants; dosage adjustment may be necessary.

■ **Stavudine** (Zerit; Bristol-Myers Squibb Oncology)

How Supplied: *PO:* 15, 20, 30, 40 mg capsules.

Administration: *PO,* at 12-hr intervals, without regard to meals. Rapidly absorbed.

Mechanism of Action: Thymidine nucleoside analog. Inhibits HIV reverse transcriptase; inhibits viral DNA synthesis by causing DNA chain termination; inhibits cellular DNA polymerase and reduces synthesis of mitochondrial DNA.

Dose: Patients ≥60 kg: 40 mg bid.

Patients <60 kg: 30 mg bid.
Adjust dose in case of renal impairment, signs of peripheral neuropathy, or elevated LFTs.

Elimination: Renal.

Indications: Advanced HIV infection when first-line therapy (e.g., Zidovudine; see p. 161) is not tolerated or significant clinical or immunologic deterioration occurred during use.

Contraindications: Hypersensitivity to stavudine; development of peripheral neuropathy (consider reinstating therapy at reduced dose if symptoms resolve). Use in pregnancy only if clearly needed; advise discontinuation of nursing. Use with caution in patients with severe hepatic/renal impairment.

Adverse effects/Toxicity: Peripheral neuropathy, usually reversible; increased LFTs (dose-related); pancreatitis (rarely fatal).

Monitor: Creatinine clearance; LFTs.

■ **Trimetrexate Glucoronate**   (Neutrexin; U.S. Bioscience, Inc.)

How Supplied:
Parenteral: 25 mg/5 ml single dose vial.

Administration: *IV:* reconstituted and diluted with D5W, infused over 60–90 min. Must be given with leucovorin (see below).

Mechanism of Action: Competitive inhibitor of dihydrofolate reductase (DHFR) in bacterial, protozoal and mammalian cells. Inhibition of DHFR leads to depletion of intracellular coenzyme tetrahydrofolate, with subsequent disruption of DNA, RNA and protein synthesis, with consequent cell death. Leucovorin (folinic acid) is actively transported into mammalian cells (but not pneumocystis carinii) and can provide a source of reduced folates necessary for normal cellular biosynthetic process. Coadministration of leucovorin thus protects normal host cells from trimetrexate cytotoxicity without inhibiting the antifolate's effect on pneumocystis.

Dose:
   Trimetrexin: 45 mg/m^2/day, single dose.
   Leucovorin: 20 mg/m^2 q6h IV over 5–10 minutes
   (80 mg/day) × 21 days, or 20 mg/m^2 q6h PO, or rounded off
   to next higher 25 mg increment × 24 days (must extend 72 hr
   past last dose of trimetrexin to avoid life-threatening toxicity).
   Adjust dose with presence of hematologic toxicity.

Elimination: Metabolized by P450 hepatic enzymes.

Indications: Alternate therapy for moderate to severe pneumocystis carinii pneumonia in immunocompromised patients,
including those with AIDS, who are refractory to or unable to
tolerate trimethoprim-sulfamethoxazole.

Contraindications: Sensitivity to trimetrexate, leucovorin, or
methotrexate; pregnancy and lactation; concomitant zidovudine.

Adverse Effects/Toxicity: Potentially fatal myelosuppression;
oral and GI mucosal ulceration; renal/hepatic dysfunction.

Monitor: CBC, absolute neutrophil counts, platelets; serum
creatinine, BUN; AST, ALT, alkaline phosphatase.

Interactions: Other drugs metabolized by P450 enzymes may
induce or inhibit elimination; e.g., erythromycin, rifampin,
rifabutin, ketoconazole, fluconazole. Metabolism also inhibited
by nitrogen-substituted imidazoles (clotrimazole, ketoconazole,
miconazole).

ANTIINFECTIVES

■ **Zalcitabine** (Hivid; Roche)

How Supplied:
PO: 0.375, 0.750 mg tablets.

Administration: *PO:* Well absorbed, but more slowly with food.

Mechanism of Action: Synthetic pyrimidine nucleoside analog. Serves as alternative substrate for HIV–reverse transcriptase
and inhibits replication of HIV–1 by inhibition of viral DNA
synthesis.

Dose: 0.75 mg q8h alone or with 200 mg zidovudine q8h; lengthen dosing interval of zalcitabine with creatinine clearance <40 ml/min.

Elimination: Renal tubular secretion.

Indications: Advanced HIV infection when either intolerant to or with disease progression while on zidovudine. Used in combination with zidovudine with advanced HIV disease and CD4 count ≤300 cells/mm^3.

Contraindications: Hypersensitivity to zalcitabine; development of severe/unremitting peripheral neuropathy. Avoid concomitant use of other potentially neurotoxic drugs (e.g., chloramphenicol, cisplatin, didanosine, disulfiram, ethionamide, hydralazine, isoniazid, metronidazole, nitrofurantoin, phenytoin, ribavirin, vincristine), other drugs potentially toxic to the pancreas (pentamidine); drugs that may slow zalcitabine renal clearance (e.g., amphotericin, foscarnet, aminoglycosides). Use with caution in patients with preexisting liver disease, abnormal LFTs, history of ethanol abuse or hepatitis.

Adverse Effects/Toxicity: Increased risk in patients with decreased CD4 cell counts:
  Peripheral neuropathy (22%–35%); sensorimotor numbness, burning dysesthesia, or sharp shooting pain, sometimes irreversible, even with drug discontinuation.
  Pancreatitis, potentially fatal; asymptomatic elevated amylase.
  Lactic acidosis, hepatomegaly, steatosis.
  Oral/esophageal ulcers; cardiomyopathy/CHF; anaphylaxis.

Monitor: Baseline and periodic CBC, SMA20, amylase.

Interactions: See contraindications, above.

■ **Zidovudine** (Retrovir; Burroughs Wellcome)

How Supplied:
PO:
  100 mg capsules
  50 mg/ml syrup

Parenteral:
   10 mg/ml, 20 ml vial.

Administration:　*PO:* rapidly absorbed; slow IV infusion over
1 hr.

Mechanism of Action:　Thymidine analog, formerly called azi-
dothymidine (AZT). Interferes with HIV viral RNA dependent
DNA polymerase (reverse transcriptase), thus inhibiting viral
replication.

Dose:
   Symptomatic HIV infections: 100 mg PO q4h (600 mg/day).
   Asymptomatic HIV infections: 100 mg PO q4h while awake
   (500 mg/day).
   Pneumocystis carinii pneumonia or CD4 count <200/mm^3
   pretreatment:
   1–2 mg/kg IV q4h, until able to take PO; then,
   200 mg PO q4h (1200 mg/day). Reduce to 100 mg PO q4h
   (600 mg/day) after 1 mo.
   End stage renal disease on dialysis, severe anemia, or
   significant granulocytopenia: dose adjustment required.

Elimination:　Metabolized in liver by glucuronidation, then renal
excretion via glomerular filtration and active tubular secretion.

Spectrum:　Most active against HIV (also know as HTLV-III,
LAV, or ARV); some activity against other retroviruses, such as
HIV-2, HTLV-I and simian immunodeficiency virus.

Indications:
   To prolong survival and decrease the incidence of
   opportunistic infections in patient with advanced HIV
   disease.
   To delay disease progression in asymptomatic HIV–infected
   patients with evidence of impaired immunity (CD4 counts
   ≤500/mm^3).
   Symptomatic HIV infections (HIV and advanced ARC) with
   pneumocystis carinii pneumonia or CD4 count <200/mm^3
   pretreatment.

ANTIINFECTIVES

Contraindications: Life–threatening allergic reactions to any of the formulation's components. Use in pregnancy only if clearly needed; advise patients to discontinue nursing. Use with caution in patients with bone marrow compromise (granulocytes <1000/mm^3, Hb <9.5 g/dl).

Adverse Effects/Toxicity: Frequency and severity greater in patients with more advanced infections at start of therapy:
1. Hematologic (most frequent): anemia, beginning after 2–4 wk; granulocytopenia, usually after 6–8 wk. More frequent in patient with already lowered bone marrow reverse or with greater dose/duration of therapy.
2. Miscellaneous: Lactic acidosis/severe hepatomegaly; pancreatitis; anaphylaxis, vasculitis; seizures, myalgias, myositis, headache; nausea; insomnia.

Monitor: CBC, platelets, LFTs; usual HIV-disease monitoring for CD4 counts and opportunistic infections.

Interactions: Increased risk of hematologic toxicity when used with ganciclovir, interferon-alpha, or other cytotoxic drugs such as dapsone, flucytosine, vincristine, vinblastine, adriamycin. Probenecid may increase zidovudine levels. Use with phenytoin may variously affect levels of both drugs. Ribavirin may antagonize zidovudine's antiviral effects. Acyclovir may increase risk of neurotoxicity

ANTIHELMINTHICS
■ **Mebendazole** (Vermox; Janssen)

How Supplied:
Chewable tablet: 100 mg.

Administration: PO; Very little absorbed.

Dose:
1. Enterobiasis (pinworm): 100 mg × 1 dose; repeat after 2 wk.
2. Ascariasis (roundworm), trichuriasis (whipworm), *Ancylostoma duodenale,* and *Necator americanus* (hookworm): 100 mg bid × 3 days.

Mechanism of Action: Inhibits formation of worm microtubules, ultimately causing glycogen depletion and impaired glucose uptake.

Elimination: Minor absorbed portion of drug excreted in urine as decarboxylated metabolite; remainder excreted in feces.

Spectrum: Ascariasis, intestinal capillariasis, enterobiasis, trichuriasis, hookworm infections; some activity against *Strongyloides stercoralis*, trichinosis, onchocerciasis, *Tetrapetalonema perstans*, and beef and pork tapeworms.

Indication: Infection secondary to *Enterobius vermicularis*, *Trichuris trichiura*, *Ascaris lumbricoides*, *Ancylostoma duodenale*, *Necator americanus*.

Contraindications: Known drug hypersensitivity, children younger than 2 years old, pregnancy, lactation.

Adverse Effects: Abdominal pain, diarrhea; rash.

ANTIPARASITICS

ANTIMALARIAL AGENTS
General Considerations:

1. *Plasmodium* is an obligate intracellular protozoa.
2. Reproduce asexually in humans, but sexually in female *Anopheles* mosquitoes.
3. Four species:
   a. *P. falciparum* causes malignant tertian malaria. Often fatal because of fulminating infection and/or recrudescence after inadequate treatment.
   b. *P. vivax* gives rise to benign tertian malaria. Milder clinical attacks with lower mortality than *P. falciparum;* relapses can occur, however, 2 years after original infection.
   c. *P. ovale* causes a more curable but milder, less common form of malaria. Still, relapse potential similar to that of *P. vivax.*
   d. *P. malariae* causes quartan malaria, common in certain tropical areas. Low fatality risk; relapse potential exists but much rarer than with *P. vivax.*

4. Life cycle:
    a. Bite of infected mosquito transmits sporozoite form of
        parasite into circulation.
    b. Sporozoites localize in liver parenchymal cells and mul-
        tiply into tissue schizonts: asymptomatic exoerythrocytic
        or preerythrocytic phase.
    c. Schizonts rupture and release thousands of merozoites
        into circulation to invade RBCs: erythrocytic phase.
    d. Within RBCs, merozoites mature into schizonts. Rup-
        ture of these RBCs releases more merozoites into circu-
        lation and produces paroxysms of chills and fever char-
        acteristic of classic malarial attack.
    e. Released merozoites invade more RBCs to continue the
        cycle; some differentiate into male and female gameto-
        cyte forms that can reproduce sexually in the gut of
        mosquito and become the infective sporozoite.
    f. After primary-tissue schizonts of *P. falciparum* and *P.
        malariae* are released from liver, no further tissue para-
        sites remain.
    g. In *P. vivax* and *P. ovale* infections, latent hypnozoite
        forms persist in dormant fashion intrahepatically and
        may be released months to years later to produce relapse
        into erythrocytic phase.
5. Pathophysiology:
    a. Destruction of RBCs results in severe intravascular
        hemolysis with marked anemia, hemoglobinemia, and
        hemoglobinuria.
    b. Vascular obstruction from parasitized RBCs causes tis-
        sue hypoxia with ensuing organ dysfunction (i.e., hyper-
        splenism, from erythrophagocytosis), renal tubular
        necrosis, and centrilobular liver necrosis. Sympathetic
        splanchnic vasoconstriction with decreased hepatic and
        renal blood flow may compound problem.

■ Chloroquine Phosphate (Aralen; Winthrop)

How Supplied:
PO: 500 mg tablets (phosphate salt; equivalent to 300 mg base,
respectively).
IM: 50 mg/ml in 5 ml ampule (hydrochloride salt; equivalent to
40 mg base/ml).

Administration:
PO: Rapidly and almost completely absorbed.
IM: Switch to oral form as soon as can be tolerated.

Dose for malaria:
1. PO suppression: Ideally begin 2 wk before exposure and continue weekly (on same day of week) until 8 wk after leaving endemic area. If unable to start preexposure, administer loading dose as twice usual dose in 2 divided doses, 6 hr apart; then continue therapy at usual weekly dose.
2. Oral treatment of acute attack (concomitant primaquine [e.g., Aralen], required for radical cure of *P. vivax* and *P. malariae*): 1 gm (= 600 mg base) PO, then 500 mg (= 300 mg base) after 6–8 hr, then 500 mg/day × 2 days.
3. Parenteral (see specific indications below): 160–200 mg base IM, ½ in each buttock; repeat q6h, if necessary, to maximum of 800 mg base/24 hr.

Dose for extraintestinal amebiasis (*Entamoeba histolytica*):
1. PO: Combine Rx with an effective intestinal amebicide (e.g. emetine or dihydroemetine): 1 gm (= 600 mg base) q24h × 2 days, then 500 mg (= 300 mg base) q24h × 2–3 wk.
2. Parenteral (see specific indications below): 160–200 mg base IM q24h × 10–12 days.

Mechanism of Action: 4-Aminoquinoline structure. May act via inhibition of DNA polymerase and (to a certain extent) RNA polymerase. Another factor may be drug uptake and concentration within plasmodium-infected erythrocytes with resultant membrane damage and lysis.

Elimination: Excreted by kidneys. Avidly tissue bound, thus long half-life of 6–17 days.

Spectrum: Erythrocytic forms of *P. vivax* and *P. malariae* and most strains of *P. falciparum,* but not effective against exoerythrocytic malarial forms. Also amebicidal for trophozoites of *Entamoeba histolytica*.

Indications: Suppressive treatment and acute attacks of malaria secondary to *P. vivax, P. malariae, P. ovale,* and susceptible strains of *P. falciparum;* hepatic amebiasis unresponsive to metronidazole or when metronidazole contraindicated (less

ANTIINFECTIVES

effective for intestinal amebiasis because of poor tissue drug uptake and concentration in large bowel). Parenteral therapy indicated only when PO therapy cannot be tolerated (e.g., coma caused by falciparum malaria).

Contraindication: Retinal or visual field changes; known drug hypersensitivity. Psoriasis (may precipitate severe attack); porphyria (may exacerbate). Use with caution in hepatic disease, alcoholism, or concurrent hepatotoxic drug therapy (since drug is concentrated in liver); also in presence of severe gastrointestinal, neurologic, or blood disorders including G–6–PD deficiency. Although some data suggest potential teratogenic effect on fetal vestibular apparatus, generally drug is considered safe for use as suppressive therapy and for treatment of acute attacks. Not significantly excreted in breast milk.

Toxicity: Usual doses may cause GI upset, pruritus, headache, and visual changes (blurring, difficulty accommodating). Prolonged treatment at these doses may result in reversible lichenoid skin eruptions, neuropathy, blood dyscrasias, skin/mucosal pigmentary changes, and nerve deafness. Long–term therapy with excessive doses (>250 mg phosphate form/day) can cause irreversible retinopathy.

Monitor: Baseline and periodic ophthalmologic examination, periodic knee and ankle reflex testing (to rule out muscle weakness), CBC.

Interaction: Concomitant use of gold or phenylbutazone may exacerbate tendency to produce dermatitis; may potentiate side effects of hepatotoxic agents.

■ Quinine Sulfate (Quinamm; Marion Merrell Dow).

How Supplied:
PO:
    260 mg tablet.
Parenteral: Available in United States only through Malaria Branch, Division of Parasitic Diseases, Center for Infectious Diseases, CDC, Atlanta (specific indications only, see p.167).

Administration: *PO;* well and nearly completely absorbed.

Dose:
1. Malaria: 650 mg PO after meals tid × 10–14 days.
2. Nocturnal leg muscle cramps: 260 (to 520) mg PO qhs × several nights, then as needed.

Mechanism of Action: "General protoplasmic poison"; toxic to many bacteria and other unicellular organisms.

Elimination: Extensively metabolized in liver; excreted in urine. Half–life 4–5 hr.

Spectrum: "Cidal" for schizonts (erythrocytic forms) of all *Plasmodium* species; gametocidal for *P. vivax* and *P. malariae*.

Indications:
1. Administer with primaquine to achieve radical cure in relapsing vivax malaria.
2. Administer with pyrimethamine and sulfonamide or with tetracycline to achieve suppressive cure in multidrug–resistant falciparum malaria.
3. Parenteral form only indicated for emergencies; e.g., fulminant or cerebral malaria caused by chloroquine-resistant or multidrug-resistant *P. falciparum*.
4. Recumbency leg muscle cramps.

Contraindications: Pregnancy, G–6–PD deficiency, known drug hypersensitivity, tinnitus, optic neuritis. Use with caution in lactating women.

Toxicity: Cinchonism: Tinnitus, headache, nausea, visual changes; more common with repeated doses or overdosage. Also eighth nerve damage with vertigo and impaired hearing; blurred vision and possible optic atrophy; blood dyscrasias; rash; CNS changes such as delirium; renal damage with hemolysis, hemoglobinemia and hemoglobinuria (more common in pregnancy), hypoprothrombinemia.

Interaction: May increase plasma levels of digoxin and digitoxin or potentiate effects of oral anticoagulants and neuromuscular blocking agents. Urinary alkalizers (acetazolamide, sodium bicarbonate) may decrease quinine excretion and thus increase risk of toxic blood levels.

ANTIINFECTIVES

CHAPTER 5

ANTICOAGULANTS

The most commonly used anticoagulants are heparin and warfarin derivatives. Parenteral heparin has an immediate onset of action and causes the formation of various proteases, including antithrombin III, that result in the reduction of fibrin and clot formation. Warfarin derivatives block the coagulation cascade by impairing vitamin K–dependent reactions. These orally administered compounds take about 72 hours to reach their maximum anticoagulant effect.

ANTICOAGULANTS

Warfarin Derivatives

■ **Warfarin** (Coumadin; Du Pont): 2, 2.5, 5, 7.5, 10 mg tablet.

Dose: Must be individualized and adjusted based upon results of prothrombin time (PT). Commonly used initial dosage is 2–5 mg/day for 2–4 days with daily dosage based on PT results (1.2–1.5 × nl pt is optimal range).

Indication: Prophylaxis or treatment of venous thrombosis; pulmonary embolism; atrial fibrillation with embolization.

Contraindications: Pregnancy (drug passes placental barrier and may cause fetal hemorrhage); hemorrhagic tendencies; bleeding tendencies associated with active ulcers; regional or spinal anesthesia.

Adverse Effects: Hemorrhage from any tissue or organ; necrosis of skin; alopecia, dermatitis.
Overdosage: Treat with oral or parenteral Vitamin K.

Monitor: Prothrombin time.

Heparin

■ **Heparin Sodium Injection, USP** (Upjohn):
1000 U/ml in 10, 30 ml vial.
5000 U/ml in 1, 10 ml vial.
10,000 U/ml in 1, 4 ml vial.

■ **Heparin Lock Flush Solution** (Wyeth-Ayerst):
Not for use as anticoagulant. Use only for maintenance of
patency of IV injection devices.

■ **Heparin sodium injection, USP** (Wyeth-Ayerst):
1000, 2500, 5000, 7500, 10,000, 20,000 U in 1 ml Tubex
syringe.

Dose: Initial dosage: 5000–10,000 U SC, intermittent IV or
continuous IV infusion.
Maintenance dosage must be individualized depending on
needs of patient and condition treated.

Indication: Prophylaxis or treatment of venous thrombosis
(including during pregnancy), pulmonary embolism, or arterial
embolism; pelvic thrombophlebitis; atrial fibrillation with
embolization; disseminated intravascular coagulation (DIC).

Contraindications: Severe thrombocytopenia; active bleeding,
except DIC.

Adverse Effects: Hypersensitivity, hemorrhage, thrombocytopenia.

Monitor: PTT, platelets.

Protamine Sulfate (Lilly)

For use only in treatment of heparin overdose. Rapid administration can cause severe hypotension and anaphylactoid reaction.

Dose: Each milligram protamine sulfate neutralizes about 90
USP units heparin. Give slow intravenous injection over 10 min,
and do not exceed 50 mg (5 ml ampule).

ANTICOAGULANTS

CHAPTER 6

ANTICONVULSANTS

Pregnancy has an unpredictable effect on epileptic seizures, although in most cases there is increased frequency. Many reasons for this deterioration have been suggested, including the changing physiology of the pregnant woman. Probably the most important reason is the decrease in therapeutic serum levels of the anticonvulsant drug, which may be due to dilutional effects of expanding blood volume, increased hepatic and renal clearance, and patient noncompliance.

Consultation with appropriately trained specialists in maternal-fetal medicine should be obtained before initiation of anticonvulsant medication during pregnancy.

ANTICONVULSANTS

Selected anticonvulsants are listed in Table 6-1.

■ Phenytoin Sodium (Dilantin; Parke-Davis)

How Supplied:
PO:
   30, 100 mg capsule.
   125 mg/5 ml suspension.
Parenteral:
   50 mg/ml in 2 ml ampule or syringe.

Dose:
Initial: 100 mg tid.

Maintenance: Individualized based on therapeutic serum levels of drug.

TABLE 6-1
SELECTED ANTICONVULSANTS

Drug	Brand Name	Daily Dose (mg)	Therapeutic Level (µg/ml)	Manufacturer
Phenytoin	Dilantin	300–500	10–25	Parke-Davis
Carbamazepine	Tegretol	200–1000	4–12	Geigy
Clonazepam	Klonopin	0.5–1.5	0.02–0.08	Roche
Ethosuximide	Zarontin	500–1500	40–100	Parke-Davis
Mephenytoin	Mesantoin	300–600	10–25	Sandoz
Methsuximide	Celontin	300–1500	40–100	Parke-Davis
Primidone	Mysoline	750–1500	5–12	Wyeth-Ayerst
Trimethadione	Tridione	900–1800	5–12	Abbott
Valproic acid	Depakene	1000–3000	50–120	Abbott

Mechanism of Action: Inhibits spread of seizure activity in motor cortex by stabilizing the neuronal threshold against hyperexcitability. After PO administration, half-life is about 22 hr (range 7–42 hr). Optimum serum levels are between 10–20 µg/ml.

Indication: Control of tonic-clonic and psychomotor seizures.

Contraindications: Hypersensitivity; severe liver or renal dysfunction.

Adverse Effects:
1. Effects on lactation are unknown. Use during pregnancy may be associated with an increase in birth defects, neonatal hemorrhage, prematurity, intrauterine growth retardation, congenital heart disease, microcephaly and carcinogenicity (neuroblastoma).
2. CNS: Ataxia, slurred speech, nystagmus, other.
3. GI: Nausea, vomiting, constipation.
4. Skin: Minor/major allergic reactions.
5. Other: Gingival hyperplasia, coarsening of facial features, hirsutism, systemic lupus erythematosus (SLE), toxic liver changes.
6. Drug interactions: May cause decreased efficacy of oral steroid contraceptives, usually spotting or bleeding.

■ Carbamazepine (Tegretol; Geigy)

How Supplied: *PO:* 100 mg chewable tablet; 200 mg tablet.

Dose: 200 mg bid initially, then individualize.

Indication: Epilepsy; trigeminal neuralgia.

Contraindications: Previous blood dyscrasias; sensitivity to other tricyclic compounds.

Adverse Effects: Bone marrow depression. See also Phenytoin, above.

■ Clonazepam (Klonopin; Roche)

How Supplied: *PO:* 0.5, 1, 2 mg tablet.

Dose: 1.5 mg/day divided.

Indication: Adjunct therapy in petit mal seizures.

Contraindications: Hypersensitivity to benzodiazepines, hepatic dysfunction.

Adverse Effects: See Phenytoin, p. 172. Major side effects are CNS depression, behavioral changes, and GI symptoms.

■ Ethosuxamide (Zarontin; Parke-Davis)

How Supplied: *PO:* 250 mg tablet.

Dose: 500 mg/day initially, then individualize.

Indications: Petit mal seizures.

Contraindications: Hypersensitivity to succinamides.

Adverse Effects: See Phenytoin, p. 172.

■ Mephenytoin (Mesantoin; Sandoz)
Mechanism of Action: Hydantoin homologue of the barbiturate mephobarbital; exhibits effects of diphenytoin and barbiturates.

How Supplied: 100 mg tablet.

Dose: 2–6 tab/day initially; maintenance individualized.

Indication: Grand mal seizures, psychomotor seizures.

Contraindications: Hypersensitivity to hydantoin.

Adverse Effects: See Phenytoin, p. 172.

■ **Methsuximide** (Celontin; Parke-Davis)

How Supplied: *PO:* 300 mg capsule.

Dose: 300 mg/day for first week, then alter dose depending on response and side effects.

Indication: Petit mal seizures refractory to other drugs.

Contraindications: Hypersensitivity; abnormal liver or renal function.

Adverse Effects: See Phenytoin, p. 172.

■ **Paramethadione** (Paradione; Abbott)

How Supplied:
PO: 150 mg capsule.
 300 mg/ml suspension.

Dose: 300–600 mg/day in divided doses.

Indications: Petit mal epilepsy.

Contraindications: Hypersensitivity.

Adverse Effects: See Phenytoin, p. 172.

■ **Phenacemide** (Phenurone; Abbott)

How Supplied: *PO:* 500 mg tablet.

Dose: 500 mg tid.

Indication: Severe epilepsy refractory to other antiepileptics.

Contraindications: Should not be used as primary therapy.

Adverse Effects: Aplastic anemia, CNS effects, hepatic and GI disturbances. Very toxic drug.

■ Primidone (Mysoline; Wyeth-Ayerst)

How Supplied: *PO:* 50, 250 mg tablets; 250 mg/5 ml suspension.

Dose: 50 mg tid initially, then individualize.

Indication: Grand mal, psychomotor seizures.

Contraindications: Hypersensitivity to phenobarbital.

Adverse Effects: See Phenytoin, p. 172.

■ Trimethadione (Tridione; Abbott)

How Supplied: *PO:* 150 mg chewable tablet; 300 mg tablet.

Dose: 300–600 mg tid initially.

Indication: Petit mal seizures refractory to other therapy.

Contraindications: Hypersensitivity.

Adverse Effects: See Phenytoin, p. 172.

■ Valproic Acid (Depakene; Abbott)

How Supplied: *PO:* 250 mg capsule.

Dose: 15 mg/kg/day initially; maintenance depends on desired effect and toxic effects.

Indication: Control of petit mal seizures.

Contraindications: Abnormal liver function.

Adverse Effects: Hepatic failure. Increased incidence of congenital birth defects has been reported. See also Phenytoin, p. 172.

■ **Barbiturates**
See Chapter 26.

■ **Diazepam** (Valium; Roche)
See Chapter 26.

■ **Clorazepate Dipotassium** (Tranxene; Abbott)
See Chapter 26.

CHAPTER 7

ANTIEMETICS

PHENOTHIAZINES

■ **Chlorpromazine HCl**(Thorazine; Smith-Kline Beecham)

How Supplied:
PO:

    10, 25, 50, 100, 200 mg tablet.

    30, 75, 150 mg sustained-release capsule.

    30 mg/ml and 100 mg/ml concentrate.

    10 mg/5 ml syrup.

Parenteral:

    1, 2 ml (25 mg/ml) ampule.

    10 ml (25 mg/ml) multiple dose vials.

Rectal: 25, 100 mg suppository.

Administration:
PO: Well absorbed.

Rectal: Variable absorption.

Undiluted deep IM injection or slow IV infusion diluted to 1 mg/ml.

Mechanism of Action: Dimethylamine derivative of phenothiazine group with psychotropic, sedative, and antiemetic activity. Acts at all CNS levels (especially subcortical); effects on multiple organ systems include strong antiadrenergic and lesser peripheral anticholinergic activity.

Adult Dose:
Antiemetic:

    PO: 10–25 mg q4–6h prn; increase if necessary.

    IM: 25–50 mg q3–4h prn. Watch for hypotension. Switch to PO when vomiting stops.

    Rectal: 50–100 mg q6–8h prn.

    Intraoperatively: 12.5 mg IM; repeat in 30 min prn and no hypotension. Or 2 mg IV q2 min, max 25 mg.

Psychosis:

> *Acute:* 25 mg IM, then 25–50 mg in 1 hr prn; increase gradually. Usual maintenance 500 mg/day, max 2000 mg/day.
>
> *Less acute:* 25 mg PO tid; increase gradually. Usual maintenance 400 mg/day.

Intractable hiccups: 25–50 mg PO tid–qid. If ineffective after 2–3 days, 25–50 mg IM. If still no effect, slow IV infusion of 25–50 mg in 500–1000 ml normal saline solution (NS); keep patient flat to avoid hypotension.

> Acute intermittent porphyria: 25–50 mg PO or IM tid–qid.
>
> Tetanus: 25–50 mg IM tid–qid, usually with barbiturates; or 25–50 mg IV diluted to at least 1 mg/ml and given at 1 mg/min.

Elimination: Oxidation by hepatic microsomal enzymes; half–life 30 hr.

Indication: Psychosis; moderate to severe vomiting; to control presurgical restlessness and apprehension; acute intermittent porphyria, tetanus; manic-phase manic-depression; psychiatric/movement disorder (e.g., Gilles de la Tourette's syndrome), intractable hiccups; severe behavioral problems in children (e.g., explosive or combative hyperexcitable behavior). Use in pregnancy only in psychotic patients requiring continued medication; discontinue 1–2 wk before delivery to avoid neonatal symptoms.

Contraindications: Comatose states; presence of high levels of other CNS depressants (e.g., alcohol, barbiturates, narcotics); Reye's syndrome. Use with caution in pregnancy, lactation, cardiovascular or liver disease (risk of increased sensitivity to CNS effects, i.e., impaired cerebration and abnormal EEG slowing), chronic respiratory disease (e.g., severe asthma or emphysema, especially in children).

Toxicity:

1. Tardive dyskinesia: Potentially irreversible, involuntary dyskinetic movements (higher risk in elderly women).
2. Neuroleptic malignant syndrome: Potentially fatal (in 10%) complex of catatonia hyperpyrexia, muscle rigidity, altered mental status, autonomic instability.
3. Also motor restlessness, dystonias, pseudoparkinsonism, akasthesia, perioral tremor, other extrapyramidal (neuromuscular) reactions.

4. Miscellaneous: Cholestatic photosensitivity, leukopenia, agranulocytosis, hyperthermia, heat stroke. More frequent with chlorpromazine: orthostatic hypotension from α-adrenergic blockade (especially with mitral insufficiency, pheochromocytoma), jaundice, hypercholesterolemia malformations.

5. Pregnancy (some risk with all phenothiazines): Maternal hypotension with uteroplacental insufficiency; neonatal extrapyramidal effects and respiratory depression (in some studies), jaundice, sedation followed by motor excitement, agitation, hypertonicity, and depression; small left colon syndrome (i.e., decreased intestinal motility, abdominal distention, failure to pass meconium).

6. Overdosage: CNS depression to point of coma, convulsions, cardiac dysrhythmias, α-adrenergic blockade.

Monitor: Serial CBC (especially in patients with URTI).

Interaction: Potentiates effects of CNS depressants (e.g., alcohol, anesthetics, narcotics) and atropine; accentuated orthostatic hypotension with thiazides; diminishes or inhibits effects of direct dopaminergic agonists, levodopa, oral anticoagulants, and epinephrine; may precipitate phenytoin toxicity or lower seizure threshold and thus require anticonvulsant dosage adjustment. In particular, may augment respiratory depression caused by meperidine and meiotic or sedative effects of morphine. May block antihypertensive effect of guanethidine.

■ Perphenazine (Trilafon; Schering)

How Supplied:
PO.
    2, 4, 8, 16 mg tablets.
    16 mg/5 ml concentrate.
Parenteral: 5 mg/ml in 1 ml ampule.

Administration:
PO.
Parenteral: Deep IM injection preferred (watch for hypotension).
IV infusion: Only very few indications; dilute to 0.5 mg/ml, not more than 1 mg/injection at not less than 1–2 min intervals; switch to PO as soon as possible.

Mechanism of Action: Piperazine-type phenothiazine derivative; acts at all CNS levels, especially hypothalamus.

Dose:
Antiemetic:
> *PO:* 8–16 mg/day, divided; max 24 mg/day. Early dose reduction desirable.
>
> *IM:* 5 or 10 mg × 1 dose.

Antipsychotic, less severe:
> *PO:* 4–24 mg/day divided bid–qid; reduce to minimum effective dosage as soon as symptoms controlled; max 24 mg/day except in inpatients.
>
> *IM:* 5 mg q6h; max 15 mg/day in outpatients, 30 mg/day in inpatients.

Antipsychotic, severe:
> *PO:* 8–16 mg bid–qid; max 64 mg/day.
>
> *IM:* 5–10 mg qh; max 15 mg in outpatients, 30 mg/day in inpatients. Switch to PO (at slightly increased dose to maintain efficacy) as soon as feasible.

Indication: Severe nausea and vomiting; psychosis.

Contraindications: See Chlorpromazine, pp. 178, and Prochlorperazine p. 181. Also not for use in patients with subcortical brain damage (risk of hyperthermic reaction).

Toxicity: See Chlorpromazine, pp. 178. Compared with less potent antipsychotics, sedation and hypotension less likely and extrapyramidal symptoms more likely.

Interaction: See Chlorpromazine, p. 179. Most important, potentiates CNS depressants, anticholinergics (e.g., atropine); partially blocks or reverses epinephrine effect; moderately epileptogenic.

■ **Prochlorperazine** (Compazine; Smith-Kline Beecham)

How Supplied:
PO:
> 5, 10, 25 mg tablets.

10, 15 mg spansule.

5 mg/5 ml syrup.

Parenteral:

5 mg/ml in 2 ml and 10 ml vials.

5 mg/ml, 2 ml disposable syringes.

Rectal: 2.5, 5, 25 mg suppositories.

Administration:

PO, rectal: Well absorbed.

Parenteral: Deep IM injection, undiluted slow IV push, or diluted isotonic infusion, not faster than 5 mg/min.

Mechanism of Action: Phenothiazine derivative of piperazine group. Works as an antiemetic (chief indication) via central effect on chemoreceptor trigger zone. As a neuroleptic, reduces agitation, anxiety, restlessness, aggressive behavior, and psychotic symptoms of hallucinations, delusions, disorganized thoughts; however, other member of phenothiazine class preferable for these states because of side effects.

Dose:

Antiemetic:

PO: 5–15 mg tid, max 40 mg/day.

Rectal: 25 mg bid.

IM: 5–10 mg q3–4h prn, max 40 mg/day.

IV: 2.5–10 mg IV; max single dose 10 mg, or 40 mg/day (watch for hypotension).

Perioperatively: 5–10 mg IM 1–2 hr before induction of anesthesia; repeat in 30 min or later if needed.

Nonpsychotic disorders:

5 mg PO tid–qid, or 15 mg slow-release spansule every AM and 10 mg q12h. Maximum duration 12 wk for doses over 20 mg/day (risk of persistent or irreversible tardive dyskinesia).

Psychosis:

Mild: 5–10 mg PO tid–qid.

Moderate to severe (i.e., hospitalized patients): 10 mg PO tid–qid; for maximum improvement, increase dose gradually to avoid significant side effects (i.e., q2–3 days). Usual maintenance 50–75 mg/day, max 150 mg/day. For immediate effect in uncontrollable patient, give 10–20 mg/day IM, repeat q1–4h prn × 3–4 doses. If unable to switch to PO, maintain on 10–20 mg q4–6h.

Indication: Severe nausea and vomiting; short-term therapy for generalized nonpsychotic anxiety (but not as first-line drug). May be used in pregnancy only to treat severe nausea and vomiting refractory to conservative measures.

Contraindications: Coma; patients with high levels of CNS depressants (e.g., alcohol, barbiturates, narcotics), including withdrawal syndromes; children younger than 2 years old or less than 20 lb body weight; Reye's syndrome (drug effects may mimic encephalopathic symptoms). Exercise extreme caution in acutely ill or dehydrated children (higher risk extrapyramidal syndromes, especially dystonias), cardiovascular impairment (risk of hypotension), glaucoma, bone marrow depression, or prior phenothiazine hypersensitivity reactions.

Toxicity: See Chlorpromazine p. 178.

Monitor: Serial CBC (especially if patient has URTI) to detect impending agranulocytosis.

Antidote: Antiparkinson drugs, barbiturates, or diphenhydramine (Benadryl); norepinephrine bitartrate (Levophed) or phenylephrine HCl (Neo-Synephrine) if vasoconstrictor required.

Interactions: See Chlorpromazine p. 179.

■ **Promethazine HCl** (Phenergan; Wyeth-Ayerst)

How Supplied:
PO: 12.5, 25, 50 mg tablet.
    6.25, 25 mg/5 ml syrup.
Parenteral: 25, 50 mg/ml in 1 ml ampule.
Rectal: 12.5, 25, 50 mg suppository.

Administration:
PO, rectal: Well absorbed.
Parenteral: Deep IM injection preferred; or IV, diluted to at least 25 mg/ml and no faster than 25 mg/min. Inadvertent intraarterial injection may give rise to severe arteriospasm with gangrene; chemical irritation from subcutaneous injection may cause necrotic lesions.

Mechanism of Action:
Phenothiazine derivative with antihistaminic, sedative, antiemetic, antimotion sickness, and anticholinergic effects.

Dose (Adult):
Allergy:
> *IM:* 25 mg; repeat in 2 hr prn.
> *PO, rectal:* 25 mg qhs or 12.5 mg qid.

Sedation:
> *IM:* 25 mg qh.
> *PO, rectal:* 25–50 mg qhs.

Antiemetic:
> *IM, IV:* 12.5–25 mg q4h.
> *PO, rectal:* 12.5–25 mg q4–6h.

Obstetrics:
> *IM, IV:* 25–75 mg q4h; max 100 mg/day.

Motion sickness:
> *PO, rectal:* 25 mg bid, begin 30–60 min before travel.

Indication: Transfusion (allergic) reactions; adjunctive therapy in anaphylaxis (with epinephrine); motion sickness, preoperative, postoperative, and intrapartum sedation; antiemetic; IV as an adjunct to analgesics for pain postoperatively and intraoperatively (e.g., bronchoscopy, ophthalmic surgery, and poor-risk patients [to reduce amount of narcotic needed]); allergic and vasomotor rhinitis and conjunctivitis.

Contraindications: Comatose states; high present levels of CNS depressants (e.g., alcohol, sedative hypnotics, barbiturates, general anesthetics, narcotics); known drug hypersensitivity. Use with caution in patients with bone marrow depression (risk of leukopenia, agranulocytosis), sulfite sensitivity, asthmatic attacks, narrow-angle glaucoma, prostatic hypertrophy, stenosing peptic ulcer, pyloroduodenal and bladder neck obstruction. Also, exercise caution in children: greater risk of dystonias, masked signs of Reye's syndrome; large doses may incite hallucinations, convulsions, and sudden death. Further caution urged with cardiovascular or hepatic dysfunction and in the elderly (reduce dose).

Toxicity: See Prochlorperazine, p. 182. Most commonly, sedation; extrapyramidal reactions mostly at high doses or in children. Overdose manifested as hyperexcitability, abnormal movements, delirium, and respiratory depression.

Interactions: Additive CNS depression with narcotics (reduce narcotic dose by ¼–½), barbiturates (reduce barbiturates dose by ½), alcohol, sedative hypnotics, general anesthetics. Further sedative effects and increased pressor response with tricyclic antidepressants. Hypertensive crisis or extrapyramidal reactions with MAO inhibitors. Tachycardia or dysrhythmias with sympathomimetics; blocks cardiostimulating effects of β-blockers; epinephrine may further lower BP in patients with hypotension from excessively high drug levels.

■ Thiethylperazine Maleate (Torecan; Roxane)

How Supplied:
PO: 10 mg tablet.
Parenteral: 10 mg/2 ml in 2 ml ampule.

Administration: *PO; deep IM injection.*

Mechanism of Action: Piperazine-type phenothiazine derivative with direct action on chemoreceptor trigger zone and vomiting center. Also has dopaminergic antagonist activity.

Dose: 10–30 mg/day; may divide tid.

Indication: Nausea and vomiting.

Contraindications: Coma, severe CNS depression, previous phenothiazine hypersensitivity reaction, pregnancy, lactation.

Toxicity: See Prochlorperazine, p. 182.

Interactions: Potentiates CNS depressants and atropine; reverses epinephrine effect. Contains sodium metabisulfite: May cause allergic/anaphylactic reaction.

BENZAMIDES

■ **Metoclopramide Hydrochloride** (Reglan; Robins)

How Supplied:
PO:
 5, 10 mg tablets.
 5 mg/5 ml syrup
Parenteral:
 5 mg/ml, 2, 10, 30 ml single dose vial.
 2 ml, 10 ml ampule

Administration: Rapidly and well absorbed orally.

Mechanism of Action: Antiemetic effects result from antagonism of central and peripheral dopamine receptors, thus blocking chemoreceptor trigger zone.

 Relieves reflux by stimulating mobility of upper GI tract without enhancing gastric, biliary or pancreatic secretions. Also increases antral contractions while relaxing pyloric sphincter and duodenal bulb and increasing duodenal and jejunal peristalsis, resulting in accelerated gastric emptying and intestinal transit. Increases resting tone of lower esophageal sphincter.

Dose:
As antiemetic:
 10–20 mg IM; or
 1–2 mg/kg IV over 15–30 min; repeat q2–3h prn.
 For reflux: 10–15 mg qid 30 min before meals and qhs.
 Elderly patients or those with renal impairment: Reduce dose.

Elimination: Excreted in urine.

Indications: Nausea and vomiting (postoperative, associated with chemotherapy); symptomatic gastroesophageal reflux; diabetic gastroparesis.

Contraindications: GI hemorrhage, mechanical obstruction, perforation (excess GI motility should be avoided); pheochromocytoma (may precipitate hypertensive crisis); epileptic or patients on other drugs known to cause extrapyramidal reactions (possible increased seizures or side effects).

Adverse Effects/Toxicity: See Chlorpromazine p. 178. Also, depression, galactorrhea/amenorrhea; methemoglobinemia.

Monitor: Serum prolactin (in patients with amenorrhea/ galactorrhea).

Interactions: GI motility effects lessened by anticholinergics and narcotics. Additional sedation when given with alcohol, sedatives, hypnotics, narcotics or tranquilizers.

■ **Granisetron Hydrochloride** (Kytril; Smith-Kline Beecham)

How Supplied:
PO: 1 mg tablet
Parenteral: 1 mg/ml, 1 ml single-use vial

Administration: *PO; IV,* diluted in 0.9 NS or D5W to 20–50 ml total volume

Mechanism of Action Selective 5–hydroxytryptamine$_3$ (5-HT$_3$) receptor antagonist. Blocks serotonin stimulation of 5–HT$_3$ receptors on vagal nerve terminals and in chemoreceptor trigger zone. (Chemotherapy causes vomiting via serotonin released from mucosal enterochromaffin cells.)

Dose:
PO: 1 mg bid during chemotherapy, starting up to 1 hr before.
IV: 10 µg/kg IV over 5 min, starting up to 30 min before chemotherapy.

Elimination: Hepatic metabolism by N–demethylation and aromatic ring oxidation, then by conjugation.

Indications: Prevention of nausea/vomiting caused by initial and repeat courses of emetogenic cancer therapy (e.g., high–dose cisplatin).

Contraindications: Known drug hypersensitivity. Avoid use in pregnancy unless clearly needed; discourage nursing during administration.

Adverse effects: Headache (14%–21%); constipation, diarrhea, abdominal pain, asthenia. Rarely: HTN, cardiac dysrhythmias, fever, allergic reactions.

Interactions: Theoretically, other drugs that induce or inhibit hepatic cytochrome P–450 enzymes may change clearance and half–life.

■ Ondansetron HCL (Zofran; Cerenex)

How Supplied:
PO:
   4, 8 mg tablets.
Parenteral:
   2 mg/ml, 2 ml vial.
   20 ml multidose vial.

Administration: Well absorbed orally (better with food); IV.

Mechanism of Action: Selective blocking agent of the 5–HT_3 receptor type, with probable (indirect) inhibition of vomiting reflex.

Dose:
PO: 8 mg tid; 1st dose 30 min before chemotherapy and continued 1–2 days after completion
IV: Starting 30 mins before chemotherapy: single 32 mg dose or 0.15 mg/kg dose × 3, diluted in 50 ml D5W or 0.9NS, infused over 15 min.
   For prevention of postoperative nausea/vomiting: 4 mg over 2–5 min., undiluted.
   Severe hepatic insufficiency: maximum dose 8 mg/day.

Elimination: Metabolized via hydroxylation on the indole ring, then subsequent glucuronide or sulfate conjugation.

Indications: Nausea and vomiting associated with emetogenic chemotherapy; prevention of postoperative nausea and vomiting expected to be severe.

ANTIEMETICS

Contraindications: Known drug hypersensitivity; avoid use in pregnancy and lactation (insufficient data).

Adverse Effects: Diarrhea/constipation; headache; fever.

Toxicity: Rare risk of liver failure in patients receiving hepatotoxic drugs concurrently; isolated reports of sudden blindness, hypotension, transient second-degree heart block, seizures.

Monitor: LFTs; serum potassium.

Interactions: See Granisetron p. 187.

■ Trimethobenzamide (Tigan; Smith-Kline Beecham)

How Supplied:
PO: 100, 250 mg capsule.
Parenteral:
    100 mg/ml in 2 ml ampule and disposable syringe.
    20 ml multiple-dose vial.
Rectal: 100, 200 mg suppository.

Administration: 60% of PO and rectal dose absorbed; deep IM undiluted injection.

Mechanism of Action: Depresses chemoreceptor trigger zone in medulla oblongata; direct impulses to vomiting center not blocked. Only weak antihistamine activity.

Dose: 200–250 mg tid–qid (PO, rectally, IM).

Elimination: Partially metabolized in liver; partially excreted unchanged in urine.

Indication: Nausea and vomiting. Considered safe in pregnancy.

Contraindications: Use extreme caution in pediatric, elderly, or debilitated patients with acute febrile illnesses, encephalitides, gastroenteritis, or dehydration with electrolyte imbalance, because of risk of opisthotonos, seizures, coma, extrapyramidal symptoms, and Reye's syndrome.

Toxicity: Sedation, hypersensitivity reactions, parkinson-like syndrome, hypotension, blood dyscrasias.

Interaction: Potentiates CNS depressants.

ANTIEMETICS

ANTIHISTAMINES: H$_1$-BLOCKING AGENTS

■ **Dimenhydrinate** (Wyeth-Ayerst. Dramamine; Richardson-Vicks Health Care, Searle)

How Supplied:
PO:
    12.5 mg/4 ml liquid.
    30 mg tablet, chewable tablet.
Parenteral:
    50 mg/ml in 1, 5 ml vial.

Administration:
PO, IM, IV: 50–100 mg q4–6h prn; max 400 mg/day.

Mechanism of Action: Ethanolamine-type H$_1$ blocker; depresses hyperstimulated labyrinthine function.

Indication: Motion sickness symptoms of nausea, vomiting, vertigo.

Contraindications: Pregnancy (anecdotal association with preterm labor); known drug hypersensitivity. Inadequate data on use in lactation. Use with caution in patients where anticholinergic effects are undesirable (see Diphenhydramine, p. 190).

Toxicity: See Diphenhydramine, p. 191.

Interactions: Additive effects with CNS depressants; may mask ototoxicity caused by aminoglycosides, cisplatin.

■ Diphenhydramine HCl (Benadryl; Parke-Davis. Dytuss; Lunsco)

How Supplied:
PO:
> 25, 50 mg capsule.
> 12.5 mg/5 ml elixir and syrup.
> 50 mg tablet.

Parenteral:
> 10 mg/10 ml vial; 50 mg/10 ml vial.
> 50 mg/ml disposable syringe and ampules.
> 50 mg/1 ml ampule.

Administration:
PO: Well absorbed rapidly.
IM, IV: As undiluted injection.

Mechanism of Action: Ethanolamine-type H_1 blocker with anticholinergic and sedation side effects. Competes with histamine for receptor sites on effector cells.

Dose:
PO: 25–50 mg tid–qid or 50 mg qh.
IM, IV: 10–50 mg q2–4h; max 400 mg/day.

Elimination: Mostly metabolized in liver; partially excreted unchanged in urine.

Indications: Allergic conjunctivitis or dermatitis; transfusion reactions; dermatographism; epinephrine adjunct in anaphylaxis; motion sickness; parkinsonism, including drug-induced and in the elderly (with centrally acting anticholinergics if needed), especially oculogyric crisis secondary to phenothiazines.

Contraindications: Newborns, lactation, first-trimester pregnancy (possible association with oral cleft). Because of atropine-like action, use with caution in patients with asthma, increased intraocular pressure, hyperthyroidism, cardiovascular disease, hypertension.

Adverse Effects: Sedation, disturbed coordination, epigastric distress, thickened bronchial secretions.

Toxicity: Atropine-like signs, CNS depression, or stimulation (more likely in children).

Interaction: Additive sedative effects with other CNS depressants; potentiates anticholinergic effects of MAO inhibitors.

■ Hydroxyzine HCl/Pamoate (Atarax, Roerig; Vistaril; Roerig)

ANTIEMETICS

How Supplied:
PO:
   10, 25, 50, 100 mg tablet.
   25 mg/5 ml suspension.
Parenteral:
   25 mg/ml; 10 ml vial.
   50 mg/ml; 2, 10 ml vial.

Administration:
PO: Well absorbed, rapidly.
IM: As undiluted injection, in large muscle.

Mechanism of Action: Piperazine-type H_1 blocking agent. Suppresses certain key subcortical regions of CNS, with primary skeletal muscle relaxation, bronchodilation, and antihistaminic, analgesic, and antiemetic effects.

Dose:
Anxiety:
   PO: 50–100 mg qid.
   IM: 50–100 mg q4–6h.
Pruritus:
   PO: 25 mg tid–qid.
Perioperative sedative or antiemetic:
   PO: 50–100 mg.
   IM: 25–100 mg.

Indication: Perioperative sedative/antiemetic (may permit narcotic dose reduction); anxiety and tension in psychoneurosis and organic disease states; allergic pruritus.

Contraindications: Early pregnancy, lactation, known drug hypersensitivity.

Toxicity: Infrequent, mild, and transitory: Sedation and dry mouth. Rarely, involuntary motor activity (tremors, convulsions) at excessive doses.

Interactions: Potentiates CNS depressants (e.g., meperidine, barbiturates) and requires their dosage reduction.

■ Meclizine HCl (Bonine; Pfizer Consumer Health Care; Antivert; Antivert/25; Antivert/50; Roerig)

How Supplied:
PO:
> 12.5, 25, 50 mg tablet.
> 25 mg chewable tablet.

Administration: *PO.*

Mechanism of Action: Piperazine antihistamine. Depresses labyrinth excitability and vestibular-cerebellar pathway conduction; competitively inhibits H_1 receptors to block histamine-induced increased capillary permeability and smooth muscle constriction. Anticholinergic, but without cardiovascular effects at usual doses.

Dose: 25–100 mg/day in divided doses.

Elimination: Metabolized in liver; excreted in urine.

Indication: Nausea and vomiting; vertigo resulting from motion sickness or vestibular system disease.

Contraindications: Teratogenic in rodents, but no reported malformations in humans. Not for use in children younger than 12 years; exercise caution in patients with asthma or glaucoma because of potential anticholinergic effect.

Toxicity: Sedation, dry mouth, blurred vision.

Interactions: Sedation potentiated by alcohol.

MISCELLANEOUS ANTIEMETICS
■ Benzquinamide HCL (Emete-Con; Roerig)

How Supplied: *Parenteral:* 50 mg/vial.

Administration: Deep *IM* (preferred route); slow *IV* (only without CV disease). Acts within 15 mins.

Mechanism of Action: Benzoquinolizine unrelated to phenothiazines and other antiemetics but with similar effects, including mildly anticholinergic and sedative.

Dose: *IM:* 50 mg (0.5–1.0 mg/kg) initially; repeat initial dose in 1 hr. and q 3–4 hr, prn.
IV: 25 mg (0.2–0.4 mg/kg); *IM* thereafter.

Elimination: Majority metabolized in liver; excreted in urine, bile and feces.

Indications: Nausea/vomiting caused by anesthesia, surgery.

Contraindications: Known drug hypersensitivity; pregnancy.

Adverse Effects/Toxicity: Dry mouth; BP changes; PVC's; HTN episodes after IV administration, especially if on concurrent pressor agents or epinephrine-like drugs.

Interactions: See Adverse Effects/Toxicity above.

■ Diphenidol (Vontrol; Smith-Kline Beecham)

How Supplied: *PO:* 25 mg tablet

Mechanism of Action: Specific antivertigo effect on vestibular apparatus to control vertigo; inhibits chemoreceptor trigger zone to control nausea/vomiting.

Dose: 25–30 mg q4h.

Elimination: 90% excreted in urine.

ANTIEMETICS

Indications: Peripheral (labyrinthine) vertigo and its associated nausea/vomiting; similarly, Meniere's disease, middle/inner ear surgery for labyrinthitis. Nausea/vomiting in postoperative states, malignant neoplasms.

Contraindications: Anuria; unsupervised/nonhospitalized patients; known drug hypersensitivity.

Adverse Effects/Toxicity: Auditory, visual hallucinations, disorientation, drowsiness/overstimulation; GI irritation; blurred vision.

■ **Dronabinol** (Marinol; Roxane)

How Supplied: *PO:* 2.5, 5, 10 mg capsules.

Administration: *PO,* well absorbed; however because of first-pass hepatic metabolism and high lipid solubility, only 10%–20% reaches systemic circulation.

Mechanism of Action: Orally active cannabinoid with complex effects on CNS, including central sympathomimetic activity. Exact antiemetic mechanism unknown.

Dose:
Antiemetic: 5–7.5 mg/m^2 1–3 hr. before and every 2–4 hr after chemotherapy.
Appetite stimulant: 2.5–20 mg/day divided bid, usually before lunch and supper.

Elimination: After extensive first-pass hepatic metabolism, excreted in bile, feces and urine.

Indications: Antiemetic in cancer chemotherapy, often combined with a phenothiazine for synergistic effect and reduced toxicity; as an appetite stimulant in AIDS-related anorexia and weight loss.

Contraindications: Pregnancy, lactation. Use with caution in patients with cardiac disorders (risk of BP changes, tachycardia); psychiatric conditions such as mania, depression or schizophrenia; or history of substance abuse.

Adverse Effects: Dizziness, euphoria (hallucination), paranoid reactions, somnolence, abnormal thinking; conjunctivitis; hypotension; abdominal pain, diarrhea; flushing.

Toxicity: Memory impairment, depersonalization, mood alteration, urinary retention, decreased motor coordination, lethargy, slurred speech, postural hypotension, panic reactions.

Interactions: None discovered during clinical trials, but theoretically possible based on existing cannabinoid data: Additive HTN or tachycardia with sympathomimetics, anticholinergics, tricyclic antidepressants; additive drowsiness with antihistamines, CNS depressants such as barbiturates, benzodiazepines, ethanol; decreased clearance of antipyrine and barbiturates.

■ **Droperidol** (Astra. Quad. Inapsine; Janssen)

How Supplied:
Parenteral:
    2.5 mg/ml in 1, 2, 5 ml ampule.
    10 ml multiple-dose vial.

Administration: Undiluted IM or slow IV achieves onset of action in 3–10 min.

Dose: 2.5–10 mg dose; lower doses in elderly, debilitated, or poor-risk patients.

Mechanism of Action: Tetrahydropyridine butyrophenone derivative. Neuroleptic sedative that allays anxiety, produces mental detachment but maintains mental alertness. Also, antiemetic effect, mild α-adrenergic blockade (decreased BP, temperature, pulse, and respiration).

Elimination: Metabolized in liver; excreted in urine and feces.

Indication: Perioperative sedative and antiemetic; neuroleptanalgesia with opioids.

Contraindications: Children younger than 2 years; inadequate data on use in pregnancy and lactation. Use with caution in patients with hepatic or renal dysfunction.

Toxicity: Most frequent, hypotension (treat hypovolemia aggressively), tachycardia; drowsiness. Also, extrapyramidal symptoms (dystonia, akathisia, oculogyric crisis); laryngobronchospasm; postoperative hallucinations. Overdose may cause hypoventilation or apnea in addition to the above.

Interactions: Potentiates other CNS depressants; reduce both drug dosages.

CHAPTER 8

ANTIHYPERTENSIVES

CENTRALLY ACTING AGENTS
■ **Methyldopa** (Aldomet; Merck)

How Supplied:
PO:
125, 250, 500 mg tablet.
250 mg/5 ml suspension.
Parenteral: 250 mg/5 ml vial.

Administration:
PO: Absorbed by active amino acid transport.
IV: Dilute in D_5W to 1–10 mg/ml and infuse slowly over 30–60 min (hypertensive crises).

Dose:
PO: Initially 250 mg bid–tid. Increase q2 day (at night to minimize sedation). Starting dose 500 mg/day if receiving other antihypertensives except thiazides. Usual maintenance 500 mg to 2 gm divided bid–tid; max 3 gm/day. Add a thiazide if BP not controlled with 2 gm/day.
IV: 250–500 mg q6h; max 1 gm q6h. Switch to PO when feasible.

Mechanism of Action: Metabolized to α-methylnorepinephrine, potent α_2-adrenergic agonist that decreases CNS sympathetic outflow. Reduces total peripheral resistance without much change in cardiac output or heart rate.

Elimination: Biphasic; two thirds cleared by kidney. Reduce dose if renal or hepatic dysfunction exists.

Indications: Hypertension. Effective when used with thiazides. Frequent side effects limit usefulness.

Contraindications: Active liver disease (e.g., hepatitis, cirrhosis), history of sensitivity to drug's components (including sulfites in oral suspension). Avoid use in lactation.

Adverse Effects:
Most common: sedation, orthostatic hypotension, dizziness, dry mouth, headache, decreased mental acuity, sleep disturbances, impotence, parkinsonian signs.

Toxicity: Positive direct Coombs' test (10%–20% of patients, after 6–12 months; less common with daily dose under 1 gm); hemolytic anemia in less than 5% of these. Discontinue methyldopa (treat with corticosteroids). Also, drug fever; transient liver function test changes (3%), hepatitis or hepatic necrosis (usually reversible); skin eruptions; myocarditis; retroperitoneal fibrosis; carotid sinus hypersensitivity with bradycardia and hypotension; pancreatitis; biliary carcinoma; colitis; hyperprolactinemia; choreoathetoid movements in patients with bilateral cerebrovascular disease; sudden drug cessation may precipitate HTN crisis.

Monitor: Baseline and periodic CBC; direct Coombs' test; LFTs; lithium levels if taken concurrently.

Interaction: Additive hypotensive effect with other antihypertensives, diuretics, general anesthetics, and nitroglycerine; reduced hypotensive effect with tricyclic antidepressants, barbiturates, sympathomimetic amines. Haloperidol and lithium toxicity increased.

■ Clonidine (Catapres, Catapres-TTS; Boehringer Ingelheim)

How Supplied:
PO: 0.1, 0.2, 0.3 mg tablet.
Transdermal:
   Catapres-TTS-1, Catapres-TTS-2, Catapres-TTS-3 (delivers 0.1, 0.2, 0.3 mg/day × 1 wk) multilayered adhesive film.

Administration:
PO: Rapidly and well absorbed, with high bioavailability. Transdermal delivery based on flow via concentration gradient, with therapeutic levels achieved 2–3 days after first application.

Dose:
PO: Initially 0.1 mg bid (less in elderly patients). Increase by 0.1 mg/day until desired effect reached; usual maintenance 0.2–0.6 mg/day; max 2.4 mg/day. Dividing dose unequally with larger dose at bedtime limits drowsiness. Decrease dose in renal impairment.

Transdermal: Initially 1 Catapres–1/wk; increase after 1–2 wk to achieve desired BP. Max 2 Catapres–3/wk.

Mechanism of Action: Stimulates brainstem α-adrenoreceptors, thus lowering CNS sympathetic outflow, peripheral resistance, renal vascular resistance, heart rate, and BP. No real change in renal blood flow or GFR.

Elimination: Half degraded in liver, rest excreted unchanged in urine. Half-life 9–16 hr; up to 41 hr in renal impairment.

Indication: Hypertension, alone or with other agents (e.g., diuretics). May help blunt reflex increase in sympathetic tone produced buy vasodilators.

Contraindications: Known drug or component (e.g., adhesive film) hypersensitivity. Use with caution in severe coronary insufficiency, recent MI, cerebrovascular disease, chronic renal failure. Remove transdermal form before defibrillation or cardioversion (may cause arcing). Avoid use in pregnancy unless clearly necessary; advise discontinuation of nursing.

Adverse Effects:
1. Xerostomia and sedation in up to 50% of patients; lessens in 2–4 wk. Discontinuation rate 10% because of above and GI distress, impotence or dizziness.
2. Fluid retention, weight gain, and loss of hypotensive effect may occur if used as single-agent HTN therapy.
3. CNS effects: Sleep disturbances, depression, and anxiety.
4. Skin problems: Rash, angioneurotic edema, urticaria, alopecia, pruritus.
5. Miscellaneous: Hyperglycemia, elevated CPK, gynecomastia, urinary retention, increased sensitivity to alcohol.
6. Sudden drug withdrawal may give rise to HTN crisis with sympathetic overactivity (headache, abdominal pain, tachycardia), especially in patients receiving β-blockers (e.g., propranolol).

ANTIHYPERTENSIVES

Toxicity: Hypotension, bradycardia, lethargy, irritability, somnolence, miosis, vomiting and hypoventilation; rarely, cardiac dysrhythmias, apnea, seizures and transient HTN.

Interaction: Reduced effect on BP with tricyclic antidepressants. Alcohol, barbiturates, hypnotics, sedatives, and methyltestosterone enhance CNS depression. May augment insulin-induced hypoglycemia. Rarely, sinus bradycardia and AV block with digitalis.

■ Guanabenz Acetate (Wytensin; Wyeth-Ayerst)

How Supplied:
PO: 4, 8 mg tablet.

Administration:
PO: 75% absorbed.

Dose: Initially 4 mg bid; increase by 4–8 mg/day q1–2wk; max 32 mg bid.
    Reduce dose in patients with cirrhosis.

Mechanism of Action: See Clonidine p. 199.

Elimination: Metabolized extensively in liver. Half-life, 4–6 hr.

Indication: Hypertension, alone or with thiazide diuretic.

Contraindications: Pregnancy, lactation, children younger than 12 years old, known drug hypersensitivity. Exercise caution in patients with severe coronary insufficiency, recent MI, cerebrovascular disease, serious liver or kidney failure.

Adverse Effects/Toxicity: See Clonidine, p. 199.

Interaction: Potential for increased sedation with other CNS depressants.

■ Guanfacine HCl (Tenex; Robins)

How Supplied: *PO:* 1, 2 mg tablets.

Administration: *PO.*

Dose: 1 mg qhs (to minimize somnolence). Increase to 2 mg/day after 3–4 weeks if necessary; max 3 mg/day (higher risk of adverse effects at this dose). Use lower dosing range if renal impairment.

Mechanism of Action: See Clonidine p. 199.

Elimination: Renal excretion, 50% as unchanged drug.

Indications: HTN, alone or with other agents; e.g., thiazides.

Contraindications: See Guanabenz Acetate p. 200.

Adverse Effects: Sedation, xerostomia, asthenia, dizziness, constipation, impotence. "Rebound" with abrupt drug cessation: nervousness, anxiety, HTN.

Toxicity: Bradycardia, hypotension.

Interactions: See Guanabenz Acetate p. 200.

GANGLIONIC BLOCKING AGENTS
■ **Trimethaphan Camsylate** (Arfonad; Roche)

How supplied:
Parenteral: 500 mg/10 ml ampule.

Administration: *IV,* appropriately diluted; not to be infused with any other drug.

Mechanism of Action: Produces ganglionic blockade by occupying receptor sites on ganglion cells and by stabilizing postsynaptic membranes against the action of acetylcholine liberated from presynaptic nerve endings. Also has a direct peripheral vasodilator effect, thus lowering BP by causing pooling of blood in the dependent periphery and the splanchnic system.

Dose: 0.3–6 mg/min, using lower dosage range in patients under deeper planes of anesthesia, the elderly, or debilitated patients.

Indications: Controlled hypotension during surgery; acute control of BP in hypertensive emergencies (e.g., aortic dissection); emergency treatment of pulmonary edema when pulmonary HTN coexists with systemic HTN.

Contraindications: Where hypotension will cause significant risk: uncorrected anemia, hypovolemia, shock, asphyxia, uncorrected respiratory insufficiency. Use with extreme caution in patients with arteriosclerosis; cardiac, hepatic or renal disease; degenerative CNS disease; Addison's disease, diabetes, concurrent steroids; pregnancy (crosses placenta and causes meconium ileus in fetus).

Adverse Effects: Related to ganglion blockade: paralytic ileus, bladder dysfunction, dry mouth, blurred vision.

Toxicity: Respiratory arrest.

Drug Interaction: Additive hypotensive effect when given with other antihypertensive drugs, anesthetic agents (especially spinal anesthetics), procainamide. Ganglionic blockade enhanced by diuretics. Concomitant administration prolongs neuromuscular block resulting from tubocurarine or succinylcholine.

ADRENERGIC BLOCKING AGENTS
■ **Guanethidine Monosulfate** (Ismelin; CIBA)

How Supplied:
PO: 10, 25 mg tablet.

Administration:
PO: 3%–50% absorbed.

Dose: Initially 10 mg/day as single dose; increase q2wk; average daily dose 25–50 mg. For hospitalized patients, may begin with 25–50 mg/day and increase qod. Max 400 mg/day.

Mechanism of Action: Inhibits neurotransmitter (norepinephrine) release presynaptically, blocking responses mediated by α- and β-adrenoreceptors. Drug accumulates in and displaces norepinephrine at sympathetic nerve terminal. Venodilatation causes lowered peripheral resistance; inhibition of cardiac sympathetic nerves lowers cardiac output; thus systolic and diastolic BP lowered. Renal blood flow and GFR modestly decreased.

Elimination: Fifty percent metabolized by hepatic microsomal enzymes; rest excreted unchanged in urine. Half-life, 5 days.

Indication: Moderate to severe HTN, always with a diuretic, and for renal HTN, including that caused by pyelonephritis, renal amyloidosis, and renal artery stenosis.

Contraindications: Pheochromocytoma, hypersensitivity, severe CHF not caused by HTN, MAO inhibitor therapy. Exercise caution in patients with bronchial asthma (more sensitive to catecholamine depletion), renal dysfunction and nitrogen retention or rising BUN (decreased BP may further compromise renal function), coronary insufficiency, recent MI, cerebrovascular disease, peptic ulcer (relative increase in parasympathetic tone may aggravate), pregnancy.

Adverse Effects/Toxicity: Postural hypotension, at times with symptoms of cerebral or myocardial ischemia; weakness; diarrhea, nausea and vomiting; fluid retention and edema if not receiving adjuvant diuretic, may progress to heart failure (drug inhibits adrenergic myocardial effects); HTN crisis in pheochromocytoma.

Interaction: *Rauwolfia* derivatives (e.g., reserpine) may exaggerate postural hypotension, bradycardia, and mental depression. Digitalis can slow heart rate further. Thiazides enhance hypotensive effect. CNS agents such as amphetamines, tricyclic antidepressants, and phenothiazines, and oral contraceptives may lessen hypotensive effect. Discontinue MAO inhibitor therapy at least 1 wk before starting guanethidine.

■ Guanadrel Sulfate (Hylorel; Fisons)

How Supplied:
PO: 10, 25 mg tablets

Administration: *PO:* rapidly absorbed.

Mechanism of Action: See Guanethidine Monosulfate p. 204.

Elimination: 85% eliminated in urine; half-life, 10 hr.

Indications: HTN with inadequate response to thiazides; administer with diuretic.

Contraindications: See Guanethidine Monosulfate p. 205.

Dose: Initially 5 mg bid; adjust q wk/mo. until BP controlled. Usual dose 25–75 mg/day, divided bid–qid; max 400 mg/day. Reduce dose and/or lengthen interval with creatinine clearance < 60 ml/min.

Adverse Effects/Toxicity: See Guanethidine Monosulfate p. 205. Lower incidence of diarrhea with guanadril.

Drug Interaction: Concurrent α- and β-adrenergic blockers, reserpine, and (theoretically) vasodilators can potentiate guanadril, increasing risk of postural hypotension and bradycardia. Tricyclic antidepressants, indirect acting sympathomimetics (e.g., ephedrine, phentolamine, some OTC allergy medicines) can lessen hypotensive effect. Discontinue MAO inhibits at least 1 wk prior.

■ **Reserpine** (Diupres, Hydropres; Merck. Ser-Ap-Es; CIBA. Demi-Regroton, Regroton; Rhone Poulenc Rorer. Diutensin-R; Wallace)

How Supplied:
PO: 0.1, 0.125, 0.25 mg in tablets combined with diuretic or other antihypertensive agent.

Administration:
PO: Well absorbed.

Dose:
Hypertension: Initially 0.5 mg/day × 1–2 wk. Reduce for maintenance to 0.1–0.25 mg/day, divided bid; max 1.0 mg/day (higher doses increase side effects).

Mechanism of Action: Depletes stores of catecholamines and 5-hydroxytryptamine in central and peripheral adrenergic neurons. Depression of sympathetic functions causes reduction in heart rate and peripheral vascular resistance. Depletion of brain neurotransmitters accounts for sedative and tranquilizing effects.

Elimination: Extensively bound to plasma proteins; half–life may be days.

Indication: Mild essential HTN, rarely for initial therapy.

Contraindications: History of mental depression, peptic ulcer, ulcerative colitis, concurrent electroconvulsive therapy. Use with caution in patients with gallstones (may precipitate biliary colic), renal insufficiency. Relatively contraindicated in pregnancy (other agents preferable); observe neonate for respiratory difficulty secondary to nasal congestion.

Adverse Effects/Toxicity:
1. CNS (most common): Sedation, inability to concentrate, nightmares, depression.
2. GI: Abdominal cramps and diarrhea (increased GI tone, acid secretion, and motility).
3. CV: Dysrhythmias if used with digitalis or quinidine; syncope; bradycardia and hypotension during surgical anesthesia.
4. Miscellaneous: Weight gain, impotence, flushing, nasal stuffiness.

Interaction: Digitalis or quinidine can provoke cardiac dysrhythmias. Do not give with MAO inhibitors. Barbiturates enhance CNS depression.

β-ADRENERGIC ANTAGONISTS: Nonselective

Table 8-1 lists common combination agents.

■ Propranolol HCl (Inderal, Inderal LA; Wyeth-Ayerst)

How Supplied:
PO:

    10, 20, 40, 60, 80 mg tablet.
    60, 80, 120, 160 mg sustained-release capsule.

Table 8-1

COMBINATION AGENTS*: ANTIHYPERTENSIVE/DIURETIC

Brand Name (Pharm. Co.)	How Supplied	Antihypertensive Agent (mg)	Diuretic (mg)	Usual Dosage Range
Aldochlor (Merck)	Tablets: 150	Methyldopa, 250	Chlorthiazide, 150	1–2 Tab bid-qid
	250	Methyldopa, 250	Chlorthiazide, 250	1 Tab bid-tid; 2 Tab qid max
Aldoril (Merck)	Tablets: 15	Methyldopa, 250	HCTZ, 15	1 Tab bid-tid
	25	Methyldopa, 250	HCTZ, 25	1 Tab bid-tid
	D30	Methyldopa, 500	HCTZ, 30	1 Tab bid-tid
	D50	Methyldopa, 500	HCTZ, 50	1 Tab bid-tid
Apresazide (CIBA)	Capsules: 25/25	Hydralazine, 25	HCTZ, 25	1 Tab bid
	50/50	Hydralazine, 50	HCTZ, 50	1 Tab bid
	100/50	Hydralazine, 100	HCTZ, 50	1 Tab bid
Capozide (Bristol-Myers Squibb)	Tablets: 25/15	Captopril, 25	HCTZ, 15	1 Tab qd-tid
	25/25	Captopril, 25	HCTZ, 25	1 Tab qd-bid
	50/15	Captopril, 50	HCTZ, 15	1 Tab qd-tid
	50/25	Captopril, 50	HCTZ, 25	1 Tab qd-bid
Combipres (Boehringer)	Tablets: 0.1	Clonidine, 0.1	Chlorthalidone, 15	1–2 Tab bid
	0.2	Clonidine, 0.2	Chlorthalidone, 15	1–2 Tab bid
	0.3	Clonidine, 0.3	Chlorthalidone, 15	1–2 Tab bid
Demi-Regroton (Rorer)	Tablets:	Reserpine, 0.125	Chlorthalidone, 25	1–2 Tab qd
Diupres (Merck)	Tablets: 250	Reserpine, 0.125	Chlorthiazide, 250	1–2 Tab qd or bid
	500	Reserpine, 0.125	Chlorthiazide, 500	1 Tab qd or bid
Diutensin-R (Wallace)	Tablets	Reserpine, 0.1	Methyclothiazide, 2.5	1 Tab–IV/day
Esimil (CIBA)	Tablets	Guanethidine, 10	HCTZ, 25	1 Tab qd or bid
Hydromox-R (Lederle)	Tablets	Reserpine, 0.125	Quinethazone, 50	1–2 Tab qd
Hydropres (Merck)	Tablets: 25	Reserpine, 0.125	HCTZ, 25	1–2 Tab qd
	50	Reserpine, 0.125	HCTZ, 50	1 Tab qd

Inderide (Wyeth-Ayerst)	Tablets: 40/25	Propranolol, 40	HCTZ, 25	1 Tab bid–qid
	80/25	Propranolol, 80	HCTZ, 25	1 Tab qd–bid
Lopressor-HCT (Geigy)	Tablets: 50/25	Metoprolol, 50	HCTZ, 25	1–2 Tab qd or 1 Tab bid
	100/25	Metoprolol, 100	HCTZ, 25	1 Tab–2 Tab qd or divided
	100/50	Metoprolol, 100	HCTZ, 25	1 Tab qd or bid
Prinizide (Merck)	Tablets: 10–12.5	Lisinopril, 10	HCTZ, 12.5	1 Tab qd
	20–12.5	Lisinopril, 20	HCTZ, 12.5	1 Tab–2 Tab qd
	20–25	Lisinopril, 20	HCTZ, 25	1 Tab–2 Tab qd
Regroton (Rhone Poulenc Rorer)	Tablets	Reserpine, 0.25	Chlorthalidone, 50	1 Tab–2 Tab qd or divided
Ser-Ap-Es (CIBA)	Tablets	Reserpine, 0.1	HCTZ, 15	1 Tab–2 Tab tid
		Hydralazine, 25		
Tenoretic (Zaneca Pharma)	Tablets: 50	Atenolol, 50	Chlorthalidone, 25	1 Tab qd
	100	Atenolol, 100	Chlorthalidone, 25	1 Tab qd
Timolide (Merck)	Tablets: 10–25	Timolol, 10	HCTZ, 25	1 tab bid or 2 Tab qd
Trandate-HCT (Allen and Hamburys)	Tablets: 100/25	Labetalol, 100	HCTZ, 25	1 Tab bid; 2 Tab bid max
	200/25	Labetalol, 200	HCTZ, 25	1 Tab bid; 2 Tab bid max
	300/25	Labetalol, 300	HCTZ, 25	1 Tab bid; 2 Tab bid max
Vaseretic (Merck)	Tablets: 10–25	Enalapril, 10	HCTZ, 25	1 Tab–2 Tab qd
Zestorectic (Stuart)	Tablets: 10–12.5	Lisinopril 10	HCTZ, 12.5	1 Tab–IV qd
	20–12.5	Lisinopril 20	HCTZ, 12.5	1 Tab–2 Tab qd
	20–25	Lisinopril 20	HCTZ, 25	1 Tab–2 Tab qd

HCTZ, Hydrochlorothiazide.
*Fixed combination drugs listed here not indicated for initial Rx of HTN.

Parenteral: 1 mg/ml in 1 ml vial.

Administration:

PO: Almost completely absorbed, but interindividual variation in presystemic first pass through liver accounts for wide plasma concentration variability. Therapy discontinuation requires gradual weaning over several weeks to avoid "rebound"-like effect of sympathetic activity and exacerbation of angina and possible myocardial infarction (MI).

IV: Slow infusion (not more than 1 mg/min) during continuous ECG monitoring.

Dose:

PO:

1. Hypertension: Initially 40 mg bid or 80 mg sustained-release capsule/day, either alone or with diuretic. Increase gradually; may need days to weeks to see full therapeutic response. Usual maintenance 120–240 mg/day, max 640 mg/day.
2. Angina: 80–320 mg/day, divided bid–qid.
3. Dysrhythmias: 10–30 mg tid–qid before meals and qhs.
4. MI: 180–240 mg/day divided bid–qid. Coexistent HTN or angina may require higher doses.
5. Migraine prophylaxis: Initially 80 mg/day as single dose or divided bid. If no effect, increase slowly; usual effective dose 160–240 mg/day. If no benefit in 4–6 wk, wean gradually.
6. Essential tremor, including prevention of acute panic symptoms: Initially 40 mg bid.

     Usual dose for optimum control of symptoms 120 mg/day, sometimes 240–300 mg/day.
7. Hypertrophic subaortic stenosis: 20–40 mg tid–qid before meals and qhs.
8. Pheochromocytoma:
     a. Preoperative: 60 mg/day, divided doses, after an α-adrenergic blockade has been established (to avoid acute BP increase from blockade of skeletal muscle vasodilatation).
     b. Inoperable tumor: 30 mg/day in divided doses.

IV:

1. Life-threatening dysrhythmias: 1–3 mg; repeat after 2 min if necessary; do not repeat again in less than 4 hr. Switch to PO as soon as feasible.

Mechanism of Action: Nonselective β-adrenergic receptor blocker. Lowers BP by decreasing heart rate and cardiac output, inhibiting renin release from kidneys, and lowering CNS tonic sympathetic outflow. Antianginal effect also caused by decreased myocardial O_2 requirement and consumption.

Elimination: Metabolized in liver and excreted in urine. Half-life, 4 hr.

Indication:

1. Hypertension: For daily management (not HTN emergency), alone or with other agents (especially thiazide diuretics). Use with a vasodilator minimizes reflex tachycardia and compensatory increase in cardiac output.
2. Angina pectoris: Long-term management.
3. Dysrhythmias:
   a. Supraventricular: Paroxysmal atrial tachycardia, especially catecholamine or digitalis induced or associated with Wolff-Parkinson-White (WPW) syndrome (watch for sudden severe bradycardia during therapy or WPW). Also, persistent noncompensatory sinus tachycardia including that associated with thyrotoxicosis; persistent atrial extrasystoles; atrial flutter and fibrillation not controlled with digitalis.
   b. Ventricular: Ventricular tachycardias (not usually first drug of choice, because need to avoid possible total sympathetic block to failing heart); persistent premature ventricular extrasystoles.
   c. Resistant tachydysrhythmias caused by catecholamine overstimulation during anesthesia.
4. MI: To reduce size of infarct and reinfarction rate.
5. Hypertrophic subaortic stenosis: Especially with angina, palpitations, and syncope.
6. Migraine prophylaxis (not acute attack).
7. Essential tremor (but not in Parkinson's syndrome); acute panic symptoms.
8. Pheochromocytoma: Adjunct to control tachycardia after primary therapy with α-adrenergic blocker preoperatively, intraoperatively, and postoperatively if inoperable or metastatic.

Contraindications: Cardiogenic shock, sinus bradycardia, second- and third-degree block; bronchial asthma; congestive heart failure (unless caused by a tachydysrhythmia treatable with propranolol). Use with caution in patients prone to hypoglycemia, with insulin-dependent diabetic patients, or impaired renal or hepatic function. Use in pregnancy only for life-threatening situations; exercise caution during lactation.

Adverse Effects/Toxicity:
1. CV: Bradycardia, impaired myocardial contractility, AV block, congestive failure, hypotension.
2. Miscellaneous: Bronchospasm, GI distress, fatigue/lethargy, depression.
3. Obstetric: During long-term therapy, watch fetus for intrauterine growth retardation (IUGR) and neonate for hypoglycemia and bradycardia.

Antidote:
1. Bradycardia: 0.25–1.0 mg atropine; cautious isoproterenol if no response.
2. Cardiac failure: Digitalis and diuretics.
3. Hypotension: Vasopressors (e.g., epinephrine, levarterenol).
4. Bronchospasm: Isoproterenol and aminophylline.

Interactions: Aluminum hydroxide decreases propranolol absorption. Chlorpromazine in increases both drugs' levels; cimetidine increases propranolol levels. T_3 levels less than expected with thyroxine. Prolongs insulin-induced hypoglycemia. Use with catecholamine-depleting drugs (e.g., reserpine) can result in excessive antisympathetic effects of hypotension, bradycardia, and syncope. Concomitant calcium-channel blockers (e.g., verpamil) can depress myocardial contractility or AV conduction, especially in patients with cardiomyopathy, congestive heart failure (CHF), or recent MI. Reduces clearance of antipyrine, lidocaine, and theophylline. Phenytoin, phenobarbital, and rifampin speed propranolol clearance.

■ **Timolol Maleate** (Blocadren; Merck)

How Supplied:
PO: 5, 10, 20 mg tablets.

Administration: *PO:* Rapidly absorbed.

Mechanism of Action: See Propranolol p. 209.

Dose:
  HTN: 10 mg bid; alone or with diuretic. Increase at weekly or greater intervals to usual dose 20–40 mg/day; maximum 60 mg/day divided bid.
  MI: 10 mg bid.
  Migraine: 10–30 mg/day, single dose or divided bid.
  Discontinue gradually if no response after 6–8 weeks.
  Reduce dose if significant hepatic/renal insufficiency exists.
  Avoid abrupt discontinuation: may precipitate angina and myocardial infarction.

Elimination: Metabolized extensively (including moderate pass) in liver. Half-life, 4 hours.

Indications: HTN, alone of with other agent (e.g. thiazide); to reduce CV mortality and reinfarction risk after acute phase of myocardial infarction; migraine prophylaxis.

Contraindications: Bronchial asthma; severe COPD; sinus bradycardia; second- and third-degree AV block; overt cardiac failure (may slow AV conduction); cardiogenic shock. Use with caution in diabetic patients, on insulin or oral hypoglycemics (may mask signs of acute hypoglycemia) and in patients with cerebrovascular insufficiency. Abrupt withdrawal may precipitate thyroid storm in patients at risk of thyrotoxicosis. Use in pregnancy only if absolutely necessary; advise discontinuation of breastfeeding.

Adverse Effects: Bradycardia; fatigue; dizziness; dyspnea; pruritus; bronchial spasm.

Toxicity: Heart block, dysrhythmia, hypotension, bronchospasm, acute cardiac failure.

Drug Interaction: Use with oral calcium antagonists (e.g., nifedipine, verapamil, diltiazem) in patients with impaired cardiac function may precipitate hypotension, AV conduction disturbances, and left ventricular failure. IV calcium antagonists or digitalis may also prolong AV conduction. Catecholamine-depleting agents (e.g.

ANTIHYPERTENSIVES

reserpine) may potentiate hypotension, bradycardia, vertigo or syncope. NSAIDs may blunt antihypertensive effect.

■ Pindolol (Visken; Sandoz)

How Supplied:
PO: 5, 10 mg tablets.

Administration: *PO:* Rapidly absorbed; no significant first pass effect.

Mechanism of Action: See Propranolol p. 209.

Dose: Initially, 5 mg bid. Increase q 2–4 wk by 10 mg/day up to maximum 60 mg/day.

Elimination: One third excreted unchanged in urine; remainder metabolized mostly to hydroxymetabolites and excreted as glucuronides and ethereal sulfate.

Indications: HTN, either alone or with other agents (e.g., thiazides).

Contraindications: See Timolol p. 211. Also, in severe bradycardia. Consider gradual discontinuation several days before major surgery to avoid hypotension and low cardiac output.

Adverse Effects: Reversible mental depression progressing to catatonia, disorientation, short-term memory loss, emotional lability; intensified AV block; laryngospasm.

Toxicity: See Timolol p. 211.

Drug Interaction: See Timolol p. 211.

■ Labetalol HCl (Normodyne; Schering. Trandate; Allen and Hanburys)

How Supplied:
PO:
    100, 200, 300 mg tablet.

Parenteral:
    5 mg/ml in 20, 40 ml vial.
    4, 8 ml prefilled disposable syringe.

Administration:
PO: Well absorbed. First-pass effect metabolizes considerable fraction in liver.

Dose:
PO: Initially 100 mg bid, alone or with diuretic. May increase by 100 mg bid q2–3 days, using standing BP to judge response. Usual maintenance 200–400 mg bid; max 1200–2400 mg/day. Lower dose in the elderly or those on additional diuretic therapy.
    IV: 20 mg over 2 min, then check supine BP at 5–10 min to evaluate response. Repeat 40–80 mg q10 min until BP corrected or maximum 300 mg. Alternatively, give appropriately diluted drug at controlled infusion rate of 2 mg/min. Switch to PO as soon as possible.

Mechanism of Action: Selective α_1-and nonselective β-adrenergic blocker. α receptor blockade relaxes arterial smooth muscle and vasodilates, thus reducing total peripheral resistance and BP, more while standing than supine. β_1 blockade also blocks reflex sympathetic stimulation of heart, but without significant change in HR and CO.

Elimination: Hepatic conjugation to glucuronide metabolites; excreted in urine (55% unchanged), bile, and feces.

Indications: Hypertension, alone or in combination therapy (especially thiazide and loop diuretics). IV form for hypertensive emergencies (Table 8-2).

Contraindications: Overt cardiac failure, second- or third-degree heart block, cardiogenic shock, severe bradycardia; bronchial asthma. Use with caution in presence of liver disease, history of heart failure, pheochromocytoma (may see paradoxical hypertensive response), diabetes (hypoglycemic tachycardia may be masked). No reported birth defects, but adequate data during first trimester and lactation lacking; observe neonate for signs of β–blockade.

ANTIHYPERTENSIVES

Table 8-2

HYPERTENSIVE CRISIS IN PREGNANCY—INDUCED HYPERTENSION*

Agent	Class	Dose/Administration	Onset (min)	Peak (min)	Duration	Additional Effects	FDA Pregnancy Category
Captopril	ACE inhibitor	25 mg sublingual	5	60	4 hr	Postpartum only because of possible oligohydramnios, fetal renal failure, and death	C/D*
Labetalol	Nonselective β-adrenergic blocker	20 mg–80 mg IV bolus (0.25 mg/kg), then 2 mg/min infusion or repeat bolus q10 min	5	5–60	4–6 hr	↓ HR reduces myocardial O_2 requirements; drug also blocks dysrhythmias caused by high circulating catecholamines	C
Nifedipine	Calcium channel blocker	10 mg PO q4–6 hr	10	30	6–8 hr	Direct coronary artery vasodilator; reduces afterload by ↓ TPR	C

Table 8-2
HYPERTENSIVE CRISIS IN PREGNANCY—INDUCED HYPERTENSION*—cont'd

Agent	Class	Dose/Administration	Onset (min)	Peak (min)	Duration	Additional Effects	FDA Pregnancy Category
Sodium nitroprusside	Vasodilator (arterioles and venules)	0.5–1.0 µg/kg/min IV infusion	0.5	2	3 min after infusion stopped	↓TPR while maintaining renal blood flow; ↓myocardial O₂ requirements; watch cyanide levels in mother and newborn.	

Modified from Usta IM, Sibai BM: Emergent management of puerperal eclampsia, *Obst Gynecol Clin N Am*, 22(2):315, 1995.
HR, Heart rate; *TPR*, total peripheral resistance.
*First trimester/second and third trimester.

215

Adverse Effects: Paresthesias (especially scalp tingling); fatigue; nausea; dizziness; nasal stuffiness; impotence; increased ANA titer; skin rash. Most adverse effects mild, transient and occur early in treatment.

Toxicity: Postural hypotension; severe bradycardia; cardiac failure; seizures; rare but sometimes fatal hepatocellular necrosis.

Monitor: Liver function tests.

Interaction: Increased incidence of tremor when used with tricyclic antidepressants. Cimetidine increases labetalol bioavailability. Halothane anesthesia intensifies hypotensive effect. Catecholamine depletors (e.g., reserpine) may intensify sympathetic block, with resultant hypotension or bradycardia.

β-ADRENERGIC ANTAGONISTS: SELECTIVE

■ Metoprolol Tartrate (Lopressor; Geigy)

How Supplied:
PO: 50, 100 mg tablet.
Parenteral: 5 mg/ml ampules.

Administration:
PO: Well absorbed rapidly, especially if taken around meals, but only 40% reaches systemic circulation after first-pass metabolism in liver. Therapy discontinuation requires gradual dosage reduction over 1–2 wks to avoid possible exacerbation of angina and myocardial infarction.

Dose:
1. Hypertension: Initially 100 mg/day as 1 dose or divided, alone or with a diuretic. Increase weekly until desired BP achieved. Usual effective dose 100–450 mg/day; higher doses should be divided.
2. Angina: Initially 100 mg/day divided bid, with meals. Increase weekly until symptoms relieved or bradycardia occurs. Usual dose 100–400 mg/day.

3. MI:
   a. Early: Initiate therapy as soon as possible with 5 mg bolus IV q2min × 3. If tolerated, after 15 min switch to 50 mg PO q6h × 2 days; then maintain on 100 mg PO bid. If full 15 mg initial IV dose not tolerated, after 15 min switch to 25–50 mg PO q6h, or discontinue if intolerance severe.
   b. Late: if start of therapy is delayed because of intolerance or other contraindications, start with 100 mg bid × 3–36 mo.

Mechanism of Action: β–Adrenoreceptor blocker, preferential for $β_1$ (cardiac muscle), except at higher doses also inhibits $β_2$ (bronchial and vascular muscle). Reduces heart rate and cardiac output by competitive catecholamine antagonism at peripheral adrenergic sites (e.g., heart muscle). Also reduces systolic BP and reflex tachycardia by a central effect leading to decreased sympathetic outflow to the periphery; also suppresses renin activity.

Elimination: Metabolized in liver. Half-life, 3 hr.

Indications: Mild to moderate HTN alone or in combination therapy; long-term control of angina pectoris, in acute MI to reduce mortality and incidence of recurrence or fatal dysrhythmia and to reduce the size of the infarct.

Contraindications:
1. CV: Sinus bradycardia or heart rate less than 45 beats/min, second- or third-degree heart block, cardiogenic shock, overt heart failure, systolic BP <100. Exercise caution in patients with heart failure controlled with digitalis (both drugs slow AV conduction).
2. Bronchospastic disease: Relative contraindication unless unresponsive to other therapy; use lowest possible metoprolol dose divided tid and concomitant $β_2$-stimulator.
3. Miscellaneous: Use with caution in hyperthyroidism and diabetes (may mask tachycardia of thyrotoxicosis or hypoglycemia) and in liver disease. Inadequate data on use in pregnancy and lactation; no congenital malformations reported, but observe neonate for bradycardia if recent use before delivery.

ANTIHYPERTENSIVES

Adverse Effects: Fatigue and dizziness (10%), depression (5%), headache, insomnia, bronchospasm, GI upset.

Toxicity: Bradycardia, hypotension, precipitation or exacerbation of AV block or congestive heart failure.

Antidote:
1. Bradycardia: Atropine; isoproterenol if no response.
2. Hypotension: Vasopressors (e.g., levarterenol, dopamine).
3. Bronchospasm: β_2–stimulator or theophylline derivative.
4. Cardiac failure: Digitalis glycoside and diuretic; if with inadequate contractility, use dobutamine, isoproterenol, or glucagon.

Interaction: May see additive antisympathetic effects (e.g., hypotension, bradycardia, syncope) when used with catecholamine-depleting agents (e.g., reserpine).

■ Atenolol (Tenormin; Zeneca)

How Supplied:
PO: 25, 50, 100 mg tablet.

Administration:
PO: Rapidly but incompletely absorbed. Do not discontinue abruptly to avoid exacerbation of angina, myocardial infarction and ventricular dysrhythmias.

Dose:
1. Hypertension: Initially 50 mg/day as single dose, either alone or with diuretic. If no response after 1–2 wk, increase to 100 mg/day, single dose.
2. Angina: Initially 50 mg/day, single dose. May increase after 1–2 wk to 100 mg/day; max 200 mg/day.
3. Reduce dose in elderly patients or those with renal impairment.

Mechanism of Action: Selective β_1 (cardiac muscle) adrenoreceptor blocker; also blocks β_2 (bronchial and vascular muscle) at higher doses. Reduces heart rate, cardiac output, systolic and diastolic BP; reduces cardiac oxygen requirements; inhibits reflex orthostatic tachycardia. Also see Labetalol p. 213.

Elimination: Primarily renal excretion. Half-life 6–7 hr. Reduce dose in patients with renal dysfunction (creatinine clearance < 35 ml/min).

Indication: Hypertension, alone or with other antihypertensives (e.g., thiazide diuretic); angina pectoris, long-term management; to reduce CV mortality in hemodynamically stable with myocardial infarction.

Contraindications: Sinus bradycardia, second- or third-degree heart block; cardiogenic shock; overt cardiac failure. Use with caution in patients with bronchospastic disease (give lowest possible dose, divided, with bronchodilator), diabetes (may mask tachycardia of hypoglycemia but does not delay glucose return to normal as with other nonselective β–blockers); hyperthyroidism. No adequate data on use in pregnancy and lactation; no reported birth defects, but observe newborn for signs of β–blockade bradycardia).

Adverse Effects: Dizziness, fatigue, hypoglycemia, diarrhea, nausea.

Toxicity: Bradycardia, postural hypotension, CHF, bronchospasm.

Interaction: Possible additive effect with other antihypertensives, catecholamine depletors (e.g., reserpine) and calcium channel blockers resulting in hypotension or marked bradycardia. Exposure to allergens may produce unusually severe anaphylactic reaction. Anesthetic agents that depress myocardium may induce vagal dominance (correct with atropine).

■ Esmolol HCl (Brevibloc; Oclassen)

How Supplied:
Parenteral: 100 mg/10 ml single-dose vial.
2.5 gm/10 ml ampule.

Administration: IV; short duration of action. Ampule form must be appropriately diluted.

Dose:

Supraventricular tachycardia: Usually 50–200 µg/kg/min; maximum 300 µg/kg/min.

Intraoperative and postoperative tachycardia and/or HTN:
Immediate control: 80 mg bolus over 30 sec, then 150 µg/kg/min. Adjust up to max 300 µg/kg/min.
Gradual control: Loading dose 500 µg/kg/min × 1 min, then 50 µg/kg/min × 4 min. If suboptimal response, repeat loading dose, followed by maintenance infusion 50–100 µg/kg/min. Rarely, postoperative HTN may require doses of 250–300 µg/kg/min.

Mechanism of Action: Selective β_1 antagonist. Also see Atenolol p. 218.

Elimination: Rapidly hydrolyzed by esterases in RBCs; half–life 8 min.

Indications: Short-term rapid control of ventricular rate in patients with atrial fibrillation/flutter in perioperative/postoperative or other emergent circumstances, especially where tachycardia needs immediate control.

Contraindications: See Labetolol p. 213.

Adverse Effects/Toxicity: Thrombophlebitis, extravasation, skin necrosis secondary to local reaction; hypotension; dizziness; bronchospasm; nausea.

Drug Interaction: Additive effect with catecholamine-depleting drugs (e.g., reserpine). Titrate drug with caution in patients on digoxin, morphine, succinylcholine, or warfarin, because of theoretical risk of increased hypotensive or other CV effect.

■ **Acebutolol Hydrochloride** (Sectral; Wyeth-Ayerst)

How Supplied:
PO: 200, 400 mg capsules.

Administration: *PO,* well absorbed. Extensive first-pass hepatic biotransformation; major metabolite diacetolol is pharmacologically active.

Mechanism of Action: Cardioselective β-adrenoreceptor blocker. Reduces HR, CO and systolic and diastolic BP at rest and after exercise. Also delays AV conduction time and increases refractoriness of AV node without significantly affecting sinus node recovery time, atrial refractory period, or AV conduction time. Less bronchoconstriction and less reduction of β2 bronchodilatation (than nonselective agents such as propranolol).

Dose:
HTN: 200–800 mg/day, max 1200 mg/day; higher doses divided bid.
Ventricular dysrhythmias: 200 mg bid; increased gradually until optimal response obtained, usually at 600–1200 mg/day.
Elderly: Avoid doses over 800 mg/day.
Renal insufficiency: Reduce dose by 50%–75% if creatinine clearance < 50 ml/min.

Elimination: One third renal elimination; two thirds by excretion into bile and direct passage through intestinal wall.

Indications: HTN, either alone or combined with another agent (e.g., thiazides). Ventricular dysrhythmias: PVCs, including paired, multiple, and R-on-T.

Contraindications: See Labetalol p. 213. Also, use with caution in patients with peripheral or mesenteric vascular disease (may precipitate symptoms of arterial insufficiency). Unlike Labetalol, low doses may be used with caution in patients with bronchospasm who do not respond to or who cannot tolerate alternative treatment.

Adverse Effects: Dizziness, fatigue, insomnia, GI distress, reversible elevated ANA.

Toxicity: See Labetalol p. 216.

Interactions: Possible additive effect with other catecholamine–depleting drugs (e.g., reserpine). Exaggerated hypotensive effect with α–adrenergic stimulants (e.g., OTC cold remedies, vasocon-strictive nose drops). Blunted antihypertensive effect with NSAIDs.

■ Carteolol Hydrochloride (Cartrol; Abbott)

How Supplied:
PO: 2.5 mg tablets.

Administration: *PO,* well absorbed.

Mechanism of Action: Long-acting nonselective β–adrenergic receptor blocker. Competes with β-adrenergic receptor agonists for $β_1$ cardiac muscle receptors and $β_2$ bronchial and vascular musculature receptors, blocking the chronotropic, inotropic and vasodilator responses to β-adrenergic stimulation. Also lowers response to sympathetic outflow from brain vasomotor centers, renin release, and CO.

Dose: Initially 2.5 mg/day; increase gradually to 5–10 mg/day. Reduce dose or lengthen interval if creatinine clearance <60 ml/min.

Elimination: 50%–70% eliminated unchanged by kidneys.

Indications: HTN, either alone or in combination with other agents (e.g., thiazides).

Contraindications: Bronchial asthma, severe bradycardia; sec-ond- or third-degree heart block; cardiogenic shock; CHF. Use with caution in patients undergoing major surgery (beta blockade impairs heart's ability to respond to reflex stimuli); DM (may block signs of acute hypoglycemia and inhibit reflex glycogenol-ysis); hyperthyroidism (may block signs of thyrotoxicosis).

Adverse Effects: Asthenia, muscle cramps, somnolence; GI dis-tress, impotence; angina or myocardial infarction if drug is sud-denly discontinued.

Toxicity: See Atenolol p. 219.

Drug Interaction: See Atenolol p. 219. Also, NSAIDs may blunt antihypertensive effect.

α-ADRENERGIC BLOCKING AGENTS
■ **Phenoxybenzamine HCl** (Dibenzyline; Smith-Kline Beecham)

How Supplied:
PO: 10 mg capsule.

Administration:
PO: Incompletely absorbed (20%–30% in active form).

Dose: Initially, 10 mg bid. Increase gradually qod, observing for desired BP or troublesome side effects. Usual dosage 20–40 mg bid–tid.

Mechanism of Action: Haloalkylamine-type long-acting α-adrenergic receptor blocker. Blockage of α-adrenergic receptors in smooth muscle lowers peripheral resistance; cardiac output increases because of reflex sympathetic stimulation. Lowers supine and erect BP; improves blood flow to abdominal viscera, mucosa, skin.

Elimination: Highly lipid soluble; large doses may accumulate in fat. Half-life 12–24 hr.

Indications: Pheochromocytoma: preoperatively, intraoperatively to avoid paroxysmal hypertension (HTN); postoperatively if malignant or unresectable. Excessive tachycardia may require adjunctive β-blocker.

Contraindications: Hypovolemia (inhibition of vasoconstrictor reflex can result in shocklike state). Use in pregnancy and lactation restricted to oral maintenance therapy for pheochromocytoma (not for HTN crisis or intraoperative BP control). Exercise caution in patients with marked cerebral or coronary arteriosclerosis or renal damage. May aggravate symptoms of respiratory infections.

Toxicity:
1. Caused by blockade of α-adrenergic receptors: Postural hypotension, reflex tachycardia; inhibition of ejaculation; nasal congestion, miosis.
2. Miscellaneous: Fatigue, drowsiness, GI distress.

Interactions: Concomitant use of α– and β–adrenergic stimulants (e.g., epinephrine) may exaggerate hypotension and reflex tachycardia. Blocks hyperthermia produced by levarterenol; blocks hypothermia caused by reserpine.

■ **Phentolamine Mesylate** (Regitine; CIBA)

How Supplied:
Parenteral: 5 mg/vial (with 25 mg mannitol).

Administration:
IM, IV: 5 mg in 1 ml sterile water for injection.
Subcutaneous: 5–10 mg in 10 ml saline solution.

Dose:
1. 5 mg/dose IM or IV 1–2 hr preoperatively or intraoperatively until HTN controlled, then q2–4h prn.
2. Diagnosis of pheochromocytoma (blocking test): See *Physicians' Desk Reference (PDR)*.
3. Treatment of α–adrenergic agent extravasation: 5–10 mg diluted as above and injected into area within 12 hr. For prevention, add 10 mg to each liter of solution containing norepinephrine.

Mechanism of Action: Transient competitive α–adrenergic block with lesser direct positive inotropic and chronotropic effect on cardiac muscle and vasodilation of vascular smooth muscle.

Elimination: 13% excreted unchanged in urine. Half-life 19 min.

Indication:
1. Pheochromocytoma: Preoperative and intraoperative management of acute HTN episodes, including during pregnancy and cesarean. In nonpregnant patients, also used to diagnose pheochromocytoma (blocking tests; see *PDR*).
2. Prevention and treatment of dermal necrosis after IV administration or extravasation of epinephrine.

Contraindications: History of myocardial infarction or coronary artery disease, cardiac dysrhythmia, known drug hypersensitivity, lactation. Use with caution in patients with gastritis or peptic ulcer.

Adverse Effects/Toxicity:
1. Resulting from cardiac stimulation: Tachycardia, dysrhythmias, MI.
2. Resulting from vascular smooth vasodilatation: Acute, prolonged, or orthostatic hypotension, dizziness.
3. Resulting from GI stimulation: Abdominal pain, nausea, vomiting, diarrhea, peptic ulcer exacerbation.
4. Miscellaneous: Flushing, nasal stuffiness.

Interaction: In case of dysrhythmia, discontinue cardiac glycosides until rhythm returns to normal.

■ Tolazoline HCl (Priscoline HCl; CIBA)

How Supplied:
Parenteral: 25 mg/ml in 4 ml ampule.

Administration: *IV*.

Dose: Initially 1–2 mg/kg, then 1–2 mg/kg/hr.

Mechanism of Action: Moderate competitive α–adrenergic blocker and direct peripheral vasodilator. Decreases pulmonary arterial pressure, vascular resistance, and peripheral resistance; increases venous capacitance. Effects include sympathomimetic cardiac stimulation, parasympathomimetic GI stimulation (blocked by atropine), and histamine-like peripheral vasodilation and stimulation of gastric acid and pepsin secretion. BP response depends on balance of vasodilation and cardiac stimulation.

Elimination: Excreted by kidney rapidly and unchanged. Half-life 3–10 hr.

Indications: Persistent pulmonary HTN of the newborn ("persistent fetal circulation") when usual mechanical ventilation measures fail.

Contraindications: Stress ulcers, GI bleeding; mitral stenosis (may precipitate rise in pulmonary material pressure and resistance).

Toxicity:
1. CV: Hypotension, tachycardia, dysrhythmia, HTN, pulmonary hemorrhage.
2. GI: Pain, vomiting, diarrhea, GI bleeding (avoid by pretreatment with antacids), hepatitis.
3. Miscellaneous: Sweating, piloerection; thrombocytopenia, leukopenia; oliguria, hematuria.

Antidote: In cases of severe hypotension, ephedrine increases peripheral resistance, and dopamine improves cardiac output. (Do not use epinephrine: further drop in BP, then exaggerated rebound.)

Monitor: Vital signs, oxygenation, acid base and fluid status, electrolytes.

■ Prazosin HCl (Minipress; Pfizer)

How Supplied:
PO: 1, 2, 5 mg capsule.

Administration:
PO: Well absorbed.

Dose: Initially 1 mg bid–tid (give first dose at bedtime to avoid syncope); increase slowly. Usual therapeutic doses 6–15 mg/day divided bid–tid; max 20 mg/day (40 mg/day in special cases).

Mechanism of Action: Potent and selective blocker of postsynaptic α_1-adrenoreceptors, causing a decrease in total peripheral resistance without reflex tachycardia and relatively little change in cardiac output or renal blood flow.

Elimination: Metabolized by demethylation and conjugation, and excreted in bile and feces.

Indications: Hypertension, alone or in combination therapy with diuretics or β-adrenergic blockers.

Contraindications: No data available on use in pregnancy or lactation.

Adverse Effects: Headache, drowsiness, fatigue, nausea, anticholinergic effects.

Toxicity:
Syncope, postural hypotension, sometimes with loss of consciousness, most often 30–90 min after initial dose (especially with doses >2 mg) or with rapid dosage increase, addition of another antihypertensive agent or β–blocker (e.g., propranolol), or with alcohol ingestion.

Interaction: Additive hypotensive effect with β–blockers, diuretics, other antihypertensive agents (minimize risk by reducing prazosin dosage to 1–2 mg tid).

■ Terazosin Hydrochloride (Hytrin; Abbott)

How Supplied:
PO: 1, 2, 5, 10 mg tablets.

Administration: *PO;* well absorbed.

Mechanism of Action: Highly specific α_1–adrenoreceptor blocker. Lowers BP by decreasing total peripheral vascular resistance. Also relaxes smooth muscle by blockade of α_1–adrenoreceptor in bladder neck and prostate.

Dose: Initially 1 mg at bedtime; then slowly increase depending on BP to 1–5 mg/day, single dose; maximum 20 mg/day.

Elimination: Minimal hepatic first-pass metabolism; 40% of administered dose excreted in urine and 60% in feces.

Indications: HTN, alone or with other antihypertensives (e.g., diuretics, β-adrenergic blockers), also, symptomatic benign prostatic hyperplasia.

Contraindications: Any known hypersensitivity; avoid use in pregnancy and lactation.

Adverse Effects: Asthenia, blurred vision, dizziness, nasal congestion, nausea, peripheral edema, palpitations, somnolence.

Toxicity: See Prazosin p. 227.

Drug Interaction: Additive hypotensive effect and increased risk of syncope with other antihypertensives.

VASODILATORS: Arterial

■ Hydralazine (Apresoline; CIBA)

How Supplied:
PO: 10, 25, 50, 100 mg tablet.

Administration:
PO: Quickly and well absorbed; significant first-pass metabolism in liver. Slow acetylators achieve higher plasma concentrations and need lower doses for BP control.

Dose: Initially 10 mg qid × 2–4 days, then increase to 25 mg qid for first week. Increase to 50 mg qid in second wk. Max 300 mg/day (lower in slow acetylators).

Mechanism of Action: Direct relaxation of arteriolar smooth muscle with compensatory increase in heart rate, stroke volume, and cardiac output. Decreases diastolic more than systolic BP by preferential dilatation of arterioles, thus lowering total peripheral resistance and minimizing postural hypotension. Reflex sympathetic discharge may increase renin and angiotension II, thus stimulating aldosterone with sodium and fluid retention.

Elimination: Hepatic acetylation; metabolites excreted in urine. Half-life 3–7 hr.

Indication: Essential HTN, especially with a diuretic (to limit fluid retention) and β-blocker or other sympatholytic (reflex tachycardia and other side effects limit use as single agent).

Contraindications: Coronary artery disease (may provoke angina or signs of myocardial ischemia), mitral valvular rheumatic heart disease (may increase pulmonary artery pressure), drug hypersensitivity. Use with caution in patients with cerebral vascular accidents or advanced renal disease.

Adverse Effects/Toxicity: Overall incidence 20%:
1. Most frequent: Headache, GI upset, tachycardia, postural hypotension.
2. Less common: Diarrhea, constipation, anxiety, sleep disturbances, angina, nasal congestion, paresthesias (treat with pyridoxine).
3. Less than 10%: Reversible lupuslike syndrome with arthralgia, fever, antinuclear antibodies, and rarely, rash, lymphadenopathy, hepatosplenomegaly. Mostly occurs after 2 mo of therapy, in summer, and with doses over 200 mg/day.
4. Intrapartum: fetal distress caused by overshoot hypotension.

Interaction: Adding other potent parenteral antihypertensives (e.g., diazoxide) may cause profound hypotension. Pressor responses to epinephrine reduced. Avoid use with MAO inhibitors.

■ Minoxidil (Loniten; Upjohn)

How Supplied:
PO: 2.5, 10 mg tablet.

Administration:
PO: Rapidly and well absorbed. Must be given with β-blocker to prevent tachycardia and myocardial workload and with a diuretic to avert fluid retention.

Dose: Initially 5 mg, single daily dose. Increase q3 days to 10, 20, then 40 mg as single or split dose. Usual dose 10–40 mg/day; max 100 mg/day. Loading dose (if faster response required) 5–20 mg; additional doses 2.5–10 mg q4–6h if needed and patient is carefully monitored. Use with diuretic (usually loop agent) and β-adrenergic blocker or methyldopa.

Mechanism of Action: Direct peripheral arteriolar vasodilatation: lowers systolic and diastolic BP by decreasing total peripheral resistance, with reflex-increased heart rate and cardiac output (minimize with β–blocker), and salt and water retention from increased renin (minimize with loop diuretic).

Elimination: Conjugated to glucuronide in liver; metabolites excreted in urine. Half-life 4 hr.

Indication: Severe HTN refractory to usual three-drug regimens with maximum doses of diuretic, sympatholytic, and another vasodilator (side effects limit usefulness in milder forms of HTN).

Contraindications: Pheochromocytoma (drug may stimulate tumor catecholamine release), MI in preceding 1 mo (may further limit blood flow to myocardium), pregnancy, lactation. Use with caution in patients with renal failure or receiving dialysis.

Toxicity: Up to 70% of patients stop therapy because of adverse reactions:
1. Most common: Fluid retention (minimize with loop diuretic); reflex sympathetic stimulation with tachycardia and palpitations (avoid with β–blocker). Pericardial effusion (up to 15% of patients), at times progressing to tamponade, exacerbation of angina, and myocardial fibrosis.
2. Skin: Reversible hypertrichosis in 80% of patients.
3. Allergic: Rashes, bullous eruptions, Stevens-Johnson syndrome.

Monitor: Fluid and electrolyte balance and body weight. Any abnormal lab test results at start of therapy should be followed up periodically: Urinalysis (UA), renal function tests, ECG, chest x-ray (CXR), and so on.

Interaction: Profound orthostasis with guanethidine.

■ **Diazoxide** (Hyperstat; Schering. Proglycem; Baker Norton)

How Supplied:
PO: 50 mg capsules.
     50 mg/ml suspension.
Parenteral: 300 mg/20 ml ampule.

Administration:

PO: (for control of hypoglycemia only).

IV: Minibolus undiluted injection over 30 sec into peripheral vein with patient recumbent, avoiding extravasation.

Dose: HTN: 1–3 mg/kg IV, repeated q5–15 min until diastolic BP less than 100 mm Hg; maximum single injection 150 mg; usual therapy 4–5 days, maximum 10 days. Repeat at 4–24 hr intervals until BP stabilized and PO therapy feasible. (For hypoglycemia: 3–8 mg/kg/day divided q8–12 hr).

Mechanism of Action: Directly relaxes arteriolar smooth muscle and increases heart rate and cardiac output. Some antidiuretic action with no effect on venous capacitance; hypotensive effect thus lessened by reflex sodium and water retention unless diuretic added. Coronary blood flow maintained, renal blood flow increased (after initial decrease). Hypoglycemic action caused by inhibition of insulin release from pancreas.

Elimination: Twenty–50% eliminated by kidney; remainder metabolized in liver.

Indication: Short-term emergency use for malignant and nonmalignant HTN in hospitalized patients. (Oral form for treatment of hypoglycemia caused by hyperinsulinism from inoperable islet cell adenoma or carcinoma, or extrapancreatic malignancy).

Contraindications: Compensatory HTN (e.g., caused by aortic coarctation, dissection, or arteriovenous shunt); pheochromocytoma (ineffective); known hypersensitivity to diazoxide; other thiazides or sulfonamide-derived drugs. Use with caution in patients with impaired cerebral or cardiac circulation, or acute pulmonary edema. Use in pregnancy only for severe acute HTN; may give rise to fetal bradycardia (from hypotension) and hyperglycemia and cause uterine relaxation with interruption of labor.

Adverse Effects: GI distress, flushing, local reactions after extravasation, dizziness, weakness.

Toxicity: Repeated injections may lead to sodium retention, edema and even dysrhythmia, angina, CHF, or MI, more often in patients with limited cardiac reserve. Isolated report of optic

ANTIHYPERTENSIVES

nerve infarction after too rapid lowering of BP; cerebral ischemia with possible infarction, unconsciousness, convulsions. Mild transient hyperglycemia may require treatment in diabetics.

Monitor: CBC, platelets, SMA-20, serum osmolality, creatinine clearance, ECG.

Interaction: Potentiates effects of other antihypertensives and should not be given within 6 hr of hydralazine, reserpine, alphaprodine, methyldopa, β–blocker, prazosin, minoxidil, the nitrites, and other papaverine–like compounds. Thiazides can add to their hyperuricemic and antihypertensive effect.

VASODILATORS: ARTERIAL AND VENOUS
■ Sodium Nitroprusside (Elkins-Sinn)

How Supplied:
Parenteral: 50 mg single–use vial.

Administration:
IV: For infusion with D_5W only (not direct injection).

Dose: (0.5–10 µg/kg/min); lower dose if on other antihypertensives; increase for controlled hypotension in normotensive patient under surgical anesthesia. Stop infusion if BP not lowered in 10 min; avoid too precipitous a drop in BP.

Mechanism of Action: Direct, immediate peripheral vasodilator, both arteriolar and venous. Decreases preload and afterload by venous pooling and reduced arterial impedance, thus lowering total peripheral resistance. Also causes mild increase in heart rate and decrease in cardiac output in patients with normal left ventricular function; in patients with impaired left ventricular function and diastolic ventricular distention, net effect causes a rise in cardiac output. Maintains renal blood flow and GFR.

Elimination: Rapidly converted to cyanide in RBCs; further degraded in liver to thiocyanate and excreted by kidneys. Drug half–life, minutes; duration of action continues only as long as infusion maintained. Thiocyanate half-life 3 days if renal function is normal.

Indication: HTN crisis for short-term reduction in cardiac preload and/or afterload; e.g., acute aortic dissection, to increase CO in CHF, to lower oxygen demand in acute MI (begin β–adrenergic antagonist concurrently). Also used to achieve controlled hypotension intraoperatively to reduce bleeding in certain surgical procedures.

Contraindications: Compensatory HTN (arteriovenous shunt, coarctation of aorta); inadequate cerebral circulation. Use with caution in patients with renal or hepatic insufficiency (impairs thiocyanate clearance) and hypothyroidism (thiocyanate inhibits uptake and binding of iodine). May worsen arterial hypoxemia in patients with COPD because drug interferes with hypoxic pulmonary vasoconstriction, thus promoting ventilation/perfusion mismatch. Do not use in pregnancy or lactation except in HTN emergency unresponsive to IV hydralazine or diazoxide (risk of cyanide toxicity in fetus even when mother asymptomatic). Also see Table 8-2.

Toxicity:
1. Acute: Excessive vasodilation and hypotension if BP lowered too quickly, with nausea, vomiting, headache, palpitations, chest pain; quick resolution with slowing of infusion rate.
2. Chronic: Thiocyanate toxicity: anorexia, nausea, tinnitus, blurred vision, toxic psychosis, convulsions.

Monitor: Acid-base balance (cyanide toxicity); daily thiocyanate levels for therapy longer than 48 hr (do not allow > 0.1 mg/ml), especially with renal dysfunction.

Antidote (Cyanide Poisoning): Amyl nitrite inhalation; sodium nitrite to induce methemoglobin formation and convert cyanide to cyanmethemoglobin; sodium thiosulfate to further convert to sodium thiocyanate.

Interaction: Hypotensive effect augmented by ganglionic blocking agents, volatile liquid anesthetics (halothane, enflurane), antihypertensives, and most circulatory depressants.

CALCIUM CHANNEL BLOCKERS

■ **Diltiazem Hydrochloride** (Cardizem, Cardizem CD, Cardizem SR; Marion Merell Dow. Dilacor XR; Rhone Poulenc Rorer)

How Supplied:
PO:
>120, 180, 240, 300 mg capsules.
>60, 120, 180, 240 mg extended release capsules.
>30, 60, 90, 120 mg tablets.

Parenteral: 25 mg/5 ml vial.

Administration: *PO,* well absorbed; *IV,* as bolus or continuous infusion.

Mechanism of Action: Benzothiazepine–type calcium ion influx inhibitor. Selectively inhibits influx of calcium ions during membrane depolarization of cardiac and vascular smooth muscle. Lowers BP by relaxation of vascular smooth muscle with resultant decrease in peripheral vascular resistance. Exerts antianginal effect by dilatation of epicardial and subendocardial coronary arteries, inhibition of coronary artery spasm with subsequent increase in coronary blood flow, thus reducing heart rate and myocardial oxygen demand.

Dose:
PO:
1. HTN: 180–240 mg/day, single dose; increase q2 wk to usual dose 240–360 mg/day; maximum 480 mg/day.
2. Angina: 120–180 mg/day, single dose; increase q1–2 wk to maximum of 480 mg/day.

IV:
1. Bolus: 0.25 mg/kg body weight over 2 min (e.g., 20 mg for average patient); followed in 15 min by 0.35 mg/kg body weight over 2 min (e.g., 25 mg) if needed.
2. Continuous infusion: After single dose bolus as above with decrease in HR, 5–15 mg/hr.

Elimination: Extensive first-pass hepatic metabolism by cytochrome P-450 mixed-function oxidase; excreted by kidneys and in bile.

Indications:
PO: HTN, along or with other antihypertensives. Chronic stable angina caused by coronary artery spasm.

IV: Temporary control of rapid ventricular rate in atrial fibrillation or flutter, rapid conversion of paroxysmal supraventricular tachycardia to sinus rhythm.

Contraindications: Sick sinus syndrome or second or third-degree AV block, except in the presence of a functioning ventricular pacemaker; hypotension (systolic BP < 90) or cardiogenic shock; acute MI and pulmonary congestion, atrial fibrillation/flutter associated with an accessory bypass tract; e.g., WPW or short PR syndrome; recent administration (within few hrs) of IV β-blockers. Use caution in patients with CHF or impaired ventricular function, especially if on β-blockers; and in patients with impaired renal or liver function. Avoid use in pregnancy and lactation.

Adverse Effects:
PO: Edema, headache, dizziness, hypotension, asthenia, first-degree AV block, bradycardia, flushing, nausea, rash.
IV: The above, plus injection site reactions, dysrhythmia, premature ventricular beats.

Toxicity: Bradycardia, hypotension, high-degree heart block, cardiac failure.

Drug Interaction: Additive prolongation of AV conduction with β–blockers or digitalis. Competitive inhibition of metabolism with other drugs that undergo cytochrome P-450 oxidative biotransformation (e.g., cyclosporin), especially in the presence of hepatic/renal dysfunction. Concurrent propranolol, digitalis, and carbamezapine levels increased; cimetidine increases diltiazem levels. Anesthetics may further depress cardiac contractility, conductivity and automaticity.

Monitor: LFTs, bilirubin, creatinine clearance; continuous EKG, BP measurement if on IV fusion.

■ **Nifedipine** (Adalat, Adalat CC; Miles. Procardia, Procardia XL; Pratt)

How supplied:
PO: 10, 20 mg capsules.
 30, 60, 90 mg extended release tablets.

Administration: *PO,* well absorbed.

Mechanism of Action: See Diltiazem p. 234. Exerts antianginal effect by dilating peripheral arterioles, thus reducing arterial pressure and TPR (afterload), with net reduction in myocardial energy consumption and O_2 requirements. Also dilates main coronary arteries and arterioles and inhibits spasm, thus increasing myocardial O_2 delivery.

Dose: Initially 10 mg tid; then increase q7–14 days (unless hospitalized or under close observation) to usual dose of 10–20 mg tid–qid; maximum 180 mg/day. In severe postpartum preeclampsia, doses of up to 10 mg q3–4 hr have been used safely.

Elimination: Highly bound to plasma protein, undergoes hepatic biotransformation; metabolites eliminated by kidney.

Indications: Vasospastic and chronic stable (effort-associated) angina. HTN, including the severely preeclamptic/hypertensive postpartum patient unresponsive to the traditional therapy (e.g., hydralazine, methyldopa) (see Table 8-2).

Contraindications: Known drug hypersensitivity. Patients on β–blockers may develop severe hypotension if undergoing surgery using high-dose fentanyl anesthesia, and may develop heart failure if they have aortic stenosis; exacerbation of angina if β–blockers have been recently withdrawn. Use with great caution in pregnancy and lactation (see below).

Adverse Effects: Peripheral edema (in patients with CHF, must distinguish this from worsening left ventricular dysfunction); dizziness; nausea; headache; flushing.

Toxicity: Severe hypotension requiring cardiovascular and respiratory support.

Monitor: LFTs, CPK, bleeding time; digoxin level; PT if on coumadin; BUN, serum creatinine if there is renal insufficiency.

Drug Interaction: See Contraindications above. Possible increased digoxin levels; increased PT on coumadin; increased nifedipine levels if on cimetidine; decreased quinidine levels.

■ Nicardipine Hydrochloride (Cardene, Cardene SR; Syntex. Cardene IV; Wyeth-Ayerst)

How Supplied:
PO:
    20, 30 mg capsules.
    30, 45, 60 sustained-release capsules.
Parenteral:
    25 mg/10 ml ampules.

Administration: *PO,* completely absorbed; *IV* by slow continuous infusion.

Mechanism of Action: See Diltiazem p. 234 and Nifedipine p. 235.

Dose:
PO:
1. Angina: Initially 20 mg tid; increase q3 days to usual dose 20–40 mg tid.
2. HTN: Initially 60 mg/day, divided bid–tid; usual effective dose 20–40 mg tid. Titrate dose careful with renal/hepatic insufficiency or CHF.

IV:
1. HTN in drug-free patient: 0.1 mg/ml concentration, at 50 ml/hr (5.0 mg/hr) rate. Increase by 25–50 ml/hr q15 min up to maximum 150 ml/hr. Decrease to 30 ml/hr when desired BP achieved.

Elimination: First-pass hepatic metabolism; 60% excreted in urine and 35% in feces.

Indications: Chronic stable effort-associated angina, alone or in combination with β-blockers; HTN, alone or in other agents. (Sustained release form for HTN only).

Contraindications: See Nifedipine p. 236.

Adverse Effects: See Nifedipine p. 236.

ANTIHYPERTENSIVES

Toxicity: Marked hypotension, bradycardia, drowsiness, confusion, slurred speech.

Drug Interaction: Cimetidine increases in cardipine levels; use of fentanyl anesthesia and a β-blocker may cause severe hypotension; increased cyclosporine levels.

■ Nimodipene (Nimotop; Miles)

How Supplied:
PO: 30 mg capsules.

Administration: *PO,* rapidly absorbed, but more slowly with food.

Mechanism of Action: See Diltiazem p. 234 and Nifedipine p. 235. Greater effect on cerebral arteries than elsewhere, since it is highly lipophilic.

Dose: 60 mg q4h × 21 days, 1 hr before or 2 hr after meals; begin within 96 hr of subarachnoid hemorrhage. Lower dose to 30 mg q4h with hepatic cirrhosis.

Elimination: 95% bound to plasma proteins; high first-pass metabolism.

Indications: To improve neurologic outcome by reducing incidence/severity of ischemic deficits in patients with subarachnoid hemorrhage from ruptured congenital aneurysm. Investigational use ongoing for treatment of cerebral vasospasm and status epilepticus in eclampsia.

Contraindications: None known.

Adverse Effects: Hypotension; edema; diarrhea; headache; ileus.

Toxicity: Peripheral vasodilatation with marked hypotension.

Drug Interaction: Potentiation of added calcium channel blockers; increased nimodipene levels if also on cimetidine.

■ **Verapamil Hydrochloride** (Calan, Calan SR;
Searle. Isoptin, Isoptin SR; Knoll. Verelan;
Lederle, Wyeth-Ayerst)

How Supplied:
PO:
  40, 80, 120 mg tablets.
  240, mg sustained release caplets.
  120, 180, 240 mg sustained release tablets and capsules.

Administration: *PO,* well absorbed.

Mechanism of Action: Modulates calcium ion influx across
arterial smooth muscle and myocardial cell membranes. Exerts
antianginal effect by increasing myocardial oxygen supply,
reducing myocardial oxygen consumption and inhibiting coronary artery spasm. Also prolongs effective refractory period of
AV node and slows AV conduction in rate-related manner, thus
slowing ventricular rate in chronic atrial flutter/fibrillation; lowers BP by decreasing systemic vascular resistance, usually without orthostatic BP decrease or reflex tachycardia.

Dose:
  Angina: 80–120 mg tid; titrated q1–7day.
  Chronic atrial fibrillation, digitalized: 240–320 mg/day
  divided tid–qid.
  Prophylaxis of PSVT, nondigitalized: 240–480 mg/day,
  divided tid–qid.
  HTN monotherapy: 80–120 mg tid, titrated weekly.
  Lower dose in the elderly, small stature, or patients with
  hepatic insufficiency.

Elimination: Rapid biotransformation during first pass through
portal circulation; majority of metabolites excreted in urine.

Indications: Angina at rest, including vasospastic (Prinzmet-
al's), unstable (crescendo, preinfarction); chronic stable angina,
with digitalis for control of ventricular rate at rest and during
stress in patients with chronic atrial flutter/fibrillation; prophylaxis of PSVT, essential HTN.

Contraindications: Severe left ventricular dysfunction (after-load may not be reduced enough to counter negative inotropism, and CHF or pulmonary edema may result); hypotension (systolic BP <90) or cardiogenic shock; sick sinus syndrome or second- or third-degree AV block (except with functioning artificial ventricular pacemaker, atrial fibrillation or flutter with an accessory bypass tract (e.g., WPW syndrome). Use caution in patients with hepatic insufficiency (elimination prolonged), attenuated neuromuscular transmission (e.g., Duchenne's muscular dystrophy; impaired renal function/dialysis).

Adverse Effects: Constipation, dizziness, nausea, hypotension, headache.

Toxicity: CHF, pulmonary edema bradycardia, AV block.

Monitor: Periodic LFTs; digoxin, carbamazepine, theophylline levels.

Drug Interaction: β-blockers and flecainide may add negative effect on HR, AV conduction and/or cardiac contractivity; increased serum digoxin, theophylline, cyclosporin, or carbamazepine levels; additive BP lowering effect with other antihypertensives; or with quinidine in patients with hypertrophic cardiomyopathy; increased risk of neurotoxicity with lithium; rifampin may reduce verapamil bioavailability; phenobarbital may increase verapamil clearance; increased risk CV depression with inhalation anesthetics.

ANGIOTENSIN-1 CONVERTING ENZYME (ACE) INHIBITORS

■ Captopril (Capoten; Squibb)

How Supplied:
PO: 12.5, 25, 50, 100 mg tablet.

Administration:
PO: Rapidly absorbed. Take 1 hr before meals to improve bioavailibility; restrict sodium if used as single agent.

Dose:
1. Hypertension: Initially 25 mg bid–tid; after 1–2 wk increase to 50 mg bid–tid. If inadequate response at 50 m tid, add low dose thiazide diuretic (e.g., hydrochlorothiazide 25 mg/day); increase q1–2 wk to maximum diuretic dose. If response still is suboptimal, incrementally increase captopril to 100–150 mg bid–tid (continue diuretic). Usual dose is 25–150 mg bid–tid; max 450 mg/day. In severe cases, may increase dose q24h with careful monitoring; consider use of more potent diuretic (e.g. furosemide) and/or β–blocker.
2. Heart failure: Initially 25 mg tid; increase to 50 mg tid after several days. If response inadequate after another 2 wk, increase to 50–100 mg tid; max 450 mg/day. If BP is normal or low at start of therapy or there has been recent additional diuretic therapy with possible hypovolemia or hyponatremia, begin with 6.25–12.5 mg tid to avoid exaggerating hypotension; then increase by increments every several days to maximum 450 mg/day. Continue digitalis and diuretic prn.

Mechanism of Action: Angiotensin-converting enzyme (ACE) inhibition, resulting in decreased angiotensin II (potent vasoconstrictor) and aldosterone and increased renin (loss of negative feedback). Systemic arteriolar dilatation lowers mean, systolic, and diastolic BP and total peripheral resistance with either no change or increase in cardiac output. Afterload reduced in CHF along with stroke work, stroke volume, and heart rate. Renal blood flow increased with no change in GFR. Lowered aldosterone causes natriuresis, with contraction of excess body fluids and reduced venous return to right heart.

Elimination: 95% eliminated in urine; adjust dose in renal impairment. Half-life 2 hr.

Indication: HTN, either alone or as combination therapy with, e.g., thiazide diuretic (additive effect); used in CHF in combination with digitalis and diuretics. Also used to improve survival and reduce incidence of overt heart failure after MI in patients with left ventricular dysfunction (ejection fraction ≤40%); and to decrease the rate of progression of renal insufficiency in IDDM nephropathy (proteinuria >500 mg/day) and retinopathy.

ANTIHYPERTENSIVES

Contraindications: Known drug hypersensitivity, pregnancy. Insufficient data on use in lactation. Use with caution in patients with hypovolemia, hyponatremia, renal artery stenosis, autoimmune disease such as lupus erythematosus, collagen vascular disease (increased risk of neutropenia especially if renal function is also impaired), aortic stenosis (theoretical risk of decreased, coronary perfusion).

Adverse Effects/Toxicity: Acute BP drop if hypovolemic or hyponatremic (e.g., CHF or receiving diuretics) with tachycardia and anginal pain. Neutropenia with myeloid hypoplasia and agranulocytosis, more often in patients with renal impairment and/or collagen vascular disease, beginning 3 mo after starting drug and reversible after discontinuation. Increased BUN and creatinine or reversible proteinuria (more than 1 gm/day) and nephrotic syndrome, usually in patients with renal dysfunction or receiving doses >150 mg/day. Cholestatic jaundice with potentially fatal fulminant hepatic necrosis. Also, skin rash, dysgeusia, vertigo, headache, GI distress, and metabolic acidosis and hyperkalemia from secondary hyperaldosteronism; anaphylactoid reaction with angioedema and potentially fatal airway obstruction.

Monitor: Baseline and periodic CBC, electrolytes, BUN, creatinine for urine protein, LFTs, bilirubin; lithium levels.

Interaction: Extreme acute hypotensive episode if receiving diuretics, salt restriction, dialysis, antihypertensives that increase plasma renin, sympathetic blockers. Augmented hyperkalemia when used with potassium-sparing diuretics (e.g., spironolactone, potassium supplements or salt substitutes). Prostaglandin inhibitors may lessen effect on BP. Lithium concentrations may be increased to toxic level, especially if diuretic is also used.

■ Enalapril Maleate: Enalaprilat (Vasotec; Merck)

How Supplied:
PO: 2.5, 5, 10, 20 mg tablets.
Parenteral: 1.25 mg/ml; 1,2 ml vials.

Administration: *PO,* rapidly absorbed without regard to meals; *IV*.

Mechanism of Action: See Captopril p. 241.

Dose:
> HTN: *PO:* Initially 5 mg/day; titrate up to 10–40 mg/day, single dose or divide bid. Decrease dose with renal impairment (creatinine clearance ≤30 ml/min or serum creatinine ≥3 mg/dl).
>> *IV:* 1.25 over 5 min q6h; maximum 20 mg/day. Decrease dose with renal impairment, if on diuretics, or if at risk for hypotension.
>
> Heart Failure: *PO:* Initially 2.5 mg/day; titrate up to 2.5–20 mg bid; maximum 40 mg/day, divided. Lower dose in patients with hyponatremia (serum sodium <130 mEq/L) or serum creatinine >1.6 mg/dl.
>
> Asymptomatic left ventricular dysfunction: PO: Initially 2.5 bid, titrated up to 20mg/day, divided.

Elimination: Primarily renal excretion.

Indication: HTN, alone or with other antihypertensives (e.g., thiazides); to improve symptoms and increase survival in symptomatic CHF, usually with diuretics and digitalis; to decrease risk of overt heart failure in asymptomatic patients with left ventricular dysfunction (ejection fraction ≤35%). IV form for HTN only when PO therapy not practical.

Contraindications: Known drug hypersensitivity (including history of angioedema after prior ACE-inhibitor therapy); pregnancy. Use with caution in patients at risk for excessive hypotension; e.g., hyponatremia, aggressive diuretic therapy, renal dialysis, severe volume/salt depletion; also use with caution in patients with renal impairment especially if they also have collagen vascular disease (increased risk of agranulocytosis and bone marrow depression).

Adverse Effects/Toxicity: See Captopril p. 241.

Monitor: See Captopril p. 242.

Interaction: See Captopril p. 242.

ANTIHYPERTENSIVES

■ Fosinopril Sodium (Monopril; Bristol-Myers, Squibb)

How Supplied:
PO: 10, 20 mg tablets.

Administration: *PO,* slowly absorbed.

Mechanism of Action: See Captopril p. 241.

Dose: Initially 10 mg/day; usual effective dose 20–40 mg/day; max 80 mg/day.

Elimination: Equally by liver and kidney. Dose need not be reduced with renal/hepatic insufficiency.

Indications: HTN, alone or with thiazides.

Contraindications: See Captopril p. 241 and Enalapril p. 243.

Adverse Effects/Toxicity: See Captopril p. 241.

Monitor: See Captopril p. 242.

Interaction: See Captopril p. 242. Also, antacids may impair absorption, so dose at least 2 hr apart.

■ Lisinopril (Prinivil; Merck. Zestril; Stuart)

How supplied:
PO: 2.5, 5, 10, 20, 40 mg tablets.

Administration: *PO,* slowly and incompletely (30%) absorbed, without regard to meals.

Mechanism of Action: See Captopril p. 241.

Dose:
HTN: Initially 10 mg/day; titrate up to 20–40 mg/day, single dose; max 80 mg/day.
Heart failure: Initially 5 mg/day; titrate up to max 2 mg/day.
Use lower dose in patients already on diuretics (ideally

should discontinue diuretics 2–3 days before initiating therapy), with renal impairment (creatinine clearance <30 ml/min), hyponatremia (serum sodium <130 mEg/ml), or the elderly.

Elimination: Excreted unchanged in urine.

Indications: HTN, alone as initial therapy or with other antihypertensives; adjunctive therapy of heart failure in patients not responding to diuretics and digitalis.

Contraindications: See Enalapril p. 243.

Adverse Effects/Toxicity: See Captopril p. 241.

Monitor: See Captopril p. 242.

Interaction: See Captopril p. 242.

■ Quinapril Hydrochloride (Accupril; Parke-Davis)

How Supplied:
PO: 5, 10, 20, 40 mg tablets.

Administration: *PO;* rapidly absorbed.

Mechanism of Action: See Captopril p. 241.

Dose:
HTN: Monotherapy: Initial 10 mg/day, single dose; titrate up q2 wk to 40–80 mg/day, divided bid.
Concomitant diuretics: Initially 5 mg/day. Ideally, discontinue diuretics 2–3 days prior; restart if BP response is not controlled with quinapril alone.
Heart failure: 5 mg bid; titrate weekly to usual dose 20–40 mg/day divided bid.
Renal impairment: Decrease dose if creatinine clearance <60 ml/min.

Elimination: Primarily renal excretion.

Indications: HTN, alone or with thiazides; combination therapy for heart failure with diuretics and/or digitalis.

Contraindications: See Captopril p. 241 and Enalapril p. 243.

Adverse Effects/Toxicity: See Captopril p. 241.

Monitor: See Captopril p. 242.

Interactions: See Captopril p. 242.

■ Ramipril (Altace; Hoechst-Roussel)

How Supplied:
PO: 1.25, 2.5, 5, 10 mg capsules.

Administration: *PO,* rapidly absorbed.

Mechanism of Action: See Captopril p. 241.

Dose: Initially 2.5 mg/day, single dose, if not on diuretics; titrate up to 2.5–20 mg/day, single dose or divided bid. Decrease dose if creatinine clearance <40 ml/min or serum creatinine >2.5 mg/dl.

Elimination: 60% excreted in urine; 40% in feces.

Indications: HTN, alone or with thiazides.

Contraindications: See Captopril p. 241, and Enalapril p. 243.

Adverse Effects/Toxicity: See Captopril p. 241.

Monitor: See Captopril p. 242.

Drug Interaction: See Captopril p. 242.

CHAPTER 9

BLOOD AND BLOOD PRODUCTS

BLOOD
■ Whole Blood

How Supplied: 1 unit = approximately 450 ml whole blood + 63 ml anticoagulant (citrate-phosphate-dextrose=CPD) or anticoagulant and preservative (CPD-adenine=CDPA). Hct 30%–35%. Storage life: 3 wks for CPD blood, 5 wks for CPDA blood. At end of this period, 70%–80% RBCs still viable; WBCs and platelets nonviable; clotting factors V & VIII have low activity.

Administration: *IV:* As quickly as possible (since only given in cases of active exsanguination) via microaggregate filter; mixed and warmed if feasible.

Indication: See Table 9-1.

Adverse Effects: See Tables 9-1 to 9-3. Also, hypothermia, dilutional coagulopathy, microcirculation emboli, hypocalcemia (to avoid cardiac dysrhythmia, treat with 10 ml 10% calcium gluconate IV at site distant from transfusion), delayed hemolysis.

BLOOD PRODUCTS
■ Packed Red Blood Cells (PRBCs)

How Supplied: 1 unit = 200–250 ml RBCs. Hct 70%–90%.

Administration:
IV: Via normal saline (NS), 5% albumin, or fresh-frozen plasma (FFP); max infusion rate 350 ml/hr.

Table 9-1

BLOOD COMPONENT REPLACEMENT THERAPY

Component	Factors Contained	Indications	Major Risks
Whole Blood	RBCs; all procoagulants	Acute massive hemorrhage (e.g., GI bleed, trauma); rarely indicated	Hepatitis, allergic reaction, febrile reaction, volume overload
Packed RBCs	RBCs only	Anemia; hypovolemia from acute blood loss	Hepatitis, allergic reaction, febrile reaction
Platelets	Platelets, small amount fibrinogen, factor V and VIII	Thrombocytopenia: <50,000 preop or less than 20,000 at any time	Hepatitis, allergic reaction, febrile reaction
Fresh Frozen Plasma	All procoagulants, no platelets	Coagulation deficiency: PT >16, PTT >60, or specific factor (prothrombin precursor) deficiency	Hepatitis, allergic reaction, febrile reaction, volume overload
Cryoprecipitate	Fibrinogen; factors VIII, XIII	Hypofibrinogenemia (e.g., DIC), hemophilia, von Willebrand's factor XIII deficiency	Hepatitis (extremely low risk)
Granulocytes	WBCs	Sepsis with severe neutropenia not responding to appropriate antibiotic therapy	Hepatitis, allergic reaction, pulmonary infiltration
Factor VIII Concentrate	Partially purified pooled factor VIII	Hemophiliacs with injury or in preparation for major surgery	Coombs + hemolytic anemia; factor VIII inhibitor development; hepatitis (especially nonA nonB) allergic reaction

Modified from Creasy RK, Resnik R, *Maternal fetal medicine*, 1989; Considine T, Principles of blood replacement. In Sciarra JJ, editor: *Gynecology and obstetrics*, vol 3, 1985; Baker RJ: Blood component therapy and transfusion reactions. In Condom RE, Nyhus LM, editors: *Manual of surgical therapeutics*, 1982.

Table 9-2

TRANSFUSION REACTIONS—EARLY

Type	Components Involved	Incidence	Mechanism	Symptoms	Management
Allergic	Whole blood; packed RBCs, plasma less frequently	4% of all recipients (50% of those with past history of atopy)	Antibodies to plasma antigens	Itching, hives, fever, chills	Diphenhydramine 50 mg, antipyretics; continue transfusion
Febrile	Whole blood; packed RBCs or plasma less frequently	2% of all recipients	Antibodies to WBC and platelet antigens	Fever up to 39.4° C, flushing, headache, chills	Diphenhydramine 50 mg, antipyretics; continue transfusion
Bacteremia (severe febrile reaction)	Whole blood	0.01% of recipients	Contamination with cold-growing organisms*	Fever over 39.4° C, vomiting, diarrhea, hypotension, shock	Stop transfusion; culture donor unit and patient blood; IV fluids, antibiotics, steroids, and fresh transfusion
Hemolytic†	Whole blood, packed RBCs	0.03% of recipients	Antibodies to RBC antigens	DIC: fever, pain in flank, chest, extremities; jaundice, hemoglobinuria, shock, renal failure	Stop transfusion;‡ if laboratory tests confirm, give steroids, diuretics, heparin,§ Na bicarbonate

Modified from Considine T, Baker RJ.

*Most commonly gram-negative (sometimes gram-positive) facultative anaerobes.

†Unlike other reactions, always occurs during first 100 ml of transfusion.

‡Repeat type and crossmatch donor and recipient blood, indirect Coombs, Ab screen; test for increased free plasma Hb, methemoglobinemia, hemoglobinuria, fibrinogen, fribin split products, platelets.

§If platelets < 75,000/mm³, fibrinogen < 100 mg/100 ml; elevated fibrin split products.

BLOOD AND BLOOD PRODUCTS

249

Table 9-3
TRANSFUSION REACTIONS—LATE

Type	Components Involved	Incidence	Timing	Symptoms	Comment
Isosensitization	Whole blood, Packed RBCs		More than 2 wks later	Transfusion reaction Erythroblastosis	If given O-neg. blood in subsequent transfusion Subsequent pregnancy
Hemolytic	Whole blood, Packed RBCs	0.2–7%	3 days to several wks	Jaundice, positive direct Coombs reaction	Rarely, intramuscular hemolysis formation of antiKidd antibodies
Infectious:					
Hepatitis B	Any: Factors VIII, IX concentrate Whole blood packed RBCs, fresh-frozen plasma, cryoprecipitate	10–20%	35–120 days later	Jaundice, and so on	Higher mortality if 5 or >65 yr old; hyperimmune globulin possibly helpful
NonA/NonB hepatitis	Any	1% or less 1% (greater with multiple transfusions)		None or mild	30–50% develop chronic active hepatitis; 10% of these develop cirrhosis

Table 9-3

TRANSFUSION REACTIONS—LATE—cont'd

Type	Components Involved	Incidence	Timing	Symptoms	Comment
AIDS (HIV)	Any	1:1,000,000	Variable	Wide range	1% current AIDS cases thought to be transfusion related
Cytomegalovirus	Any		1–6 wks	Few; or spiking fever, atypical lymphocytes on peripheral smear, abnormal LFTs, + cold agglutinins	Usually self-limited, potentially fatal if immunosuppressed.

Modified from Creasy RK, Resnik R, Baker RJ, Considine T.
*Miscellaneous infections include malaria, brucellosis, and HTLV-I.

Dose: 1 unit for each desired 3% rise in Hct or 1–1.5 gm Hb.

Indication: See Table 9-1.

Adverse Effects: See Tables 9-1 to 9-3.

■ Granulocytes

How Supplied: Variable; 1 unit = 50–300 ml 10^{10} irradiated WBCs.

Administration:
IV: 2–4 hr/unit.

Indication: Sepsis with severe neutropenia not responding to appropriate antibiotic therapy.

Adverse Effects: Hepatitis, allergic reaction, febrile reaction, pulmonary infiltrates.

■ Platelets

How Supplied: 1 unit = 30–40 ml platelets (half platelet concentration of whole blood).

Administration:
IV: Without filter or warming. For preoperative prophylaxis, give 6–12 hr before surgery.

Dose: 1 unit for each desired 5000–8000/mm^3 rise in platelet count; fever, sepsis, or splenomegaly may require dose increase. Usual initial dose 6–8 units.

Indication: See Table 9-1.

Contraindications: Thrombotic thrombocytopenic purpura, immune thrombocytopenic purpura (except in near-fatal hemorrhage). No longer indicated prophylactically with massive blood transfusion or after cardiopulmonary bypass.

Adverse Effects: See Tables 9-1 to 9-3. Also Rh sensitization from contaminants (prophylax with RhoGAM [Ortho], see development of antiplatelet antibodies, HLA sensitization.

■ Cryoprecipitate

How Supplied: 1 bag = 100 units factor VIII/10–25 ml + 120–250 mg fibrinogen. Contains approximately half the factor VIII activity of fresh-frozen plasma at 1/10th the original volume. Must be stored frozen.

Administration:
IV: Reconstituted with normal saline solution. Avoid too rapid thawing.

Dose: Initial dose usually 15–20 bags (4–6 gm).

Indication: See Table 9-1.

Adverse Effects: See Tables 9-1 to 9-3. Also, development of anti–factor VIII antibodies.

■ Fresh-Frozen Plasma

How Supplied: 1 unit = 200–250 ml plasma (+ approximately 1 gm fibrinogen).

Administration:
IV: 10 ml/min immediately after thawing.

Dose: 5–20 ml/kg; repeat half dose in 4–6 hr. Minimum starting dose 4 units.

Indications: See Table 9-1. Also, to achieve immediate hemostasis in patients with multiple factor deficiencies (e.g., those receiving warfarin, and no time to allow vitamin K reversal of factor II, VII, IX, X deficiency), liver disease, DIC; antithrombin II deficiency; thrombotic thrombocytopenic purpura.

Adverse Effects: See Tables 9-1 to 9-3.

■ **Antihemophilic Factor** (Helixate, Humate-P; Armour. Koate-HP; Miles Biological)

How Supplied: *Parenteral:* 250 IU 2.5 ml single dose bottle
250, 500 IU 5 ml single dose bottle.
1000, 1500 IU 10 ml single dose bottle.

Administration: *IV,* slow infusion.

Mechanism of Action: Purified factor VIII concentrate, pooled from multiple donors; some forms prepared by monoclonal antibody and/or recombinant techniques. Lyophilizing inactivates HIV and certain other viruses (most types of CMV, herpes, hepatitis B).

Elimination: Half-life 8–12 hr.

Indications: Prevention and control of hemorrhagic episodes in hemophilia A (classic hemophilia).

Contraindication: Acquired factor VIII inhibitor level over 10 Bethesda U/ml.

Dose: 8–15 U/kg q8–24h × several days to control bleeding episode; 26–50 U/kg before major surgery.

Adverse Effects: See Table 9-1.

CHAPTER 10

BLOOD GLUCOSE REGULATORS

Insulin increases peripheral utilization of glucose, thereby lowering serum levels. A primary action is noted in the liver, where glucose production is blocked. Insulin is a protein composed of two amino acid chains linked by disulfide bonds.

Insulin is prepared from purified beef or pork pancreas by several chromatographic separation techniques. Human insulin is synthesized from recombinant DNA and is identical in structure. Pork insulin differs by one amino acid from human insulin; beef differs by three amino acids.

Insulin must be given by SC or IV injection. A variety of preparations are available and are classified by onset and duration of action (Table 10-1).

USE AND DOSAGE

The goal of insulin therapy is to maintain serum glucose at approximately normal levels throughout the 24 hr and avoid the extremes of ketoacidosis or hypoglycemic conditions. During pregnancy the increased metabolic requirements increase the need for insulin. These patients should be managed by specialists in maternal-fetal medicine.

Periodic serum glucose determinations by venipuncture or capillary methods are essential for the management of diabetic patients. Nonpregnant women may be best managed by urinary glucose determinations and occasional serum glucose measurement.

Because insulin is a protein, various types of allergic reactions can occur, especially from the animal-derived sources.

Each type of injectable insulin is available from both animal sources and recombinant human DNA. Mixtures of insulins with different durations of action are also available.

The *PDR* should be consulted for the various preparations available and their doses.

Table 10-1

CHARACTERISTICS OF INSULIN PREPARATIONS

Type and Preparation	Onset	SC Administration Peak (hr)	Duration (hr)
Rapid			
Humulin (Lilly)	0.5–1	2–5	6–8
Novolin (Novo Nordisk)	0.5–1	2–5	6–8
Intermediate			
NPH Insulin (Novo Nordisk)	1–2	7–12	24–30
Iletin, Lente (Lilly)	1–3	7–12	24–30
Long-Acting			
Humulin Ultralente (Lilly)	1–8	12–24	30–36
Ultralente (Novo Nordisk)	4–8	10–30	34–46

■ Intrapartum Use of Insulin

Management of the diabetic patient in labor requires hourly monitoring of blood glucose levels to prevent extremes in the levels of glucose. Usually the insulin requirements decrease slightly during early labor and increase slightly in late labor. The optimum type of insulin to use during labor is regular via IV infusion or SC injection. Many dosage schemes are available. Table 10-2 indicates a commonly used regimen. Table 10-3 provides glucose challenge test values during pregnancy.

OTHER AGENTS

■ Glucagon (Lilly)

Glucagon is extracted from beef and pork pancreas and chemically unrelated to insulin. It causes hyperglycemia by increased hepatic glycogenolysis. Glucagon injection is used in counteracting severe hypoglycemic states that may occur during insulin treatment.

How Supplied:

1 unit (1 mg) 1 ml vial as lyophilized powder.
Emergency kit.

Dose: 0.5–1 unit *SC, IM, IV.*

Table 10-2
INSULIN ADMINISTRATION IN LABOR

Glucose* (mg %)	IV Insulin Dose (U/hr)[†]	IV Fluid (125 ml/hr)
Less than 100	0.5	D_5 Ringer's lactate
100–140	1.0	D_5 Ringer's lactate
141–180	1.5	Normal saline
181–220	2.0	Normal saline
> 220	2.5	Normal saline

*Hourly blood determination.
[†]25 U regular insulin/250 ml NS.

Table 10-3
GLUCOSE CHALLENGE TEST VALUES DURING PREGNANCY (After 100 Gram Glucose Load)

	Serum (mg/100 ml)	Whole Blood (mg/100 ml)
Fasting	<105	<90
1 hr	190	165
2 hr	165	145
3 hr	145	125

■ Oral Hypoglycemic Agents (Table 10-4)

These synthetic agents lower blood glucose levels by stimulating the release of insulin from the pancreas. Oral agents should not be used during pregnancy because of the reported association of higher glucose levels and congenital anomalies. In Type I diabetics, better control of glucose levels is obtained with insulin. Oral agents should be reserved for Type II patients.

The administration of oral hypoglycemic agents has been associated with increased cardiovascular mortality compared with patients receiving diet alone or diet plus insulin therapy.

■ **Table 10-4.**

SELECTED ORAL HYPOGLYCEMIC AGENTS

Type and Brand Name	How Supplied	Manufacturer
Sulfonylurea		
Glybyuride; DiaBeta;	1.25, 2.5 5 mg tabs	Hoechst-Roussel
Micronase	1.25, 2.5, 5 mg tabs	Upjohn
Chlorpropamide		
Diabinese	100, 250 mg tabs	Pfizer
Glipizide	5, 10 mg tabs	Pratt
Glucotrol		

■ **Use and Dosage**

Oral hypoglycemic Agents should be used only as adjunctive therapy to diet control in Type II diabetics.

The initial starting dose and the maintenance doses cannot be fixed but must be individualized based on monitoring of patient's urinary glucose and periodic blood glucose determinations. Glycosylated Hb–A–1–C levels may be of value in monitoring.

CHAPTER 11

BLOOD SUBSTITUTES

PLASMA EXPANDERS

■ **Plasma Protein Fraction** (Plasma-Plex 5%; Armour. Plasmatein 5%; Alpha Therapeutic)

How Supplied:
Parenteral: 5% solution in 2.5 gm/50 ml, 12.5 gm/250 ml, 25 gm/500 ml bottle.

Administration:
IV: Undiluted; avoid rates over 10 ml/min because of risk of hypotension. No cross-matching required.

Dose: Usual initial dose 250–500 ml; repeat prn.

Mechanism of Action: Osmotically equivalent to plasma.

Indication: Plasma-expanding colloid for emergency treatment of shock caused by trauma, surgery, burns and infections.

Contraindications: Severe anemia, cardiac failure, patients on cardiopulmonary bypass. Use caution in patients with low cardiac reserve or without albumin deficit (rapid rise in plasma volume may lead to pulmonary edema).

Adverse Effects: Hypervolemia, allergic reaction, hypotension from kinin production. (Manufacturer heating minimizes hepatitis risk.)

■ **Albumin** (Albumarc-American Red Cross; Albuminar; Armour. Albutein; Alpha Therapeutic. Buminate; Baxter Healthcare)

How Supplied:
5% in 50, 250, 500, 1000 ml vial or bottle.
25% in 20, 50, 100 ml vial or bottle.

Administration:
IV: Undiluted or via normal saline or D_5W infusion.

Dose: 0.5–1 gm/kg/dose; max 6 gm/day.

Mechanism of Action: 5% solution osmotically equivalent to plasma; colloid effect helps treat patients with fluid sequestration (third spacing) or moderate blood loss. Hyperosmolar 25% solution may help replace protein pool in patients unable to synthesize endogenous protein or with excessive losses.

Indication:
5%: Plasma volume expander for hypovolemia resulting from operation, burns, intestinal obstruction, significant hemorrhage.

25%: Albumin pool expander in long-standing hypovolemia or hypoalbuminemia (nephrotic syndrome, liver failure, some types of hypoproteinuria).

Contraindication: History of cardiac failure, severe chronic anemia, allergic reaction to albumin. Use with caution in patients with HTN, severe pulmonary infections.

Adverse Effects/Toxicity: Hypervolemia, CHF or pulmonary edema (from albumin extravasation from pulmonary circulation), allergic reactions with hypotension (from kinin release). Contains 130–160 mEq Na/L.

■ **Dextran** (Promit, Rheomacrodex; Medi-Physics, Inc.)

How Supplied:
Parenteral:
15% dextran 1 in 0.6% NaCl; 20 ml injection.
10% dextran 40 in NS or D_5W; 500 ml bottle.

Administration: *IV.*

Dose: 500 ml rapidly; repeat prn, but more slowly and with central venous pressure monitoring to avoid circulatory overload. Max 1 L/24 hr to avoid bleeding diathesis.

Mechanism of Action: Branched polysaccharide form by action of *Leuconostoc mesenteroides* bacteria. Increases circulatory blood volume and improves hemodynamic status for 24 hr or more. Lower molecular weight form (dextran 1) improves microcirculation in addition to correcting hypovolemia; also minimizes rouleaux formation and RBC sludging that may accompany shock.

Elimination: Smaller molecular weight molecules excreted by kidney; remainder crosses capillary wall slowly and is gradually oxidized over next few weeks. Dextran 40 effect dissipated in 12 hr; dextran 70 cleared over 24–48 hr.

Indication: Moderate hypovolemia.

Contraindications: Hypofibrinogenemia, thrombocytopenia, bleeding dyscrasias. Exercise caution in patients with CHF, pulmonary edema, and renal impairment.

Adverse Effects/Toxicity: Dextran-induced rouleaux formation interferes with Rh typing and blood cross-matching; von Willebrand-like hemostatic defect; anaphylaxis, allergic reactions (with itching, urticaria, joint pains [less than 10%]). If GFR reduced, excessive tubular water and salt reabsorption may lead to high intratubular dextran concentration with increased flow impedence, viscosity and possible renal failure.

■ Hetastarch (Hespan; Du Pont)

How Supplied:
Parenteral: 6% hetastarch in NS; 500 ml bottle.

Administration: *IV;* undiluted.

Dose: Usually 500–1000 ml; maximum 1500 ml/day (20 ml/kg body weight).

Mechanism of Action: Synthetic colloid polymer; average molecular weight, 480,000 (range 400,000–550,000). Hydroxyethyl ether groups on its glucose residues retard degradation for longer effective action. Hemodynamic effects similar to albumin in management of shock and postoperative cardiac patients, with less antigenic effects than dextran.

Elimination: Molecules less than 50,000 molecular weight rapidly excreted by kidney (33% of dose in 24 hr). Higher molecular weight molecules metabolized slowly over next 2 wk.

Indications: Plasma volume expander in treatment of hypovolemia; adjunct in leukapheresis to improve harvesting and yield of granulocytes by centrifuge.

Contraindications: Bleeding disorders, CHF, renal disease with oliguria not related to hypovolemia, or when volume overload is a potential problem. No data on use in pregnancy/lactation.

Adverse Effects/Toxicity: Transient increase in PT, PTT, also bleeding time with larger doses, sometimes caused by reversible factor VIII deficiency. Volume overload; life-threatening anaphylactic reactions (wheezing, urticaria).

CHAPTER 12

CARDIAC DRUGS

Shock results from inadequate tissue perfusion of vital organs secondary to hypovolemic conditions, myocardial infarction, sepsis, or anaphylaxis. Each of these causes of shock must be treated differently, but the major aim of therapy is to restore blood flow to vital organs. Shock is accompanied by increased activity of the sympathetic nervous system, which results in the classic signs and symptoms of hypotension, pallor, tachycardia, tachypnea, mental confusion, oliguria, and metabolic acidosis.

Drug therapy is based on the precipitating cause of shock.

Hypovolemic Shock

Blood and plasma volume expanders are the primary therapy of hypovolemic shock (see Chapters 9 and 10). Secondary drug therapy may be useful, particularly sympathomimetic amines.

Cardiogenic Shock

Cardiac output is decreased, usually secondary to myocardial infarction, and this results in initial increased peripheral resistance followed by central and peripheral vascular collapse. The main aim of drug therapy is to increase coronary perfusion by increasing blood vessel resistance and diastolic pressure. In some cardiogenic shock conditions, vasodilators may be useful as adjunctive therapy to increase perfusion to vital organs, such as the kidney.

Septic Shock

Septic shock usually results from gram-negative septicemia (rarely gram-positive). Pooling of blood occurs in the venous bed and results in effective reduction of circulating blood volume. Therapy is aimed at eliminating the source of sepsis and maintaining adequate circulation. In severe septic shock states, vasopressor agents may prove useful to maintain tissue perfusion.

Anaphylactic Shock

Anaphylactic shock is an immediate hypersensitivity reaction that results in laryngeal edema and circulating collapse, caused by WBC release of prostaglandins and histamine in response to foreign protein. The goal of therapy is to maintain an adequate airway (by tracheostomy if necessary) and administer oxygen. Epinephrine is the drug of choice in an emergency. Antihistamines may be used secondarily to control the skin manifestations of the allergic response.

SYMPATHOMIMETIC AMINES: ENDOGENOUS

■ Norepinephrine (Levophed Bitartrate; Winthrop)

How Supplied:
Aqueous solution: 4 ml ampules containing 4 mg (1 mg/ml).

Dose: Administer 4 ml in 1000 ml 5% dextrose-saline solution or dextrose in water via a well-advanced intravenous catheter. Individualize total dosage based on BP response. Initial flow rate 2–3 ml/min; maintenance rate 0.5–1 ml/min.

Mechanism of Action: α-Adrenergic peripheral vasoconstrictor and inotropic stimulator of cardiac muscle with vasodilation of coronary arteries; results in increased systemic BP and improved coronary artery blood flow.

Indication: Hypotensive shock.

Contraindications: In hypovolemic shock, severe central and peripheral vasoconstriction may result if blood volume expanders are not used as primary agents.

Adverse Effects:
1. Overdose may result in dangerous elevation of BP.
2. Extreme vasoconstriction can lead to skin necrosis and gangrene of the infused extremity.
3. Extravasation ischemia. Antidote is phentolamine (Regitene; CIBA); infiltrate 10–15 ml immediately.

■ Epinephrine (Epinephrine USP; Wyeth-Ayerst, Astra, Parke-Davis)

How Supplied: 1 mg epinephrine HCl/1 ml ampule (1:1000).

Dose: Individualize.

Mechanism of Action: Activates α- and β-receptors, thus mimicking sympathetic nervous system effects.

Indication: Rapid relief in hypersensitivity reactions, bronchial asthma, prolongation of local anesthesia, hemostasis.

Contraindications: Narrow-angle glaucoma. Not to be used with local anesthetics for surgery in distal extremities. Combine with certain general anesthetic agents. Use in pregnancy only when benefits justify risks.

■ Dopamine HCl (Astra; Elkins-Sinn)

How Supplied: 5 ml ampule containing 40 mg dopamine HCl/ml single-dose syringe or vial.

Dose: Must dilute in 250 or 500 ml of any IV solution. Do not add to sodium bicarbonate solution, because drug is inactivated.

Mechanism of Action: Catecholamine that activates dopaminergic receptors in renal vasculature and positive inotropic effect on β-adrenergic receptors causes increased cardiac output.

Indication: Correct hemodynamic imbalance secondary to shock conditions; improve cardiac output.

Contraindications: Pheochromocytoma. Reduce dosage in patients treated with monoamine oxidase (MAO) inhibitors.

Adverse Effects: Extravasation may lead to necrosis and sloughing of skin. Sympathomimetic effects.

SYMPATHOMIMETIC AMINES: SYNTHETIC

■ Metaraminol Bitartrate (Aramine; Merck)

How Supplied:
Injection: 1% (10 mg Aramine) in 10 ml vial.

Dose:
SC/IM: 2–10 mg.
    IV: Dilute 15–100 mg in 500 ml normal saline solution or dextrose in water.

Mechanism of Action: Stimulates myocardium and causes peripheral vasoconstriction.

Indication: Adjunct therapy in hypotensive conditions.

Contraindications: Avoid with certain general anesthetic agents. Hypersensitivity to sulfites.

Adverse Effects: Dysrhythmias, local tissue necrosis, severe hypertension.

■ Isoproterenol HCl (Isuprel; Winthrop)

How Supplied: Ampules: 1, 5 ml containing 0.2 mg/ml.

Dose: *IV:* See *PDR*.

Mechanism of Action: Positive inotopic effect. Smooth muscle relaxant, particularly bronchial.

Indication: Bronchospasm; heart block except in ventricular tachycardia; cardiac arrest; adjunctive therapy for shock states.

Contraindications: Tachydysrhythmias.

■ Phenylephrine HCl (Neo-Synephrine; Winthrop)

How Supplied:
1% solution: 1 ml ampule contains 10 mg.
    Cartridge needle: 10 mg/ml.

Dose:
SC, IM, IV: Dose varies depending on condition being treated.
Moderate hypotension:
> *IV:* 0.2 mg.
> *SC, IM:* 2–5 mg.

Mechanism of Action: Synthetic sympathomimetic agent chemically related to epinephrine and ephedrine possessing potent α-receptor stimulation, causing peripheral vasoconstriction and reflex bradycardia.

Indication: Therapy in hypotensive conditions. Adjunct during anesthesia for BP maintenance.

Contraindications: Severe hypertension, ventricular tachycardia.

Adverse Effects: Oxytocin potentiates pressor effect, potentially resulting in persistent postpartum hypertension and predisposition to stroke. Other drug interactions are common (e.g., MAO inhibitors, anesthetic agents).

■ Dobutamine HCl (Dobutrex; Lilly)

How Supplied: 20 ml vial containing 250 mg.

Dose: See *PDR*.

Mechanism of Action: Synthetic catecholamine that has positive inotropic effect and causes peripheral vasodilation.

Indication: Short-term treatment of cardiac decompensation.

Contraindications: Valvular heart disease, hypersensitivity to sulfites.

Adverse Effects: Tachycardia, elevated BP.

CARDIAC DRUGS

VASODILATORS

Use in selected patients with acute myocardial infarction or congestive heart failure to decrease peripheral resistance, thereby increasing cardiac output. In acute situations, IV administration is preferred, although some agents may be administered by the sublingual or topical routes.

Major risk factors are hypotension, reduced coronary perfusion, and reflex tachycardia.

(See also Chapter 8.)

■ Nitroglycerin

Available agents include:
- Nitrostat tabs (Parke-Davis).
- NitroBid IV (Marion Merrell Dow).
- Nitro-Dur Transdermal (Key).

■ α-Adrenergic Blocker (Phentolamine Mesylate, Regitene IV; CIBA)

How Supplied: 5 mg ampule, lyophilized for solution.

Dose: *IV:* Infusion at 10 μg/kg/min.

Mechanism of Action: Direct relaxant of vascular smooth muscle by blocking α-receptors. Causes decreased peripheral resistance and reduces venous tone.

Indication: Acute myocardial infarction, congestive heart failure, cardiac shock.

Adverse Effects: Marked hypotension, tachycardia.

■ Digitalis Glycosides (Lanoxin; Burroughs Wellcome)

How Supplied: *IV, PO*.

Dose: See *PDR* for digitalizing dose details. Usual dose is 0.25–0.5 mg IV initially, with 0.25 mg q4–6h to total dose of 1.0 mg.

Mechanism of Action: Direct positive inotropic action that causes increased cardiac output and reduces heart size and venous pressure. Promotes diuresis. Has antidysrhythmic action.

Indications: Acute cardiac failure, chronic congestive heart failure.

Adverse Effects: Drug crosses placenta, and serum levels in newborn are similar to maternal levels.

■ Adrenocorticoid Steroids
(See Chapter 15.)

CHAPTER 13

CHEMOTHERAPEUTIC AGENTS

Although the objective of cancer chemotherapy is to achieve selective toxicity against malignant tumor cells while sparing normal cells, this selectivity is rarely achieved. Hence the goal in cancer chemotherapy is to kill malignant cells with doses that will permit the recovery of normal cells. In gynecology, the agents are mostly used as adjuncts to surgery or irradiation to eliminate metastatic tumor cells or for palliative purposes, except in trophoblastic cancer (choriocarcinoma) and germ cell tumors of the ovary, where chemotherapy has replaced surgery as the primary modality of therapy.

In all gynecologic cancers (except choriocarcinoma), combinations of various chemotherapeutic agents are used to obtain maximum tumor-killing effect while decreasing the extreme toxicity of the agents. Various combinations are used, depending on the tumor type and grade, stage of the disease, and patient response.

These agents should be used by physicians trained in oncologic chemotherapy who are totally familiar with dosage regimens, potential immediate or delayed toxic effects, and the care and treatment of women with adverse effects secondary to the chemotherapeutic agents.

Table 13-1 lists chemotherapeutic agents commonly used to treat gynecologic cancers.

ADVERSE EFFECTS

Depending on the agents used, adverse effects may include bone marrow depression, anemia, chromosomal aberrations, renal and hepatic toxicity, oral and gastrointestinal ulceration, coagulation disorders, cardiac toxicity, pulmonary fibrosis, gastrointestinal symptoms, hyperpigmentation, alopecia, fluid retention, hypercalcemia, and cholestatic jaundice, among others.

Table 13-1

CLASSIFICATION OF CHEMOTHERAPEUTIC AGENTS USED IN GYNECOLOGIC CANCER

Agent	Trade Name	Indication	Route of Administration	Manufacturer
ALKYLATING AGENTS				
Chlorambucil	Leukeran	Choriocarcinoma, ovarian	OP	Burroughs Wellcome
Cyclophosphamide	Cytoxan	Choriocarcinoma	IV, OP	Bristol-Myers
	Neosar	Ovarian, endometrial, cervical		Adria
Ifosfamide	Ifex	Ovarian, uterine, fallopian tube sarcoma	IV	Bristol-Myers
Melphalan	Alkeran	Ovarian, uterine	OP, IV	Burroughs Wellcome
Triethylenethio-phosphoramide	Thiotepa	Ovarian	IV	Immunex
ANTIMETABOLITIES				
Methotrexate	Methotrexate	Trophoblastic choriocarcinoma, cervical, ovarian	IV, OP	Immunex, Mylan
5-Fluorouracil	Fluorouracil	Ovarian, endometrial, cervical, trophoblastic	IV	Roche

Continued.

271

Table 13-1

CLASSIFICATION OF CHEMOTHERAPEUTIC AGENTS USED IN GYNECOLOGIC CANCER—Cont'd

Agent	Trade Name	Indication	Route of Administration	Manufacturer
ANTIBIOTICS				
Bleomycin Sulfate	Blenoxane	Cervical, choriocarcinoma	IV, IM	Bristol-Myers
Dactinomycin	Cosmegen	Sarcomas, ovarian	IV	Merck
Doxorubicin HCl	Adriamycin	Cervical, endometrial, ovarian, choriocarcinoma, sarcomas	IV	Adria, Astra
Mitomycin	Mutamycin	Cervical, vaginal, vulva	IV	Bristol-Myers
PLANT ALKALOIDS				
Etoposide	VePesid	Choriocarcinoma, ovarian	IV, OP	Bristol-Myers
Vinblastine Sulfate	Velban	Choriocarcinoma, ovarian, vaginal	IV	Lilly
Vincristine Sulfate	Oncovin	Choriocarcinoma, ovarian, sarcoma	IV	Lilly
HORMONES				
Medroxyprogesterone acetate	Provera Depo-Provera	Endometrial	PO, IM	Upjohn
Megestrol acetate	Megace	Endometrial	PO	Bristol-Myers
Tamoxifen citrate	Nolvadex	Ovarian, breast	PO	Zeneca

Table 13-1

CLASSIFICATION OF CHEMOTHERAPEUTIC AGENTS USED IN GYNECOLOGY CANCER—Cont'd

Agent	Trade Name	Indication	Route of Administration	Manufacturer
MISCELLANEOUS AGENTS				
Cisplatin	Platinol	Cervical, endometrial, ovarian	IV	Bristol-Myers
Carboplatin	Paraplatin	Ovarian, choriocarcinoma	IV	Bristol-Myers
Hydroxyurea	Hydrea	Cervic	OP	Bristol-Myers
Paclitaxel	Taxol	Ovarian	IV	Bristol-Myers

PREGNANCY WARNING

All of the above are classified as Category D or Category X indicating positive evidence of human fetal risk. However, the potential benefits to the pregnant woman may exceed the fetal risk. Appropriate informed consent must be obtained. Nonpregnant women of reproductive age must use effective contraception (usually oral contraceptives) before the start of chemotherapy.

CHAPTER 14

CONTRACEPTIVES

No contraceptive method is 100% effective in preventing pregnancy, completely free of side effects, or fully acceptable to all couples. Each method has its advantages and disadvantages; accordingly, the "best" contraceptive method may be the one the couple will use consistently.

EFFECTIVENESS

Contraceptive effectiveness may be expressed as theoretical effectiveness and use effectiveness. Use effectiveness measures failure rates in actual use and is always higher (less effective) than theoretical effectiveness. Contraceptive effectiveness may be measured by life-table techniques that determine the probability of pregnancy in a given time interval, and is expressed as the number of pregnancies per woman-months of use. Finally, failure rates can be expressed by a mathematical formula (Pearl index), which is defined as the number of pregnancies per 100 women-years of use.

Table 14-1 provides the approximate use effectiveness of commonly used contraceptive methods. The indicated percentages are estimates obtained from the means of many studies. The failure rates may vary considerably, depending on the motivation of the couple, the consistency of use, and the experience of the couple. With continuing use, failure rates generally decline with each method.

SAFETY

The safety of the method must be paramount in advising couples about contraceptive selection. Family planning providers must understand fully each method's potential for adverse side effects, both minor and major. In addition, known risk factors must be taken into account before a method is recommended. Table 14-2 lists potential risk factors for oral contraceptive methods.

Table 14-1

APPROXIMATE ESTIMATES OF USE-EFFECTIVENESS OF VARIOUS CONTRACEPTIVE METHODS

Method	Use-effectiveness (%)*
Male sterilization	99.8
Female sterilization	99.5
Injectable progestin	99
Implantable progestin capsules	99
Oral steroids: combination	98
IUD: copper	98
IUD: progesterone	96
Oral steroids: progestin only	95
Diaphragm and spermicide	90
Condom: male	88
Condom: female	88
Sponge with spermicide	88
Spermicide only	85
Cervical cap	80
Periodic abstinence	75
Withdrawal	70

*Indicated percentages are estimates derived from various published studies.

CONTRACEPTIVE SELECTION

Couples seeking contraceptive advice will differ educationally and economically and in lifestyle, family size preference, and pregnancy spacing requirements. Because of these differences, all couples should be provided with accurate and unbiased information regarding each contraceptive method. In concert with the history and physical examination findings, the provider will then be able to reach a decision as to the "best" contraceptive method for the particular couple.

ORAL CONTRACEPTIVES

Oral contraceptives (OCs) are highly effective in preventing pregnancy. Many formulations containing a synthetic estrogen and progestin or a progestin alone (minipill) are available. The

Table 14-2
POTENTIAL HEALTH RISK FACTORS FOR ORAL CONTRACEPTIVE USE

Risk Factor

Smoking
Hypertension
Migraine
Diabetes
Obesity
Hyperlipidemia
Sickle cell disease
History of thrombophlebitis
Coagulation disorders
Convulsive disorder
Lupus erythematosus
Liver disease
FH of vascular disease
Uterine leiomyomata
Abnormal Pap smear

estrogenic component is in the form of ethinyl estradiol (EE) or mestranol (ME). Currently available progestins include norethindrone (NET), norethindrone acetate (NETA), ethynodiol diacetate (EDDA), norgestrel (NG), levonorgestrel (LNG), desogestrel (DESO), gestodene (GEST) and norgestimate (NORG). Table 14-3 lists the available formulations and their chemical composition. Formulations include monophasic (same combination dose for 21 days), biphasic (one combination dose for 10 days plus different combination dose for 11 days), multiphasic or tricyclic (varying combination doses over 21 days), and progestin only (continuous administration). Most formulations may be obtained in cycle packs of 21 or 28 days. The latter add 7 days of inert ingredients or iron for continuous daily pill administration.

Mechanism of Action

The primary mechanism of action of the combination OC is the progestin and estrogen inhibition of hypothalamic-pituitary gonadotropins secretion, especially the midcycle surge of luteinizing hormone (LH), thereby suppressing ovulation. In addition, alterations occur in the reproductive tract that

Table 14-3
AVAILABLE ORAL CONTRACEPTIVES IN THE UNITED STATES

Trademark	Estrogen	Dose (µg)	Progestin	Dose (mg)	Manufacturer
ESTROGEN, < 50 µG					
Loestrin 1/20,21,28Fe	EE	20	NETA	1.0	Parke-Davis
Loestrin 1.5/30,21,28Fe	EE	30	NETA	1.5	Parke-Davis
Nordette 21,28	EE	30	LNG	0.15	Wyeth-Ayerst
Lo/Ovral 21,28	EE	30	NG	0.3	Wyeth-Ayerst
Levora 21,28	EE	30	LNG	0.15	Syntex
Ovcon 35,21,28	EE	35	NET	0.4	Mead Johnson
Modicon 21,28	EE	35	NET	0.5	Ortho
Ortho-Novum 1/35,21,28	EE	35	NET	1.0	Ortho
Ortho-Cyclen 21,28	EE	35	NORG	0.25	Ortho
Ortho-Cept 21,28	EE	30	DESO	0.15	Ortho
Demulen 1/35,21,28	EE	35	EDDA	1.0	Searle
Norethin 21,28	EE	35	NET	0.5	Searle
Brevicon 21,28	EE	35	NET	1.0	Syntex
Norinyl 1/35,21,28	EE	35	NET	1.0	Syntex
Levlen 21,28	EE	30	LNG	0.15	Berlex
Desogen 28	EE	30	DESO	0.15	Organon
ESTROGEN, 50 µG					
Norinyl 1/50,21,28	ME	50	NET	1.0	Syntex
Ovcon 50,21,28	EE	50	NET	1.0	Mead Johnson
Ortho-Novum 1/50,21,28	ME	50	NET	1.0	Ortho

Table 14-3
AVAILABLE ORAL CONTRACEPTIVES IN THE UNITED STATES—Cont'd

Trademark	Estrogen	Dose (µg)	Progestin	Dose (mg)	Manufacturer
ESTROGEN, 50 µG—cont'd					
Norlestrin 1/50,21,28Fe	EE	50	NETA	1.0	Parke-Davis
Norlestrin 2.5/50,21,28Fe	EE	50	NETA	2.5	Parke-Davis
Ovral 21,28	EE	50	NG	0.5	Wyeth-Ayerst
Demulen 1/50,21,28	EE	50	EDDA	1.0	Searle
Norethin 21,28	EE	50	NET	1.0	Searle
BIPHASIC					
Ortho-Novum 10/11,21,28	10—EE	35	10—NET	0.5	Ortho
	11—EE	35	11—NET	1.0	
Jenest 28	7—EE	35	7—NET	0.5	Organon
	14—EE	35	14—NET	1.0	
TRIPHASIC					
Triphasil 21,28	6—EE	30	6—LNG	0.05	Wyeth-Ayerst
	5—EE	40	5—LNG	0.075	
	10—EE	30	10—LNG	0.125	
Tri-Levlen 21,28	6—EE	30	6—LNG	0.05	Berlex
	5—EE	40	5—LNG	0.075	
	10—EE	30	10—LNG	0.125	

EE, ethinyl estradiol; ME, mestranol; NET, norethindrone; NETA, norethindrone acetate; EDDA, ethynodiol diacetate; NG, norgestrel; LNG, levonorgestrel; DESO, desogestrel; NORG, norgestimate; FE, iron.

Continued.

279

Table 14-3
AVAILABLE ORAL CONTRACEPTIVES IN THE UNITED STATES—Cont'd

Trademark	Estrogen	Dose (µg)	Progestin	Dose (mg)	Manufacturer
TRIPHASIC—cont'd					
Ortho-Novum 7/7/7 21,28	7–EE	35	7–NET	0.5	Ortho
	7–EE	35	7–NET	0.75	
	7–EE	35	7–NET	1.0	
Tri-Norinyl 21, 28	7–EE	35	7–NET	0.5	Syntex
	9–EE	35	9–NET	1.0	
	5–EE	35	5–NET	0.5	
Ortho Tri-Cyclen 21,28	7–EE	35	7–NORG	0.180	Ortho
	7–EE	35	7–NORG	0.215	
	7–EE	35	7–NORG	0.250	
PROGESTAGEN ONLY					
Micronor 28			NET	0.35	Ortho
Ovrette 28			NG	0.075	Wyeth-Ayerst
Nor-Q D 42			NET	0.35	Syntex

280

contribute to contraceptive effectiveness. These include changes in the cervical mucus that retard sperm penetration; endometrial suppression, which interferes with implantation; and changes in the motility and secretions of the fallopian tube, which may interfere with gamete transport.

The progestin-only formulations most probably prevent conception as a result of changes in cervical mucus and suppression of endometrium. Ovulation suppression may occur, however, in some women. The lack of consistent ovulation suppression may lead to a somewhat higher failure rate with the minipill.

Metabolic Effects

Both the estrogen and progestin in OC formulations have numerous metabolic effects and may cause changes in various organ systems. Most of these effects are without clinical significance, merely representing changes in laboratory values. Table 14-4 lists alterations in some laboratory values reported with OC use. In some predisposed women, the metabolic effects and accompanying laboratory value changes may be sufficiently profound to warrant OC discontinuation.

Clinical Use

Absolute contraindications to OC use are listed in Table 14-5, and relative contraindications are in Table 14-6. Careful patient selection is most important in prescribing OC. A complete history, including family history, and a complete physical examination, including a pelvic examination, must be obtained. Should any potential risk factors be present, certain baseline or confirmatory laboratory studies may be obtained.

The starting day of the cycle is specific for each formulation and varies in accordance with packaging; the instructions of the manufacturer should be closely followed.

Women should be started on OC formulations containing no more than 30-35 µg estrogen. Both monophasic and triphasic formulations are acceptable, although the monthly progestin impact is substantially reduced in the triphasic formulations. Animal experiments demonstrate different biologic effects of one or another progestin (i.e., more or less androgenic-estrogenic), but these effects have few, if any, clinical correlations, because estrogen is usually present in each formulation. All OCs have androgenic effects in women, but because of different metabolic pathways and cellular bioavailability characteristics, some

Table 14-4

ALTERATIONS IN LABORATORY VALUES REPORTED WITH ORAL CONTRACEPTIVE USE*

Test/Measurement	Increased	Decreased
Aldosterone	X	
Alkaline phosphatase	X	
Albumin		X
Amylase	X	
Angiotensinogen	X	
Antinuclear antibodies	X	
Antithrombin III		X
ACTH response	Impaired	
BSP test	Impaired	
Bilirubin	X	
Ceruloplasmin	X	
Coagulation factors II, VII, VIII, IX, X, XII	X	
17-Hydroxycorticosteroid excretion		X
17-Ketogenic steroid excretion		X
Cortisol	X	
Complement-reactive protein	X	
Cholinesterase		X
Cholesterol	X	
Erythrocyte count		X
Fibrinogen	X	
FSH (urine, serum)		X
γ-glutamyl transpeptidase	X	
Glucose tolerance test	Impaired	
Growth hormone	X	
Haptoglobin		X
Immunoglobulins (IgA, IgG, IgM)		X
Iron, transferrin	X	
LE cell preparation	Altered	
Lipoproteins		
HDL		X
HDL_2		X
LDL	X	
$ApoA_1$		X
Leucine aminopeptidase	X	
LH (urine, serum)		X
Metyrapone test	Impaired	
Plasminogen	X	

*Adapted from Zatuchni G: Known and potential complications of steroidal contraception. In Becker K, editior: *Principles and practice of endocrinology and metabolism*, 1995.

Table 14-4
ALTERATIONS IN LABORATORY VALUES REPORTED WITH ORAL CONTRACEPTIVE USE*—cont'd

Test/Measurement	Increased	Decreased
Platelet aggregability	X	
Pregnanediol excretion		X
Prolactin	X	
Prothrombin	X	
Sex steroid-binding globulin	X	
Thyroid function		
Thyroid-binding globulin	X	
PBI	X	
T_4	X	
T_3	X	
T_3 uptake		X
Triglycerides	X	
Testosterone	X	

Table 14-5
ABSOLUTE CONTRAINDICATIONS TO ORAL CONTRACEPTIVES

Thrombophlebitis or thromboembolic disorders
Past history of deep vein thrombophlebitis
Cerebral vascular disorders
Coronary artery disease
Breast carcinoma
Endometrial carcinoma
Undiagnosed abnormal uterine bleeding
Cholestatic jaundice of pregnancy
Jaundice with prior pill use
Hepatic adenoma/carcinoma
Known or suspected pregnancy

Table 14-6
RELATIVE CONTRAINDICATIONS: USE ORAL CONTRACEPTIVES WITH CAUTION

Diabetes mellitus, uncomplicated
History of gestational diabetes
History of gallbladder disease
Seizure disorders
Mitral valve prolapse, uncomplicated
Varicose veins
Hypertension, uncomplicated
Uterine leiomyomata
History of pregnancy-induced hypertension
Family history of lipid disorders
Family history of premature cardiovascular disorders
Migraine disorders
Age > 40 years
Heavy smoking

progestins are much more "potent" than others. Accordingly, norgestrel and levonorgestrel (more potent) are formulated in microgram doses, whereas norethindrone and others are in milligram doses. Desogestrel and norgestimate are reported to have reduced androgenic effects.

Initially, women should be given no more than three cycles. A return visit is essential, and if all is in order the woman may be given a prescription for 12 cycles. Annual visits are necessary to ensure that no adverse effects are present. Women with risk factors may require certain laboratory studies before OC use, and these studies may have to be repeated at 6–month intervals.

Minor Side Effects

The most common side effect is breakthrough bleeding or spotting, which results from the inability of the hormones, especially estrogen, to maintain the endometrium for the full 21–day course of therapy. This can occur secondary to hormonal formulation, missed pills, or failure to take the pill at the same time each day. Occasionally bleeding or spotting can occur because of drug interactions as a result of hepatic enzyme changes. Management includes patient reassurance and careful attention to pill use or change in prescription to a higher estrogenic OC.

Failure to have withdrawal bleeding may occur. In these cases it is essential to rule out pregnancy. When this is done, management consists of reassurance with the likelihood of normal withdrawal bleeding in subsequent cycles.

Nausea or vomiting, breast tenderness, weight gain, fluid retention, psychic changes, sleep disturbances, and other symptoms may occur, and usually are manifest in the first two or three cycles of OC use. The occurrence of these symptoms is much reduced with the low-dose formulations. Management is reassurance and symptomatic treatment. Table 14-7 lists reported adverse effects.

Serious Side Effects

Potential risks of OC use include thromboembolic disorders, deep vein thrombophlebitis, cerebrovascular disorders, myocardial infarction, optic neuritis, hepatic adenoma, hypertension, migraine headache, psychic depression, and cervical dysplasia. The most serious risks are related to the cardiovascular and cerebrovascular systems and are thought to be most related to the estrogenic component of OC. Epidemiologic investigations carried out in the late 1960s and early 1970s demonstrated significantly increased relative risks of these conditions in OC users. These studies were done when OCs contained much higher dosages of both estrogen (80–150 µg) and progestin (4–10 mg) than are used currently. In addition, patient selection was not paramount, and risk factors such as older age, smoking, and hypertension were not considered. Since the late 1970s pharmaceutical manufacturers have substantially reduced the daily dosage of both estrogen and progestin. More recent clinical and epidemiologic studies of nonsmoking women taking low-dose OCs have demonstrated no increased risks of fatal or nonfatal stroke or of myocardial infarction. It would appear that in the absence of smoking and certain other well-defined risk factors, there may be no increased risk of cardiovascular or cerebrovascular disease.

Noncontraceptive Benefits of Oral Contraceptive Use

Table 14-8 lists the known or possible benefits to the OC user.

Table 14-7

REPORTED ADVERSE REACTIONS WITH OCs

Increased Risk

Thrombophlebitis with or without embolism
Arterial thromboembolism
Pulmonary embolism
Myocardial infarction
Cerebral hemorrhage
Cerebral thrombosis
Mesenteric thrombosis
Hypertension
Gallbladder disease
Hepatic adenoma
Neuroocular disorders
Congenital anomalies

Drug-related Adverse Reactions

Nausea/vomiting
Gastrointestinal symptoms
Breakthrough bleeding/spotting
Amenorrhea
Temporary infertility after discontinuation
Edema
Chloasma (may persist)
Breast changes
Weight changes (increase/decrease)
Cervical secretion change
Cervical erosion
Cholestatic jaundice
Migraine
Uterine leiomyomata increase
Mental depression
Reduced carbohydrate tolerance
Vaginal candidiasis
Corneal curvature changes
Intolerance to contact lenses
Allergic rash

Table 14-8
NONCONTRACEPTIVE HEALTH BENEFITS OF OC USE

Decreased Incidence of:

Irregular menstrual cycles
Menorrhagia
Iron deficiency anemia
Dysmenorrhea
Functional ovarian cysts
Ectopic pregnancies
Breast fibroadenomas
Fibrocystic disorders of breast
Acute pelvic inflammatory disease
Endometrial cancer
Ovarian cancer

■ Norplant System (Levonorgestrel implants)

Norplant consists of six flexible silastic capsules, each containing 36 mg of levonorgestrel. Each capsule is 34 mm in length and 2.4 mm in diameter. The sterile capsules are inserted into the superficial plane beneath the skin. The release rates of the levonorgestrel provide for effective contraception for up to 5 years.

The mechanism of contraceptive action is similar to other oral steroid progestins.

Contraindications: Same as OCs.

Adverse Reactions: The major adverse reaction is interference with menstrual cycle control, including prolonged bleeding, spotting, amenorrhea, and irregular onset of menses. Rarely does pain or infection occur. There have been reported difficulties with removal of the capsules, especially when they are inserted deeply.

Other adverse reactions have been reported and are similar to oral contraceptive steroid users.

Insertion and Removal

The manufacturer's instructions must be followed carefully. Insertion should be performed during the early part of the menstrual cycle, to avoid an unsuspected pregnancy. Removal of the six capsules must be done at the end of 5 years, and they should be replaced with new capsules should the woman desire continuing use of this contraceptive method.

Depo-Provera
■ Depo-Provera (Contraceptive Injection)

Depo-Provera is a sterile aqueous suspension of medroxyprogesterone acetate, supplied as 150 mg in 1-ml vials. When administered every 3 months by deep intramuscular injection in the gluteal or deltoid muscle, gonadotropin secretion is inhibited and follicular maturation and ovulation does not occur.

The efficacy of this preparation depends on the woman returning every three months for re-injection. When used appropriately, the failure rate is less than 0.5%.

Contraindications: Same as OCs.

Adverse Reactions: The major adverse reaction is interference with menstrual cycle control, including prolonged bleeding, spotting, amenorrhea and irregular onset of menses. After about 12 months of use, approximately 55% of women experience amenorrhea, and after 24 months, 68% report continuing amenorrhea.

Long-term studies found slightly increased or no increased risk of breast cancer, and no increased risk of liver, cervical or ovarian cancer. These studies demonstrated a protective effect against endometrial cancer.

Use of Depo-Provera may increase the risk of development of osteoporosis. The rate of bone loss is highest in the early years of use.

Weight gain may be considerable, averaging about 5 lbs after 1 year, and 13 lbs after 4 years.

Postcoital Contraception

The administration of high-dose estrogen-containing OCs may be useful in preventing pregnancy when a woman has experienced a single unprotected or inadequately protected act of intercourse (e.g., rape). The estrogen must be administered within 72 hours of intercourse, and the patient must be followed up to ensure efficacy. Severe vomiting may occur, preventing adequate therapy. If pregnancy does occur, the patient should be offered elective abortion because of the possibility of fetal anomalies related to high-dose estrogen.

Several regimens are suggested:

- Ovral: 2 tablets stat and 2 tablets at 12 hr.
- Ethinyl estradiol: 2.5 mg bid × 5 days.
- Conjugated estrogens: 10 mg bid × 5 days.
- Estrone: 6 mg tid × 5 days.

Drug Interactions

Oral contraceptives may interact with other drugs, either decreasing the efficacy of the OC or decreasing or potentiating the pharmacologic effect of the concomitant drug. Table 14-9 lists some reported drug interactions. In general, short-term therapy should have no effect on OC use, and vice versa. Complete reference books on drug interactions should be consulted whenever OCs are considered for patients receiving long-term drug therapy.

INTRAUTERINE DEVICES

In 1985 Ortho Pharmaceutical Corp. removed the Lippes Loop from the market, and in 1986 G. D. Searle & Co. discontinued U.S. distribution of the Cu-7 and Cu-T intrauterine devices (IUDs). These voluntary actions were taken because of medicolegal and financial concerns, but these devices still have Food and Drug Administration (FDA) approval; unknown thousands of women are currently using them.

An IUD that releases the natural hormone progesterone (Progestasert, Alza Corp.) is available as a 1-year device. In 1988 GynoPharma introduced a modified Cu-T380A IUD (ParaGard), which is FDA-approved for up to 10 years of continuous intrauterine use.

Intrauterine contraception flourishes outside the United States, with an estimated 90 million women wearing one of more than 30 models available. Intrauterine contraception in the United States reached its maximum of almost 3 million women (9% of contraceptive methods) during 1968 to 1975. Because of both inadequate, inaccurate scientific reporting and nonrecognition of the epidemic of sexually transmitted diseases (STDs), pelvic infection, pelvic inflammatory disease (PID), and tubal infertility almost became synonymous with IUDs, and the Dalkon Shield in particular. It is unfortunate for U.S. women that this highly effective and highly safe method of IUD contraception has been so distorted in the minds of physicians, media, and the public.

Table 14-9
DRUG INTERACTIONS

Drug	Comment
ANTIBIOTICS Ampicillin Chloramphenicol Isoniazid Nitrofurantoin Penicillin Rifampin Sulfonamide Tetracycline	May reduce OC efficacy; spotting or contraceptive failure. Short-term therapy, use additional method. Long-term therapy, switch to another method.
ANTICONVULSANTS Barbiturates Ethosuximide Phenytoin	Liver metabolism may affect estrogen/progestin levels; may result in spotting/bleeding or contraceptive failure. Steroids may increase fluid retention.
ANTIDIABETIC AGENTS Insulin Oral hypoglycemic agents	Glucose tolerance may be impaired; use OCs with caution.
ANTIHYPERTENSIVE AGENTS Guanethidine Methyldopa	OCs may cause increased angiotensinogen; use with caution.
ANTIINFLAMMATORY AGENTS Phenylbutazone	May interfere with OC efficacy. OCs may accentuate agent's effects.
β–BLOCKERS	Estrogen decreases response.
HYPNOTICS	Same effects as anticonvulsants.
TRANQUILIZERS Phenothiazine Reserpine Tricyclics	Effect potentiated by OCs. May require dosage adjustments.

The Progestasert and ParaGard are safe and effective IUDs in certain highly selected women. Each of the two devices has different characteristics regarding effectiveness, complications and side effects, approved duration of use, and cost.

Mechanism of Action

1. Intrauterine devices cause a sterile inflammatory leukocytic response that is spermatotoxic and interferes with sperm transport.
2. Intrauterine devices cause many physiologic changes in the endometrium, which cumulatively prevent the implantation of the blastocyst should fertilization occur.
3. Copper IUDs increase local prostaglandin secretion, which increases uterine contractions, making blastocystic implantation less favorable.
4. The Progestasert IUD releases 65 µg/day progesterone into the intrauterine cavity, with resulting endometrial glandular suppression and inappropriate proliferative response, making implantation unlikely.
5. Daily intrauterine progesterone release suppresses both uterine and tubal muscular activity, which may interfere with gamete transport.

Effectiveness

The rates of effectiveness and continuation of use depend on the type and size of IUD, experience of the inserter, appropriate intrauterine placement, and individual characteristics such as age, parity, and cultural determinants. The Cu-T380A IUD has a 1–year failure rate of less than 1%, and the progesterone-releasing IUD about 2%–3%.

The IUD event rates include pregnancy, expulsion, medical removals related to bleeding, pain, infection, and other reasons; and elective removal (desire for pregnancy). These events are usually portrayed as a life-table analysis for each year of use, a 12 mo rate, and for more than 1 year/cumulative. The event rates per woman-months of use are given in Table 14-10, and represent figures drawn from many studies.

Patient Selection

A major concern with IUDs is their association with PID. However, IUDs do not cause PID; only certain bacteria and other

▎Table 14-10
▎**IUD EVENT RATES**

	Progestesert*		ParaGard (Cu-T380A)†			
	12 Months		Months of Use (Annual Rates)			
EVENT	PAROUS	NULLIPAROUS	12	36	60	120
Pregnancy	1.3	2.1	0.7	0.6	0.3	0.0
Expulsion	2.7	7.6	5.7	1.6	0.3	0.4
Med? removal, bleeding/pain	9.3	12.0	11.9	7.0	3.7	3.7
Med? removal, other	4.2	4.9	2.5	1.6	0.1	0.3
Total continuation	81.2	73.4	76.8	81.2	89.0	91.8

*Data from Alza Corp, Palo Alto, Calif, 1986.
†Combined Population Council and WHO Studies.

organisms do. It is essential that the physician determine the relative risk of the woman for STDs, and if she is at high risk, an IUD should not be advised.

IUD Insertion

Absolute and relative contraindications to IUD insertion are given in Tables 14-11 and 14-12, respectively.

Informed Consent

Each patient must be provided the extensive information regarding IUD contraception prepared by the manufacturer. At the return visit, all questions and concerns must be addressed. Documentation (for medicolegal purposes) of informed consent to this procedure is mandatory and requires patient acknowledgment and signature that she has read, understands, and discussed all of the risks with her physician.

Insertion Technique

The manufacturer's instructions to the physician must be read before IUD insertion, because each of the two currently available IUDs requires somewhat different insertion steps.

Table 14-11
ABSOLUTE CONTRAINDICATIONS TO IUD INSERTION

1. Known or suspected pregnancy
2. Acute/subacute pelvic infection, lower/upper reproductive tract
3. History salpingitis or PID, regardless of etiology
4. Untreated acute cervicitis/vaginitis, until infection is controlled
5. History of ectopic pregnancy
6. Impaired response to infection (e.g., diabetes, corticosteroid treatment)
7. Multiple sexual partners
8. Coagulation disorders (anticoagulation therapy)
9. Endometrial cavity less than 6.5 cm measured by sound
10. Uterine cavity distortion (e.g., fibroids, congenital anomaly)
11. Allergy to copper (or Wilson's disease)
12. Cervical or endometrial malignancy
13. Abnormal Pap smear or cervical dysplasia
14. Valvular heart disease
15. Unexplained genital tract bleeding
16. Previously inserted IUD that has not been removed

Table 14-12
RELATIVE CONTRAINDICATIONS TO IUD INSERTION

1. Severe dysmenorrhea/menorrhagia
2. Anemia
3. Endometriosis
4. Endometrial cavity greater than 9.0 cm measured by sound
5. Multiple (2 or more) cesarian sections
6. Previous myomectomy procedure
7. Cervical stenosis
8. History of pelvic actinomycosis
9. History of severe vasovagal reaction
10. History of herpes genitalis or syphilis
11. Nulliparity

Precautions:

1. Insertion of an IUD always introduces cervical bacteria and other organisms into the endometrial cavity, although postinsertion (up to 4 months) pelvic infection is unlikely to occur unless the dose and virulence of the organism is capable of overcoming natural defense mechanisms. Some recommend the administration of prophylactic antibiotics (e.g., doxycycline) 100 mg bid × 3 days, starting about 12 hours before insertion. Other regimens may be equally useful.

2. The recommended time of insertion is just after menstrual flow has stopped. To obviate the possibility of menstrual blood serving as a culture medium, some physicians perform insertions during the second week of the cycle. In the postpartum period, IUD insertion should be delayed until the eighth week because of the higher risk of uterine perforation if done earlier.

3. Careful bimanual examination must be accomplished to ascertain the presence of abnormalities contraindicating IUD insertion and to determine the uterine axis.

4. Sterile techniques, including preinsertion cervical antisepsis, must be observed.

5. Intracervical and paracervical block with local anesthetic is desirable to assist cervical dilation and prevent vasovagal reaction.

6. The anterior lip of the cervix is grasped with a single-tooth tenaculum to obtain traction, thereby straightening the endocervical canal and lower uterine segment. This is essential to prevent uterine perforation, especially with an anteriorly flexed or posteriorly retroflexed fundus.

7. The uterus must be sounded gently; perforation can occur. The measurement should be noted, and if it is less than 6.5 cm (top of fundus to external cervical os), the IUD should not be inserted. Inappropriate fitting may lead to expulsion, cramping pain, infection, or pregnancy.

8. All IUDs must be placed high in the uterine fundus in the horizontal axis, never in the lower uterine segment or intracervical canal.

9. The tailstring requires cutting, leaving approximately 5–6 cm (or longer with postpartum insertion). The tail serves the dual purposes of patient reassurance that the IUD has not been expelled or perforated and provides easy physician removal of the IUD when necessary.

Table 14-13
POTENTIAL ADVERSE EFFECTS OF IUD USE

1. Syncope secondary to IUD insertion causing a vasovagal response
2. Partial/complete expulsion
3. Severe cramping pain
4. Abnormal uterine bleeding, especially menorrhagia
5. Uterine perforation (partial or complete)
6. Cervical perforation by vertical arm of IUD
7. Chronic cervicitis (inflammatory Pap smear)
8. Intermittent leukorrhea from chronic endometritis/cervicitis
9. Spontaneous abortion with/without sepsis
10. Genital actinomycotic infection
11. Salpingitis (PID)
12. Tubal infertility
13. Ectopic pregnancy

10. Contraceptive protection may not be assured in the first
    month of IUD use. It is recommended, therefore, that an
    additional barrier method be used. Some women desiring
    even greater long-term effectiveness may be advised to use
    an additional barrier method during ovulation.

Complications of IUD Use

Approximately 20% of patients will require IUD removal
during the first year, primarily because of irregular or heavy
bleeding and cramping pain, another 5%–7% will expel the IUD.

Potential adverse effects of IUD use are given in Table 14-13.

"Missing" IUD Tailstring

If the string cannot be felt by the patient or seen by the physician, it is mandatory that an investigation be done to ascertain the
status of the IUD. Several possibilities include unnoticed expulsion, perforation, retraction of the string into the uterus or endocervical canal, or pregnancy. Ultrasound localization is easily
accomplished.

Perforation of the Uterus

Perforation of the uterus is most likely to occur at the time of
insertion and may be partial (embedment) or complete. If perforation is partial, the IUD can be removed blindly by grasping

techniques or may require hysteroscopy. If the uterus is completely perforated, mandatory removal of the IUD is necessary and may be accomplished through a laparoscope.

Intrauterine Pregnancy

There is a significantly increased risk of spontaneous abortion during the first trimester, and about 50% of IUD wearers abort. An IUD increases somewhat the risk of a second-trimester abortion, and the IUD has been associated with premature labor in the early third trimester.

As pregnancy advances, the IUD tailstring may be pulled up into the endometrial cavity, potentially introducing pathogenic organisms, especially anaerobes. Should this occur (every pregnant woman is at risk), septic abortion may ensue with its significant risk of mortality. Accordingly, women determined to have an intrauterine pregnancy with an IUD in situ should be advised to have an elective termination. Intrauterine devices have been successfully removed from a pregnant uterus, under ultrasound guidance, when the IUD was located inferior to the fetal sac.

The IUD has not been associated with any congenital anomaly formation.

Ectopic Pregnancy

There is no question that ectopic pregnancies occur more frequently among all IUD wearers. It has been reported that among all IUDs, the Progestasert carries the highest risk of associated ectopic pregnancy, a sixfold to tenfold frequency of ectopic pregnancies compared with copper IUDs. Whether IUDs are causally related is still somewhat controversial; however, the physician must have a high index of suspicion for ectopic pregnancy in every past or present IUD user.

Pelvic Infection

Upper tract pelvic infection occurring during the first 4 months of IUD use most probably is the result of the inadvertant introduction of pathogenic organisms. After this period, the occurrence of upper tract pelvic infection most likely is due to a sexually transmitted organism, such as gonococcus, *Chlamydia,* or anaerobes. The role of the IUD tail in the possible transmission of bacteria from the vagina and cervix to the endometrium and endosalpinx is highly controversial.

When pelvic infection occurs, appropriate bacteriologic studies should be accomplished, broad-spectrum antibiotics administered, and the IUD removed within about 24 hours. Close monitoring of the patient is required, especially for the increased risk of pelvic abscess formation.

Actinomyces *Infection*

Actinomyces, an anaerobic gram-positive bacteria, is occasionally reported on a cytologic Pap smear from IUD wearers. Should this occur, appropriate antibiotic therapy (e.g., ampicillin, 250 mg qid × 14 days) is applied. If results of repeat cytology are still positive, the IUD should be removed.

Fertility After IUD Discontinuation

Most recent studies indicate that pregnancy rates after IUD termination are similar to non-IUD users. Nevertheless, "asymptomatic" salpingitis can occur among IUD users as it does among nonusers. Tubal infertility may be the end result of this previously unrecognized sexually transmitted infection.

VAGINAL CONTRACEPTION

Vaginal insertion of various substances or devices intended to act as a barrier to sperm (semen) or to render the semen "harmless" has been practiced by women since 1500 BC. Efficacy of these substances is unknown, but many have spermicidal properties. Contraceptive sponges were used by the Egyptians, Hebrews, Chinese, and Greeks before the Christian era. In 1564 AD, Fallopius (Italian anatomist) described a linen sheath for men as protection against syphilis. During the 19th century, the cervical cap, condom, and diaphragm were invented and marketed as contraceptives in Europe. Goodyear patented the process of rubber vulcanization in 1884 and began providing condoms. The first contraceptive suppository was marketed in England in 1885, and in 1906 the first commercially produced spermicidal jelly was introduced in Germany.

Effectiveness

Published studies of effectiveness of vaginal contraceptive methods provide numbers that cover the entire range from "highly effective" to "not very effective." Because all of these methods are user dependent, their efficacy will be determined by the motivation of the couple and the appropriate and correct use of the methods. Although Table 14-1 provides a comparison of estimated use-effectiveness rates for various contraceptive methods, it must be emphasized in the use of barrier methods that the individual couple's experience may be far better or far worse than the indicated percentages.

Condom

The condom, or sheath, the only available, effective, and reversible male contraceptive method, was first introduced as a method for preventing the transmission of syphilis (hence the name prophylactic). Recent surveys indicate that the condom is used by about 20% of couples. Manufacturing standards and quality control have reduced the theoretical failure rate to less than 1% (condom holes or breakage during use). The use-effectiveness rate is considerably higher, varying from 4% to 12% failure, and is highly dependent on appropriate and proper use.

Except for a rare individual who is allergic to latex rubber, there are no contraindications. Table 14-14 lists the indications for condom use.

The condom, unlike other methods, is highly effective for preventing the spread of STDs including gonorrhea, syphilis, *Chlamydia,* herpes, *Trichomonas,* and *Gardnerella.* Recently, it has been shown that the acquired immunodeficiency syndrome (AIDS) virus cannot pass through the pores of a latex condom, but the virus may pass through the larger pores of a "natural" condom made of processed tissue from animal intestines.

Spermicidal substances in the form of surfactants have been shown (in vitro) to kill most organisms responsible for STDs, including the viruses of herpes and AIDS. Since 1982, several condom manufacturers have packaged condoms in spermicidal solution (nonoxynol-9), both for added contraceptive protection and STD prevention.

Manufacturing and Packaging

Condoms produced in the United States must meet vigorous FDA standards, including quality control. Except for two products made of lamb intestine (Fourex, Schmid Labs.; Naturalamb, Carter-Wallace), all condoms are made of latex rubber or

Table 14-14
INDICATIONS FOR CONDOM USE

Contraindications to OC or IUD use
High-risk situations for STD
Aversion to manipulating genitalia
Infrequent sexual intercourse
    Premarital
    Older reproductive age
Additional contraceptive protection required
    First OC cycle
    Missed pills
    First month IUD use
    Midcycle IUD use
    First 1 or 2 cycles vaginal diaphragm use
Early postpartum/postabortal period
Additional backup for less-effective methods (foam, suppository)
Presence of active genital infections under treatment
Intercourse during menstruation
Psychological aversion to semen contact
Enhance sexual response
Premature ejaculation
Penile sensitivity to vaginal secretions/spermicides
Infertility secondary to sperm antibody formation
Postvasectomy until semen free of sperm

CONTRACEPTIVES

polyurethane. Approximately 70 varieties are made of thin, opaque or transparent rubber, with a blunt or teat end (reservoir), cylindrical or contoured, ribbed or textured, choice of color, and lubricated with spermicidal silicone solution or powdered. Packaged in aluminum foil, they have a shelf life of about 2 years, especially if kept in a cool place.

Female Condom

This device consists of a polyurethane sheath with two flexible rings; one at the closed end is similar to a diaphragm ring; the second ring remains outside the vagina covering the labia. The failure rate averages about 12%, although FDA labeling indicates a 25% failure rate.

The device may be useful in preventing the transmission of disease-producing organisms, including viruses. However, no clinical studies are available to support this concept.

Vaginal Diaphragm

The diaphragm is a latex dome-shaped device that is inserted into the vagina before intercourse. Spermicidal preparations must be used in conjunction with the diaphragm to obtain maximum effectiveness.

Effectiveness

The diaphragm-plus-spermicide method is a highly effective means of preventing pregnancy, provided the diaphragm is properly fitted and consistently used. Reported use-failure rates vary from 2% to 18%; effectiveness is highly dependent on the motivation of the couple to use the method at all times of sexual exposure and in the correct manner.

Indications

The diaphragm-plus-spermicide should be used when there is desire for female fertility control. Some women desiring intercourse during menses use the diaphragm as a menstrual cup.

Contraindications

1. Allergy to latex or spermicide
2. Anatomic abnormalities of the vagina or uterus that prevent correct fitting
3. Postpartum period (to 8 weeks)
4. Inability to learn correct placement
5. History of repeated urinary tract infections
6. History of toxic shock syndrome

Available Types

Currently four types of diaphragms are available in sizes 50 to 105 mm in diameter, in 5 mm increments.

Flat Spring.   The flat spring consists of a flat, narrow spring-steel band forming a ring covered by latex rubber shaped into a dome. The steel ring permits compressibility in one plane only, thus facilitating insertion and lateral compression against the vaginal wall.

Coil Spring.   The coil spring is identical to the flat spring type except the ring is made of corded wire that allows flexibility in both lateral and frontal planes.

Arcing Spring.   The circumference of the diaphragm is a dual spring within a spring, allowing elasticity in all directions. It is especially recommended for women with minor degrees of uterine or vaginal wall prolapse or in women with retroverted uterus.

Wide Seal Rim. A flexible latex flange is attached to the inner edge of the diaphragm rim. Two models, the coil spring and arcing spring, are available. The wide seal (flange) theoretically creates a better seal at the vaginal walls and also serves to hold the spermicide in place.

Fitting

Adequate protection is ensured by selecting the type and size of the diaphragm according to the woman's individual measurements and her anatomic vaginal configuration. Although each type has its own particular advantages, satisfactory results may be obtained with all types. The appropriate diaphragm is the largest one that fits snugly into the plane between the posterior fornix of the vagina and the retropubic groove without being "noticed" by the woman. Table 14-15 lists available contraceptive diaphragms.

Safety Concerns

1. Toxic shock syndrome has been reported among women who did not remove the diaphragm within 24 hr.
2. Repeated urinary tract infections may be associated with diaphragm use.
3. Ulcerations of the vagina and cervix have been reported after prolonged continuous use of the diaphragm.
4. Allergic dermatitis in women and men has been reported because of either the latex rubber or spermicidal ingredient.
5. Use of the diaphragm plus spermicide may prevent sexually transmitted infections in women, including herpes and AIDS.

Cervical Cap

The cervical cap is a minidiaphragm that fits over the cervix, and when properly fitted and used with spermicide can be a relatively effective method of contraception. Varying models have been used in Europe for many years, but only recently (1988) has one been approved for use in the United States, Prentif Cavity Rim Cervical Cap (Lamberts).

The cap is available in four different sizes (22, 25, 28, and 31 mm internal rim diameter), and must be fitted by a trained individual. The intended user must receive detailed instructions on how to insert and remove the cap. The FDA has approved 48-hour continuous use. Extensive experience with the method is not yet available. A research study conducted in the United States indicated a 1–year failure rate of 17.4 for 100 women-years of use, and a continuation rate of 59% at 12 months.

▌Table 14-15
VAGINAL DIAPHRAGM

Trade Name	Type	Sizes (mm)	Manufacturer
Koroflex Arcing Spring diaphragm	Arcing spring	60–95	Schmid
Koromex Coil Spring Diaphragm	Coil spring	60–95	Schmid
Ortho Diaphragm Kit, All Flex	Arcing/dual spring	55–95	Ortho
Ortho Diaphragm Kit, Coil Spring	Coil spring	50–105	Ortho
Ortho Diaphragm Kit, Flat Spring	Flat spring	55–95	Ortho
Wide Seal Arcing Diaphragm	Arcing	60–95	Milex
Wide Seal Omniflex Diaphragm	Coil	60–95	Milex

Indications

1. Women who are unable or unwilling to use more effective methods.
2. Where anatomic changes may preclude diaphragm use (e.g., mild vaginal prolapse, narrow vagina).

Contraindications

1. Allergy to latex rubber or spermicide.
2. History of repeated urinary tract infections.
3. Abnormal Pap smears or previous cervical dysplasia.
4. Acute or subacute cervicitis or vaginitis.
5. Postpartum period up to 8 weeks.
6. Anatomic configuration of the cervix that precludes satisfactory fitting.
7. Inability of the woman to insert or remove the cervical cap correctly.
8. History of toxic shock syndrome.

Vaginal Spermicides

Table 14-16 indicates the effects of the vehicle on time and duration of effectiveness of spermicidal preparations. They include foams, creams, gels, jellies, suppositories, film, and sponge. All preparations have a chemical surfactant (nonoxynol-9

Table 14-16
CHARACTERISTICS OF VAGINAL SPERMICIDAL AGENTS

Vehicle	Time to Effectiveness	Duration of Effectiveness
Cream	Immediate	1–2 hr
Foam	Immediate	1–2 hr
Jelly (gel)	Immediate	1–2 hr
Foaming tablet	10–15 min	1–2 hr
Suppository	10–15 min	1–2 hr
Film	10 minutes	1–2 hr

CONTRACEPTIVES

or octoxynol-9) as the principal spermicidal agent. These surfactants have long-chain alkyl groups that penetrate the lipoprotein membrane of sperm, increasing its permeability and leading to loss of motility and destruction. Many of the spermicidal preparations can be used alone or in combination with diaphragm, cervical cap, or condom.

Table 14-17 provides some examples of each category of spermicidal preparations. The use-effectiveness rates vary considerably, depending primarily on their appropriate use and consistency of use, factors that are entirely consumer dependent. Published series indicate failure rates from 3% to 20%.

Indications

1. Primary method of contraception.
2. Backup method (e.g., first month of OC or IUD use, postpartum period, breast feeding).
3. Additional contraception required (e.g., IUD use, condoms, time of ovulation).
4. Some preparations can be used with a diaphragm or cervical cap.
5. Woman at risk of contracting a STD.

Contraindications

1. Allergy to spermicidal ingredient.

Special Considerations

Nonoxynol-9 is a potent detergent that in vitro has been shown to destroy bacteria, viruses, and other organisms, in particular those that can cause STDs (e.g., gonococcus, *Chlamydia,*

Table 14-17

EXAMPLES OF VAGINAL SPERMICIDAL PRODUCTS

Trade Name	Active Ingredient (Amount)	Manufacturer
CREAM		
Ortho-Creme	Nonoxynol–9 (2%)	Ortho
Koromex Cream	Octoxynol–9 (9%)	Schmid
JELLIES		
Conceptrol Gel	Nonoxynol–9 (100 mg)	Ortho
Gynol-II	Nonoxynol–9 (2%)	Ortho
Koromex Jelly	Nonoxynol–9 (3%)	Schmid
Ortho-Gynol	Octoxynol–9 (1%)	Ortho
FOAMS		
Because	Nonoxynol–9 (8%)	Schering
Delfen	Nonoxynol–9 (12.5%)	Ortho
Emko	Nonoxynol–9 (8%)	Schering
Koromex	Nonoxynol–9 (12.5%)	Schmid
SUPPOSITORIES		
Encare	Nonoxynol–9 (100 mg)	Thompson Medical
Intercept	Nonoxynol–9 (100 mg)	Ortho
Semicid	Nonoxynol–9 (100 mg)	Whitehall

Gardnerella, Trichomonas, Treponema, Pallidum [syphilis], herpes, and human immunodeficiency virus). Accordingly, spermicidal preparations may provide increased protection against STDs and should be recommended as an additional method whenever there is a high-risk situation.

Several studies have investigated the possible role of spermicidal use and the development of congenital anomalies and chromosomal defects after the publication of a study done by telephone interviews of supposed spermicidal users. At least two recent epidemiologic investigations that included large numbers of women reporting various birth defects demonstrated convincingly that spermicidal use during the time of conception, implantation, and early pregnancy was not associated with any known birth defect.

CHAPTER 15

DIURETICS

MECHANISM OF ACTION

All diuretics interfere with the reabsorption of sodium, chloride, or both in the renal tubules.

TYPES

Table 15-1 lists selected diuretics.

1. *Loop*: Blocks active transport of NaCI in loop of Henle.
2. *Potassium sparing:* Interferes with sodium reabsorption in the distal tubules but conserves potassium.
3. *Thiazides:* Block reabsorption of NaCI in the distal tubules; may cause kaliuresis and decrease serum potassium level.
4. *Osmotic:* Prevents reabsorption of water in the proximal tubules, thereby impairing reabsorption of sodium; increases hypertonicity in loop of Henle.
5. *Carbonic anhydrase inhibitors:* Reduce sodium bicarbonate reabsorption in the proximal tubules, thereby enhancing sodium excretion.

USES

1. Contraindicated during pregnancy unless there is a compelling medical indication (e.g., nephrotic syndrome, congestive heart failure)
2. Congestive heart failure
3. Hypertension
4. Chronic renal failure
5. Nephrotic syndrome
6. Acute renal failure
7. Other edematous conditions (e.g., cerebral edema)
8. Acute mountain (high altitude) sickness
9. Glaucoma
10. Intraocular surgery

ADVERSE EFFECTS

Adverse effects depend on specific type of diuretics. In general, loss of electrolytes may result in dizziness, fatigue, leg cramps, and potential detrimental effects of other drugs (e.g., potassium loss increases digitalis toxicity). Spironolactone carries theoretical teratogenicity (ambiguous genitalia in male fetus).

Table 15-1
SELECTED DIURETICS

Type-Drug	Brand Name (Mfr.)	How Supplied	Usual Starting Dose	Duration of Action (hr)
LOOP				
Furosemide	Lasix (Hoechst-Roussel)	20,40,80 mg tabs 10 mg/ml amp, syringe	20–80 mg single dose	Oral, 6 IV, 2
Ethacrynic Acid	Edecrin (Merck)	25,50 mg tabs, 5 mg vial	50–100 mg daily	Same as Lasix
Bumetanide	Bumex (Roche)	0.5, 1,2, mg tabs 0.25 mg/ml amp	0.5–mg daily	Same as Lasix
POTASSIUM SPARING				
Amiloride	Midamor (Merck)	5 mg tab	5 mg daily with food	
Spironolactone	Aldactone (Searle)	25,50,100 mg tabs	25–200 mg daily	
Triamterene	Dyrenium (Smith-Kline Beecham)	50,100 mg caps	100 mg bid pc	

Continued.

DIURETICS

307

Table 15-1

SELECTED DIURETICS—Cont'd

Type-Drug	Brand Name (Mfr.)	How Supplied	Usual Starting Dose	Duration of Action (hr)
THIAZIDES				
Chlorothiazide	Diuril (Merck)	50,500 mg tab; susp	500–1000 mg O.D.	6–12
Hydrochlorothiazide	Hydrodiuril (Merck)	25,50,100 mg tabs	50–100 mg O.D.	6–12
	Esidrix (CIBA)	25,50,200 mg tabs	50–100 mg O.D.	6–12
	Oretic (Sabbott)	25,50 mg tabs	25–100 mg O.D.	6–12
Hydroflumethiazide	Diucardin (Wyeth-Ayerst)	50 mg tab	50–100 mg O.D.	18–24
Methyclothiazide	Enduron (Abbott)	1,5,5 mg tabs	2.5–10 mg O.D.	24+
Quinethazone	Hydromox (Lederle)	50 mg tab	50–100 mg O.D.	18–24
OSMOTIC				
Mannitol	Mannitol	25% solution in	Individualize	
	Injection (Astra)	50 ml vial/syringe		
CARBONIC ANHYDRASE INHIBITOR				
Acetazolamide	Diamox (Lederle)	125,250 mg tabs	250 mg bid	12
		500 mg cap		

CHAPTER 16

GLUCOCORTICOIDS (ADRENAL CORTICOSTEROIDS)

Glucocorticoids are produced or derived from the adrenal cortex and are useful as antiinflammatory agents or immunomodulators. The basic mechanism of action is to decrease the inflammatory process at the molecular and cellular levels, thus attenuating the clinical response to certain inflammatory conditions. Corticosteroid therapy should be initiated only after less toxic drugs have proven ineffective.

The dosage should be based on the disease condition and severity, with the smallest amount of corticosteroid used to control the condition. The duration of therapy depends on the clinical response and the development of adverse effects.

INDICATIONS

1. Allergic disorders (e.g., rhinitis, asthma)
2. Collagen diseases (e.g., SLE)
3. Hematologic diseases (e.g., ITP)
4. Respiratory distress of newborn
5. Shock states (e.g., cerebral edema)
6. Ophthalmic diseases

ADVERSE EFFECTS

1. GI disorders, especially peptic ulcer
2. Electrolyte imbalances, especially hypokalemia, sodium retention
3. Osteoporosis (with long-term use)
4. CNS effects (euphoria, vertigo, convulsions)
5. Lipids and carbohydrate metabolic changes
6. Decreased resistance to infection
7. Fetal adrenal hypoplasia

CLASSIFICATION

Adrenal corticosteroids can be classified by their duration of activity: short-acting, intermediate, or long-acting. The drugs are also classified by their potency as glucocorticoids (Table 16-1).

AVAILABLE PRODUCTS

Glucocorticoids are available for oral, IM, IV, and IA administration and for topical use (Tables 16-2 and 16-3).

GLUCOCORTICOIDS FOR FETAL PULMONARY MATURITY

Glucocorticoids have been used up to 34 weeks gestation to lower the incidence of RDS and decrease its severity. The apparent mechanism of action is the placental transport of the drug to the fetus with resulting increased production of pulmonary surfactants. This action requires at least 24 hours. Therapy must not be started unless amniocentesis reveals pulmonary immaturity.

Table 16-1

CLASSIFICATION OF GLUCOCORTICOIDS

Drug	Potency	Equivalent Dose (mg)
SHORT ACTING		
Hydrocortisone	1	20
Cortisone	0.8	25
INTERMEDITAE ACTING		
Methylprednisolone	5	4
Prednisolone	4	5
Prednisone	4	5
Triamcinolone	5	4
LONG ACTING		
Betamethasone	25	0.60
Dexamethasone	25	0.75
Paramethasone	10	2

TABLE 16-2
SOME AVAILABLE CORTICOSTEROIDS

Drug	Brand Name (Mfr.)	How Supplied
Hydrocortisone	Hydrocortone (Merck)	Susp: 25/50 mg/ml
	Hydrocortone acetate (Merck)	Susp: 25/50 mg/ml
	Hydrocortone phosphate (Merck)	Solution: 50 mg/ml
	Hydrocortisone Na Succinate	
	Solu-cortef (Upjohn)	Powder: 100 mg
Cortisone	Cortone acetate (Merck)	Susp: 25/50 mg/ml
		Tabs: 25 mg
Methylprednisolone	Medrol (Upjohn)	Tabs: 2, 4, 8, 16, 24, 32 mg
	Depo-Medrol (Upjohn)	Susp: 20, 40 80 mg/ml
	Solu-Medrol (Upjohn)	Powder: 40, 125, 500, 1000 mg
Prednisolone	Delta-Cortef (Upjohn)	Tabs: 5 mg
	Hydeltra-T.B.A. (Merck)	Susp: 20 mg/ml
Prednisone	Deltasone (Upjohn)	Tabs: 2.5, 5, 10, 20, 50 mg
Triamcinolone	Aristocort (Abbott)	Tabs: 1, 2, 4, 8, 16 mg
	Kenacort (Bristol-Myers Squibb)	Tabs: 4, 8 mg
	Aristospan (Lederle)	Susp: 5, 20 mg/ml
Betamethasone	Celestone (Schering)	Tabs: 0.6 mg
		Syrup: 0.6 mg/5 ml
	Celestone Soluspan (Schering)	Susp: 0.6 mg/5 ml
Dexamethasone	Decadron (Merck)	Tabs: 0.25, 0.5, 0.75, 1.5, 4, 6 mg
		Elixir: 0.5 mg/5 ml
	Hexadrol (Organon)	Tabs: 0.5, 0.75, 1.5 mg

Table 16-3

SOME TOPICAL CORTICOSTEROIDS

Drug	Brand Name (Mfr.)	How Supplied
Alclomethasone dipropionate	Aclovate (Glaxo)	Cream/ung: 0.05%
Betamethasone dipropionate	Alphatrex (Savage)	Cream/ung/lotion: 0.05%
Triamcinolone acetonide	Aristocort (Fujisawa)	Cream: 0.025%, 0.1%, 0.5% Ung: 0.1%
Betamethasone valerate	Betatrex (Savage)	Cream/ung/lotion: 0.1%
Amcrinonide	Cyclocort (Fujisawa)	Cream/lotion: 0.1%
Betamethasone dipropionate	Diprolene (Schering)	Cream/ung/lotion: 0.05%
Fluocinonide	Lidex (Syntex)	Cream/ung/lotion: 0.05%
Hydrocortisone	Synacort (Syntex)	Cream: 1%, 2.5%
Fluocinolone acetonide	Synalar (Syntex)	Cream/ung/solution: 0.025, 0.01%
Desoximetasone	Topicort (Hoechst-Roussel)	Gel/ung: 0.05%, 0.25%
Desonide	Tridesilon (Miles)	Cream/ung: 0.05%

Contraindications

Absolute:

- Maternal febrile illness
- Amnionitis
- Herpes simplex virus type 2
- Imminent delivery

Relative:

Hypertension, diabetes mellitus, peptic ulcer
- Intrauterine growth retardation

Selection of Corticosteroid and Dose

The duration of corticosteroid activity is the most important parameter in drug selection. The following drugs and schedule have been suggested by various authors:

Betamethasone: *IM*, 12 mg q12h × 2 doses.

Dexamethasone: *IM*, 4 mg q8h × 6 doses.

Hydrocortisone: *IV*, 500 mg q12h × 4 doses.

CHAPTER 17

GASTROINTESTINAL PREPARATIONS

ANTACIDS

Common antacid preparations are listed in Table 17-1.

General Principles

1. Acid-neutralizing capacity (ANC): Number of mEq of 1N HCl raised to pH 3.5 in 15 min.
2. Standard ingredients:
   a. Basic anion: Hydroxide, carbonate, bicarbonate, citrate, trisilicate.
   b. Metallic cation: Aluminum, magnesium, calcium, sometimes in combination.
   c. Simethicone: Surface active agent sometimes included to disperse foam, decrease esophageal reflex and dyspepsia, and act as antiflatulent.

How Supplied:
PO: Chewable tablets and suspensions (see Table 17-1), NG tube.

Administration:
PO: Poorly and variably absorbed.

Dose: 15–45 ml q3–6h or 1 and 3 hr pc and qhs.

Mechanism of Action: Basic compounds neutralize acid in gastric contents; alkalinization also increases lower esophageal pressure and esophageal clearance.

Elimination: Fecal excretion largely as unreacted insoluble antacids.

Indication: Peptic duodenal and gastric ulcer (high doses; often given with cimetidine); reflex esophagitis; before induction

17-1
COMMON ANTACID PREPARATIONS*

Product	Content (mg per 5 ml) Metallic cation	Sodium†	ANC‡	CaCO‡
Amphojel	320 Al $(OH)_3$ gel	<2.3	10	—
Di-Gel	282 Al $(OH)_3$, 87 Mg $(OH)_2$ (20 Simethicone)	—	—	280
Gaviscon	95 Al $(OH)_3$, 358 Mg CO_3 and Na alginate	13	4	—
Gelusil§	200 Al $(OH)_3$, 200 Mg $(OH)_2$ (25 Simethicone)	1.3	12	—
Maalox	225 Al $(OH)_3$, 200 Mg $(OH)_2$	0.8	13	—
Milk of Magnesia	388 Mg $(OH)_2$	0.12	14	—
Mylanta§	200 Al $(OH)_3$, 200 Mg $(OH)_2$ (20 Simethicone)	0.7	13	—
Rolaids‖,¶	80 Mg $(OH)_2$	<0.4	11	412
Tums‖	500 $CaCO_3$ (20 Simethicone)	2–4	10–20	500

*Most compounds available in tablet form at similar concentrations.
†Sodium content in 5 ml or lower-strength tablet.
‡ANC = Acid Neutralizing Capacity (see text) in mEq/5 ml or tab.
§"‖" form designates double concentration.
‖Available in tablet form only.
¶Also available in sodium-free form.
   Modified from Gilman AG, Goodman L: The pharmacologic basis of therapeutics. In Benitz WE, Tatro DS, editors: *The pediatric drug handbook,* St. Louis, Mosby, 1988.

of anesthesia, endoscopy, or in coma to neutralize gastric acid in case of aspiration; prophylaxis of stress ulceration and acute upper GI hemorrhage. Aluminum hydroxide may be used as an antidiarrheal agent, magnesium hydroxide as a laxative and to decrease calcium oxalate nephrolithiasis risk.

Contraindications:

Calcium–containing antacids contraindicated in presence of nephrolithiasis. Aluminum compounds contraindicated in severe renal impairment because of risk of hypophosphatemia, osteodystrophy, proximal myopathy, and encephalopathy (because of higher brain aluminum concentrations).

Toxicity: Aluminum antacids can cause constipation, ileus and colonic perforation, obstruction from bezoars or fecaliths (more frequent in the elderly). Hypophosphatemia with anorexia/malaise: Calcium compounds can predispose to milk-alkali syndrome or nephrolithiasis (alkaluria causes precipitation of calcium phosphate). Magnesium compounds can cause diarrhea or hypokalemia. Release of CO_2 from carbonate compounds produces belching with possible gastroesophageal reflex, abdominal distention. Renal failure patients may exhibit toxic accumulation of magnesium or aluminum (aluminum deposits in bone termed dialysis osteomalecia).

Interactions: Gastric alkalinization decreases bioavailability of tetracyclines, iron, some antimuscarinics, phenothiazines, atenolol, propranolol, dicumarol, diflunisal, digoxin, fluoride, indomethacin, isoniazid, phosphate, prednisone, prednisolone, quinidine, ranitidine, sulfadiazine, fat-soluble vitamins (see package insert of *PDR* for individual effects). Alkalinization of urine speeds salicylate and phenobarbital elimination and slows excretion of amphetamines, ephedrine, mecamylamine, pseudoephedrine, and quinidine. Thiazides exacerbate hypercalcemia with $CaCO_3$. Increased bioavailability of metoprolol, increased absorption of sulfonamides and levodopa.

PEPTIC ULCER TREATMENT

H₂ BLOCKING AGENTS
■ **Cimetidine** (Tagamet; Smith-Kline Beecham)

How Supplied:
PO:
> 200, 300, 400, 800 mg tablet.
> 300 mg/5 ml suspension, 8 oz bottle.
> 400 mg/16.67 ml single-dose units.

Parenteral:
> 300 mg/2 ml single-dose vial and 8 ml multi-dose vial.
> 300 mg in 50 ml 0.9 NS single-dose premixed plastic container.

Administration:
PO: Well absorbed without regard to food or antacids. If PO intake is impractical, administer as undiluted IM or appropriately diluted slow IV bolus or intermittent infusion.

Dose:
PO:
1. Active duodenal ulcer: 800 mg qhs; max 1600 mg qhs if endoscopy demonstrates ulcer larger than 1.0 cm diameter and patient smokes more than 1 pack/day.
2. Maintenance duodenal ulcer therapy: 400 mg qhs.
3. Active benign gastric ulcer: 800 mg qhs or 300 mg qid (with meals and hs).
4. Pathologic hypersecretory conditions (e.g., Zollinger-Ellison syndrome): 300 mg qid (with meals and hs); max 2400 mg/day.
5. Severe renal impairment: 300 mg bid or up to tid with caution.

IM, IV: 300 mg tid–qid.

Mechanism of Action: Highly selective histamine H_2-receptor antagonist: Reversibly and competitively blocks histamine action on parietal cells, thus inhibiting daytime and nocturnal basal gastric acid secretion and acid secretion stimulated by food, histamine, pentagastrin, caffeine, and insulin. Also reduces gastric juice volume, as well as pepsin and intrinsic factor output. Has no effect on lower esophageal sphincter pressure or gastric emptying.

Elimination: Excreted by kidneys, primarily unchanged; half-life 2 hr.

Indications: Short-term (4–8 wk) at high doses for active duodenal and benign gastric ulcer; maintenance therapy for duodenal ulcer at reduced dosage after healing to lessen recurrence risk. Also, pathologic hypersecretory conditions (e.g., Zollinger-Ellison syndrome, systemic mastocytosis, multiple endocrine adenomas, basophilic leukemia with hyperhistaminemia) and conditions where reduction of gastric acid output is desired (e.g., reflex esophagitis, stress ulcers in severe burns or illnesses, preanesthetic use in emergency surgery [to lower risk of acid aspiration syndrome], short-bowel [anastomosis] syndrome).

Contraindications: Known drug hypersensitivity; lactation. No reported teratogenicity, but data on use in pregnancy are inadequate.

Toxicity: Headache, dizziness, GI upset, rash, impotence, and gynecomastia (binds to androgen receptors). Elevates prolactin when given by IV. Binds to cytochrome P-450 and decreases liver microsomal oxidases. Reversible CNS disturbances (e.g., slurred speech, lethargy, confusion, hallucinations, and seizures); more frequent in elderly patients or in those with hepatic or renal dysfunction. Rarely, thrombocytopenia, granulocytopenia, hepatotoxicity, or renal toxicity. Rapid IV bolus may cause cardiac dysrhythmia and hypotension.

Interactions: Effect on liver enzymes causes slower metabolism and thus increased levels of warfarin, phenytoin, theophyllin, phenobarbital, diazepam, chlordiazepoxide, propranolol, tricyclic antidepressants, diphylline, lidocaine, and dicumarol.

■ Ranitidine   (Zantac; Glaxo)

How Supplied:
PO:
>   150, 300 mg tablet, and capsules.
>   15 mg/ml syrup, 16 oz bottle.

Parenteral:
>   25 mg/ml, 2 ml single-dose vial, 6 ml multidose vial and 40 ml bulk package.
>   50 mg/50 ml in 0.45 NS, 100 ml premixed single-dose container.

Administration: See Cimetidine on p. 317.

Dose:
PO:
>   Active duodenal or benign gastric ulcer: 150 mg bid or 300 mg qhs with antacids to reduce pain.
>   Maintenance ulcer therapy: 150 mg qhs.
>   Pathologic hypersecretory states (e.g., Zollinger-Ellison syndrome): 150 mg bid, maximum 6 gm/day.

Renal dysfunction (creatinine clearance <50 ml/min): 150 mg/24 hr.

Mechanism of Action: See Cimetidine on p. 317.

Elimination: Renal elimination, 30% unchanged, via active tubular excretion; half-life 2.5–3 hr.

Indications/Contraindications: See Cimetidine on p. 317.

Toxicity: See Cimetidine on p. 318. Impotence, gynecomastia, hypoprolactinemia, and CNS disturbances less likely.

■ **Nizatidine** (Axid; Lilly)

How Supplied: *PO:* 150, 300 mg pulvules.

Administration: *PO:* well absorbed.

Mechanism of Action: See Cimetidine on p. 317.

Dose: 300 mg qhs or 150 mg bid. Reduce dose in severe renal insufficiency (creatinine clearance < 50 ml/min).

Elimination: Renal.

Indications: 4–8 wk treatment of active duodenal and benign gastric ulcer, then lower dose for maintenance therapy.
Up to 12 wk treatment of esophagitis, including erosive and ulcerative.

Contraindication: Known hypersensitivity to H_2–receptor antagonists.

Adverse Effects: Elevated LFTs, reversible mental confusion; anemia; sweating; urticaria; hypersensitivity reactions; hyper-uricemia.

Toxicity: Cholinergic effects: Lacrimation, salivation, emesis, miosis, diarrhea.

Monitor: LFTs, alkaline phosphatase, CBC, uric acid.

Interaction: Aluminum-magnesium-containing antacids decrease absorption.

■ Famotidine   (Pepcid; Merck)

How Supplied:
PO: 20, 40 mg tablets
   40 mg/ 5 ml suspension.

Administration:

PO: Incompletely absorbed.

Mechanism of Action: See Cimetidine on p. 317.

Dose: Usually 40 mg qhs or 20 mg bid; higher doses in pathologic hypersecretory states; lower dose in severe renal insufficiency (creatine clearance < 10 mg/ml).

Elimination: Two-thirds renal, one-third metabolic.

Indications: See Axid on p. 319. Also used for gastroesophageal reflux.

Adverse Effects: Headache, dizziness, constipation, diarrhea.

ANTIMUSCARINICS
■ Propantheline Bromide   (Pro-Banthine; Roberts)

How Supplied:
PO: 7.5, 15 mg tablet.

Administration:
PO: Absorption poor and variable.

Dose: 15 mg, 30 min before each meal and 30 mg qhs (75 mg/day); 7.5 mg tid for smaller or geriatric patients or those with mild symptoms.

Mechanism of Action: Synthetic antimuscarinic: Inhibits GI motility and decreases gastric acid secretion. Also blocks acetylcholine action at parasympathetic postganglionic sites.

Elimination: 70% excreted in urine, primarily as metabolites; half–life 1.6 hr.

Indication: Adjunctive therapy for peptic ulcer disease.

Contraindications: Glaucoma (risk of mydriasis), GI tract obstructive disease (e.g., pyloroduodenal stenosis, achalasia, paralytic ileus), obstructive uropathy (e.g., prostatic hypertrophy), intestinal atony in the elderly or debilitated, severe ulcerative colitis or toxic megacolon, unstable cardiovascular status in acute hemorrhage, myasthenia gravis. Inadequate data on use in pregnancy and lactation.

Adverse Effects: Decreased saliva and sweating (may precipitate heat stroke if in high temperature); blurred vision, mydriasis, increased ocular tension; urinary hesitancy or retention; tachycardia, palpitations; nausea, vomiting, constipation; impotence; suppression of lactation; allergic reactions.

Toxicity: Muscle weakness or paralysis (curare-like effect), CNS disturbances (varying from restlessness to psychotic behavior), and/or circulatory changes (e.g., hypotension).

Antidote: Physostigmine 0.5–2 mg IV, repeat prn to total 5 mg max; induce emesis.

Interactions: Excessive cholinergic blockade may occur with tricyclic antidepressants, atropine anticholinergics (e.g., belladonna alkaloids), phenothiazines (with potentiated sedative effect), antidysrhythmics, antihistamines. Use with steroids, atropine, or glycopyrrolate may increase intraocular pressure. May increase serum digoxin levels with slow-dissolving digoxin tablets (e.g., Lanoxin).

MISCELLANEOUS ANTIULCER MEDICATION
■ Sucralfate (Carafate; Marion Merrell Dow)

How Supplied:
PO:
    1 gm tablet.
    1 gm/10 ml suspension.

Administration:
PO: Not absorbed.

Dose: 1 gm qid on an empty stomach for 4–8 wk (no antacids 30 min before or after dose); then 1 gm bid as maintenance.

Mechanism of Action: Locally active sulfated sucrose–polya-luminum hydroxide molecule. Undergoes extensive polymerization at pH <4, with slow formation of a sticky viscid gel that adheres to epithelial cells and base of ulcer craters. Gel prevents protein exudation from crater and also absorbs pepsin, trypsin, and bile acids.

Indications: Short-term (≤8 wk) treatment of duodenal ulcer; then maintenance therapy while healing.

Contraindications: Inadequate data on use in pregnancy or lactation.

Toxicity: Constipation, dry mouth; aluminum accumulation if severe renal impairment, with aluminum osteomalacia and encephalopathy.

Interactions: Decreases absorption of tetracycline, phenytoin, digoxin, cimetidine, ciprofloxin, ketoconazole, norfloxacin, ranitidine and theophyline if taken within 2 hr of sucralfate.

■ Cisapride (Propulsid; Janssen)

How Supplied:
PO: 10, 20 mg tablets.

Administration: *PO:* rapidly absorbed.

Mechanism of Action: Enchances acetylcholine release at myenteric plexus without changing gastric acid secretion. Increases lower esophageal sphincter pressure and accelerates gastric empying.

Dose: 10–20 mg qid, at least 15 min before meals and hs.

Elimination: Extensively metabolized.

Indications: Nocturnal heartburn resulting from gastroesophageal reflux.

Contraindications: Conditions where increased gastrointestinal motility potentially harmful (GI hemorrhage, mechanical obstruction, perforation). Avoid in pregnancy and lactation.

Adverse Effects: Headache, dizziness, GI distress (more often at higher doses), pharyngitis, chest pain, fatigue, back pain, depression, myalgia.

Toxicity: Rare reports of seizures, tachycardia, elevated LFTs, hepatitis, thrombocytopenia, leukopenia, pancytopenia.

Monitor: CBC, LFTs, PT/PTT.

Interactions: Accelerates sedative effects of benzodiazepines and alcohol. Concomitant anticholinergics may compromise drug benefits. Oral anticoagulants may show increased effect.

LAXATIVES

Bulk-forming Laxatives

How Supplied:
PO: Tablet, powder, wafer (see Table 17-2 for specific products.)

Administration:
PO: Not absorbed. Usually taken with water or juice to reduce risk of esophageal and intestinal obstruction. Softening action occurs in 1–3 days.

Dose: See *PDR,* package insert of specific products.

Mechanism of Action:
1. Classification by active ingredient:
   a. Bran, whole grain, dietary fiber, malt soup extract.
   b. Psyllium/mucilloid (forms gelatinous hydrophilic mass when mixed with water).
   c. Methylcellulose, carboxymethylcellulose sodium.
   d. Polycarbophil, sodium polycarbophil (hydrophilic polyacrylic resins).
2. Binds water and ions in colonic lumen, softening feces and adding bulk. Digestion by colonic bacteria leads to formation of metabolites that add to osmotic activity of luminal fluid and also increase laxative effect and fecal mass. Reduction in intraluminal rectosigmoid pressure can relieve symptoms in irritable bowel syndrome and diverticular disease. Also binds bile acids and increases their fecal excretion; resultant enhanced hepatic synthesis of bile acids from cholesterol can help to reduce plasma cholesterol LDL levels.

Indications: Maintenance of soft feces; prevent straining in patients with hernia, or cardiovascular disease, hemorrhoids, other anorectal disorders when constipation is refractory to usual measures (adequate dietary fiber and fluid intake). Also useful in diverticular disease and irritable bowel syndrome.

Contraindications: Fecal impaction, intestinal obstruction, abdominal pain or GI bleeding of unknown cause, electrolyte imbalance, protein-losing enteropathy.

Adverse Effects: Flatulence, borborygmi; allergic reactions with certain plant gums. Carboxymethylcellulose sodium and psyllium colloid contain significant amounts of sodium and may cause sodium or H_2O retention. Calcium polycarbophil releases Ca^{++} in the GI tract; avoid in patients with calcium restriction or those taking tetracyclines. Laxative dependence may result from chronic overuse.

Interactions: Cellulose can bind and reduce the absorption of cardiac glycosides, salicylates, and nitrofurantoin. Psyllium may bind coumarin.

Saline Laxatives

How Supplied:
PO: Liquid, tablet (see Table 17-2).

Administration:
PO: Poorly and slowly absorbed. Effects a watery evacuation in 1–8 hr (time dose dependent).

Dose: See *PDR,* package insert of specific agents.

Mechanism of Action: Magnesium salts and sulfate, phosphate and tartrate salts of sodium or potassium. Draws water into gut and increases intraluminal pressure and intestinal motility. Magnesium salts also cause duodenal secretion of cholecystokinin and so stimulate GI tract fluid secretion and motility.

Indications: Constipation refractory to usual dietary measures; to induce bowel emptying before surgical, radiologic, and colonoscopic procedures. May help to remove certain toxins from the bowel in cases of drug overdose and poisoning.

Contraindications: See Bulk-forming Laxatives on p. 326.

Toxicity: Dehydration, electrolyte imbalance (hypermagnesemia, hypernatremia, hypocalcemia), especially with renal disease or CHF.

Osmotic Laxatives

How Supplied:
PO: Syrup; rectal enema, suppository (see Table 17-2)

Administration: See *PDR,* package insert.

Dose: See *PDR,* package insert.

Table 17-2

LAXATIVES/STOOL SOFTENERS: COMMON PREPARATIONS BY CLASS

Brand Name	(Co.)	Active Ingredients
I. BULK-FORMING		
Fiberall Chewable Tablets, Fiber Wafers, Powder	(CIBA)	Psyllium/mucilloid
FiberCon Tablets	(CIBA)	Calcium polycarbophil
Maltsupex Liquid, Power, Tablets	(Wallace)	Malt soup extract
Metamucil Effervescent, Powder	(Procter & Gamble)	Psyllium/mucilloid
II. SALINE		
Fleet Phospho-Soda	(Fleet)	Sodium phosphate
Phillips' Milk of Magnesia Liquid, Tablets	(Glenbrook)	Magnesium hydroxide
III. OSMOTIC		
Fleet Glycerin Laxative Rectal Applicators	(Fleet)	Glycerin

Table 17-2

LAXATIVES/STOOL SOFTENERS: COMMON PREPARATIONS BY CLASS- Cont'd

Brand Name	(Co.)	Active Ingredients
IV. STIMULANT AND COMBINATION AGENTS		
Dialose Plus Capsules	(Johnson & Johnson; Merck)	Casanthranol/docusate potassium
Dosaflex	(Richwood)	Senna concentrate
Doxidan	(Upjohn)	Phenolphthalein/docusate calcium
Dulcolax Suppositories, Tablets	(CIBA)	Bisacodyl
Fleet Bisacodyl Enema	(Fleet)	Bisacodyl
Modane, Modane Plus	(Savage)	Phenolphthalein
Peri-Colace	(Roberts)	Cascara Sagrada
Senokot Granules, Syrup, Tablets	(Purdue Frederick)	Senna concentrate
SenokotXTRA Tablets	(Purdue Frederick)	Senna concentrate
V. STOOL SOFTENERS		
Colace	(Roberts)	Docusate sodium
Dialose Capsules	(Johnson & Johnson; Merck)	Docusate potassium
Kasof Capsules	(Roberts)	Docusate potassium
Modane Soft	(Savage)	Docusate sodium
Surfak Liquigels	(Upjohn)	Docusate calcium

Mechanism of Action: Active ingredients include the disaccharide lactulose, glycerin, sorbitol. Poorly absorbed. Action of colonic bacteria on lactulose results in increased osmotic pressure and stool water content; also reduces intestinal absorption of ammonia and enhances excretion, thus lowering blood ammonia concentrations.

Indications: See Saline Laxatives on p. 325. Also for management of chronic portal hypertension and hepatic encephalopathy.

Contraindications: See Bulk-forming Laxatives on p. 324. Also, lactulose not for use in patients requiring galactose-free diet; should be used cautiously in diabetic patients.

Toxicity: GI distress; flatulence; diarrhea with hypokalemia, hyponatremia, dehydration.

Interactions: Aluminum hydroxide and calcium carbonate preparations may inhibit lactulose-induced drop in colonic pH.

Stimulant Laxatives

How Supplied: Various PO preparations, rectal enemas and suppositories (see Table 17-2).

Administration: See *PDR,* package inserts. Effect soft or semifluid stool in 6–8 hr.

Dose: See *PDR,* package inserts.

Mechanism of Action: Active agents include diphenylmethane derivatives (bisacodyl, phenolphthalein), anthraquinones (danthron and its glycosides, as in senna and cascara), castor oil. Generate accumulation of H_2O and electrolytes in colonic lumen and augment intestinal motility. Net decrease in H_2O and electrolyte absorption also increases mucosal permeability; many agents also increase prostaglandin synthesis and cyclic AMP.

Indications: See Saline laxatives on p. 325.

Contraindications: See Bulk Laxatives on p. 325. Castor oil may induce uterine contractions in pregnancy. Use in lactation may affect newborn.

Toxicity: Excess laxation with fluid and electrolyte deficit. Also, allergic reactions, fixed drug eruptions, Stevens-Johnson or lupus-like syndrome, osteomalacia, protein-losing enteropathy, laxative dependency (more common with phenolphthalein). Anthraquinones may effect nephritis or reversible melanosis coli. Phenolphthalein and anthraquinones may stain urine red.

Interactions: May decrease antacid efficacy.

Stool Softeners

How Supplied: *PO:* Capsule, tablet, solution, syrup, rectal liquid (see Table 17-2).

Administration/Dose: See *PDR,* package inserts of specific agents. Create minimal fecal softening in 1–3 days.

Mechanism of Action: Anionic surfactants (docusate compounds), bile acids (dehydrocholic acid); mineral oil; hydrate and soften stool by emulsifying feces, water and fat, and reduce water and electrolyte absorption.

Indications: Conditions in which straining at stool is to be avoided; see Bulk-forming Laxatives, p. 324.

Contraindications: See Bulk-forming Laxatives on p. 324.

Adverse Effects: Nausea; cramping. Docusate sodium may be absorbed into bile with potential hepatotoxicity. Mineral oil may cause essential fat-soluble vitamin malabsorption, intestinal mucosa, foreign body reactions, or lipid pneumonitis.

PANCREATIC ENZYMES

■ **Pancreatin** (Creon; Solvay. Donnazyme, Entozyme; Robins)

How Supplied:
PO: Enteric-coated microsphere capsule, tablet.

Administration:

PO: With meals. Enteric coatings (and supplemental H$_2$ blocking agents) avoid deactivation by acid and pepsin in stomach.

Dose: See *PDR*, package insert for individual preparations.

Mechanism of Action: Contain amylase, trypsin (protease) lipase from porcine or bovine pancreas. In alkaline duodenal environment, trypsin converts larger proteins to peptides; amylase reduces starch into maltose; lipase splits fat into fatty acids and glycerin. Various preparations also contain bile salts to enhance lipase fat–splitting action, fat emulsification, and fatty acid absorption; pepsin to aid protein breakdown to proteoses and peptones; and belladonna alkaloids or phenobarbital for spasmolysis and sedation.

Indications: Pancreatic exocrine insufficiencies (e.g., cystic fibrosis, chronic pancreatitis, pancreatectomy, post-GI bypass surgery, neoplastic ductal obstruction).

Contraindications: Pork/enzyme hypersensitivity; early acute pancreatitis. Inadequate data on use in pregnancy and lactation. (See individual constituents, e.g., belladonna alkaloids or phenobarbital, for specific indications.)

Toxicity: Nausea, diarrhea at higher doses; oral irritation if enteric-coated microspheres are chewed; steatorrhea (dependent on lipase content); hyperuricemia.

■ **Pancrelipase** (Cotazym-S, Zymase; Organon. Viokase; Robins. Kutrase, Ku-Zyme HP; Schwartz. Pancrease MT; McNeil)

How Supplied:

PO: Powder, capsule, tablet, enteric-coated microsphere.

Administration/Dose: See Pancreatin above.

Mechanism of Action: See Pancreatin above. Porcine origin; relatively more lipase activity than pancreatin.

Indications: See Pancreatin on p. 330.

Contraindications/Toxicity: See Pancreatin on p. 330.

ANTIDIARRHEALS

Common antidiarrheal medications are listed in Table 17-3.

Diphenoxylate + Atropine   (Lomotil; Searle)

How Supplied:
PO:
   2.5 mg diphenoxylate, 0.025 mg atropine/tablet.
   2.5 mg diphenoxylate, 0.25 mg atropine/5 ml liquid.

Administration:
PO: Well absorbed.

Dose: 2 tablets or 10 ml liquid qid until initial control achieved (should see some response within 48 hr), then decrease dose by 50%–75%; max 20 mg/day ×10 days.

Mechanism of Action: Diphenoxylate is a meperidine congener; constipating effect via inhibition of bowel motility and

17-3
ANTIDIARRHEALS: MISCELLANEOUS AND COMBINATION AGENTS

Brand Name	(Co.)	Active Ingredients
Donnagel	Wyeth-Ayerst	Opium, kaolin, pectin, hyoscyamine, tropine, scopolamine
Kaopectate	Upjohn	Kaolin, pectin
Parepectolin	Rhone-Pouleric Rorer	Paregoric, opium, pectin, kaolin
Pepto-Bismol	Procter & Gamble	Bismuth subsalicylate, magnesium, aluminum silicate

prolongation of transit time. Opioid-like euphoria at high doses (40–60 mg), and physical dependence after long-term intake. Subtherapeutic amount of atropine added to discourage deliberate overdosage.

Indications: Antidiarrheal adjunct.

Contraindications: Obstructive jaundice; pseudomembranous colitis or colitis caused by enteroxin-producing bacteria (e.g., certain *Escherichia coli, Salmonella, Shigella*); children younger than 2 yr. Use with extreme caution in acute ulcerative colitis (may induce toxic megacolon), advanced hepatorenal disease (incite hepatic coma). Inadequate data on use in pregnancy and lactation.

Side Effects: Numbness, confusion, lethargy; allergic rash; toxic megacolon, pancreatitis, paralytic ileus; drug dependence. Atropine effects include dryness of skin and mucous membranes, tachycardia, urinary retention.

Toxicity: Initially, overdosage may manifest as restlessness, hyperthermia, and tachycardia, then lethargy or coma, decreased reflexes, pinpoint pupils and severe, potentially fatal respiratory depression (at times delayed to 12–30 hr after ingestion).

Antidote: Naloxone HCl 0.4 mg (1 ml) IV.

Interactions: Precipitates hypertensive crisis in patients on MAO inhibitors; potentiates barbiturates, tranquilizers, and alcohol.

■ **Loperamide** (Imodium A-D; McNeil, Janssen. Pepto Diarrhea Control; Procter & Gamble)

How Supplied:
PO:
    2 mg capsule.
    1 mg/ml liquid, 2, 3, 4 oz bottle.

Administration:
PO: 40% absorbed.

Dose: Initially 4 mg, then 2 mg after each episode of diarrhea; max 16 mg/day. Effective within 48 hr. Average maintenance dose for chronic diarrhea 4–8 mg/day in single or divided doses.

Mechanism of Action: Piperidine derivative slows GI motility and inhibits peristalsis by effects on circular and longitudinal intestinal muscle, thus prolonging transit time, reducing daily fecal volume, increasing viscosity and bulk density. Acts on intestinal mucosa opioid receptors to reduce GI secretions and also diminish fluid and electrolyte loss.

Elimination: Primarily fecal excretion; half-life 9–14 hr.

Indications: Acute nonspecific diarrhea; chronic diarrhea from inflammatory bowel disease; to reduce volume of discharge with ileostomies.

Contraindications: Acute dysentery; conditions in which constipation should be avoided. Exercise extreme caution in patients with acute ulcerative and pseudomembranous colitis (risk toxic megacolon) and hepatic dysfunction (risk CNS toxicity caused by large first-pass biotransformation). Inadequate data on use in pregnancy and lactation.

Toxicity: Hypersensitivity reactions; abdominal pain, nausea, vomiting, constipation, lethargy, dry mouth. Less abuse potential than diphenoxylate.

ANTIFLATULENTS

■ **Simethicone** (Mylicon; Stuart. Mylanta Gas; Johnson & Johnson, Merck)

How Supplied:
PO:
    40, 80, 125 mg chewable tablet.
    40 mg/0.6 ml liquid.

Administration:
PO: After meals and hs; chew tablet thoroughly.

Dose: 40–125 mg qid.

Mechanism of Action: Dimethylpolysiloxanes with antifoaming and water-repellant properties. Relieves flatulence by dispersing and blocking formation of mucus-surrounded gas pockets in the GI tract; facilitates gas bubble passage by changing the bubbles' surface tension.

Indications: Painful excess GI gas conditions (e.g., postoperative gaseous distention, air swallowing, functional dyspepsia, peptic ulcer, spastic or irritable colon, diverticulosis).

CHAPTER 18

IMMUNIZING AGENTS (BIOLOGICALS)

ACTIVE IMMUNIZATION

Vaccines are suspensions of living or killed microorganisms or their components that are used to induce active immunity against the offending bacteria or virus.

Toxoids are bacterial products (toxins) that have been neutralized but still have the capability of stimulating specific antibodies.

PASSIVE IMMUNIZATION

Antiserums are preparations of preformed antibodies produced in another individual or animal (equine) that provide temporary immunity, specific or general, against infectious agents or venoms.

Immune globulin is a sterile serum solution containing antibodies pooled from human blood, primarily IgG.

Antitoxins are antibodies directed against a specific toxin (e.g., diphtheria, tetanus).

ADVERSE EFFECTS

All immunizing agents can produce local or systemic reactions that may vary from mild local inflammatory effects to severe systemic reactions, including anaphylactic shock. The physician must be prepared to manage any acute life-threatening situation when these agents are used in the office.

Immunization is generally contraindicated in pregnancy unless there is a compelling need to treat the woman (e.g., rabies,

Table 18-1

IMMUNIZATION IN PREGNANCY

Disease	Type of Immunizing Agent	Use In Pregnancy
Black Widow Spider Bite	Antivenum	Safe
Botulism	Trivalent antitoxin	Safe
Cholera	Killed bacterial vaccine	Safe
Diphtheria	Combined tetanus-diphtheria toxoids	Safe
Hepatitis A	Immune globulin	Safe
Hepatitis B	Recombinant vaccine	Safe
Influenza	Inactivated viral vaccine	Safe
Measles	Live attenuated vaccine	Contraindicated
Mumps	Live attenuated vaccine	Contraindicated
Plague	Killed bacterial vaccine	Safe
Poliomyelitis	Live attenuated vaccine	Usually contraindicated
Rabies	Immune globulin	Safe
Rubella	Live attenuated vaccine	Contraindicated
Snakebite	Polyvalent antivenum	Safe
Tetanus	Toxoid	Safe
Typhoid	Killed bacterial vaccine	Safe
Varicella-Zoster	Immune globulin	Safe
Yellow Fever	Live attenuated vaccine	Contraindicated

hepatitis B, measles). Killed vaccines, toxoids, and passive immunization agents are preferred because there is less risk of fetal damage. Table 18-1 provides a list of inmunizing agents and their use in pregnancy.

Pregnant women who must travel to other countries may require certain immunizations. The physician should request information from the Centers for Disease Control and Prevention, Atlanta.

COMMONLY USED IMMUNIZING AGENTS

■ Hepatitis B Immune Globulin (Human) (Hep-B-Gammagee; Merck)

Provides passive immunization for persons exposed to HBV. Peak serum levels of antiHBs occur 3–7 days after IM administration. Circulatory antibody persists for ≥2 mo.

How Supplied: 5 ml vial.

Dose: *IM* only: 0.06 ml/kg.

Indications: Prophylactic postexposure of any sort, including direct contact, parenteral, sexual.

Precautions: History of hypersensitivity. Do not use IV.

■ Heptavax-B (Merck)
Provides purified noninfective viral vaccine derived from surface antigen of hepatitis B virus.

How Supplied: Multidose vial: 20 μg/1.0 ml.

Dose: Immunization regimen consists of 3 doses of 1.0 ml (at initiation and 1 and 6 mo after initial dose).

Indication: Immunization against infection caused by all known subtypes of hepatitis B.

Precautions: Hypersensitivity. Do not use IV.

■ Immune Globulin (Human) (Gamastan; Miles-Cutter)

Dose: See *PDR*.

Indications: Primary humoral immunodeficiencies of idiopathic thrombocytopenia purpura.

■ Influenza Virus Vaccine
■ Flu-Immune (Lederle)
■ Fluogen (Parke-Davis)
■ Influenza Virus Vaccine (Wyeth-Ayerst)

Dose: See *PDR*.

Precautions: May be advisable to delay vaccination in pregnant women until after first trimester. However, in epidemic situations and high-risk pregnancy, probably safe in early pregnancy.

■ Tetanus Toxoid and TT Absorbed (Lederle; Wyeth-Ayerst)

■ Tetanus and Diphtheria Toxoids (Lederle, Wyeth-Ayerst)

Various vaccines for immunologic protection against tetanus and diphtheria are available for use in adults; see *PDR* for dosage and immunization schedules.

■ Rh$_o$(D) Immune Globulin
- ■ RhoGAM (Ortho)
- ■ MICRhoGAM (Ortho)
- ■ HypRho-D (Miles)
- ■ HypRho-D Mini-Dose (Miles)
- ■ WinRho SD (RH Pharmaceuticals)

These vaccines contain IgG antiRh$_o$(D) for use in preventing Rh immunization in Rh-negative individuals exposed to Rh-positive RBCs.

How Supplied: Prefilled single-dose syringes containing either 50, 120, or 300 µg.

Dose:
1. Do not give IV. WinRho SD, either IM or IV.
2. 50 µg: First trimester, tubal pregnancy spontaneous or induced abortion, chorionic villus sampling (CVS).
3. 300 µg: antepartum prophylaxis at 26–28 wk and later; postpartum (if newborn Rh positive); amniocentesis; abortion in second trimester (threatened, incomplete, complete).
4. If initial dose is given at 13–18 wk, a repeat dose should be administered at 26–28 wk.

Indications:
1. Pregnancy and other obstetric conditions, including abortion, amniocentesis, CVS, full-term delivery, IUFD, stillbirth.

2. Transfusion: Any Rh-negative woman of childbearing age who receives Rh-positive blood or components.

Contraindications: Known reaction to human globulin administration. Do not administer to previously sensitized women.

OTHER IMMUNIZING AGENTS

A broad spectrum of vaccines that provide degrees of immunity against bacteria, viruses, and toxins are available. Because of known and unknown maternal and fetal risks with vaccine administration, use during pregnancy is strongly discouraged unless there is a significant exposure to the agent. The physician must weigh the risks of acquiring the disease vs. the risks of fetal or maternal morbidity and mortality.

The manufacturer's directions for use of these vaccines must be scrupulously followed.

Additional available vaccines include:

Anthrax
Botulism
Cholera
Measles
Meningococcus
Mumps
Pertussis
Plague
Pneumococcus
Poliomyelitis
Rabies
Rubella
Snake bite
Spider bite
Tularemia
Typhoid
Varicella zoster
Yellow fever

IMMUNIZING

CHAPTER 19

IRON, VITAMINS, MINERALS, AND HEMATOPOIETICS

Tables 19-1 to 19-7 list various iron, vitamin, and mineral preparations.

■ Iron Dextran (InFeD Iron Dextran Injection; Schein)

How Supplied:
Parenteral:
   50 mg/ml,
   2 ml single-dose ampules.

Dose/Administration:
   IM: Undiluted, Z-track, deep into buttock; after test dose 0.5 ml (if anaphylaxis will occur, signs will manifest in next hour). Usual single daily dose 2 ml (100 mg Fe).
   IV: Undiluted, after test dose 0.5 ml over 30 sec, give 2 ml at maximum rate 1 ml/min.
   Calculate number of doses by formula in *PDR* or package insert, based on observed Hb deficit and body weight.

Mechanism of Action:
   After absorption, circulating iron dextran removed from plasma by reticuloendothelial system, which splits iron and dextran components. Iron is then bound as hemosiderin, ferritin, or transferrin, thus becoming available to replenish Hb and depleted Fe stores. Reticulocyte counts increase in a few days, and Hb should increase by at least 1 gm in 2 wk (if this does not occur, diagnosis of Fe deficiency as sole cause of anemia is suspect).

Table 19-1
IRON PREPARATIONS

Preparation (Co.)	Iron (mg)	Vit A (IU)	B₁ (mg)	B₂ (mg)	B₃* (mg)	B₆ (mg)	B₁₂ (µg)	C† (mg)	D (IU)	E (IU)	Folat (mg)	Docusate Sodium (mg)
Chromagen (Savage)	200	—	—	—	—	—	10	250	—	—	—	—
Feosol (Smith-Kline Beecham)	325	—	—	—	—	—	—	—	—	—	—	—
Fergon (Miles)	320	—	—	—	—	—	—	—	—	—	—	—
Fero-Folic-500 (Abbott)	525	—	—	—	—	—	—	500	—	—	0.8	—
Fero-Grad-500 (Abbott)	525	—	—	—	—	—	—	500	—	—	—	—
Fero-Gradumet‡ (Abbott)	525	—	—	—	—	—	—	—	—	—	—	—
Ferro-Sequels (Lederle)	150	—	—	—	—	—	—	—	—	—	—	100
Hemaspan (Bock)	110	—	—	—	—	—	—	200	—	—	—	20
Iberet (Abbott)	525	—	6	6	30	5	25	150	—	—	—	—
Iberet-500 (Abbott)	525	—	6	6	30	5	25	500	—	—	—	—
Iberet-Folic-500 (Abbott)	525	—	6	6	30	5	25	500	—	—	0.8	—
Irospan (Fielding)	65	—	—	—	—	—	—	150	—	—	—	—
Niferex§ (Central)	50	—	—	—	—	—	—	—	—	—	—	—
Niferex-150 Forte§ (Central)	150	—	—	—	—	—	25	—	—	—	1.0	—
Niferex with Vitamin C§ (Central)	50	—	—	—	—	—	25	100	—	—	—	—
Slow Fe (CIBA)	160	—	—	—	—	—	—	—	—	—	—	—
Slow Fe with Folic Acid (CIBA)	160	—	—	—	—	—	—	—	—	—	0.4	—
Vitron-C (CIBA)	200	—	—	—	—	—	—	125	—	—	—	—

*As ferrous sulfate, ferrous fumarate, or ferrous gluconate.
†Included to improve iron absorption.
‡Inert porous plastic matrix impregnated with ferrous sulfate as a controlled-release vehicle for patients intolerant to usual oral iron side effects.
§Elemental iron.

IRON, VIT; & MIN.

341

Indications: Treatment of documented Fe deficiency when PO administration not feasible.

Contraindications: Acute phase of infectious renal disease; known drug sensitivity. Exercise caution in patients with serious liver dysfunction, significant allergies or asthma.

Adverse Effects: Subcutaneous tissue staining or local pain at injection site, hemosiderosis. Large IV doses associated with delayed reactions: arthralgias, backache, chills, fever. IM form theoretically carcinogenic (sarcoma after repeated doses in laboratory animals).

Toxicity: Potentially fatal anaphylaxis with respiratory distress, convulsions, and/or CV collapse (0.2%–0.3% incidence), flushing, hypotension, pyrexia, exacerbation of rheumatoid arthritis symptoms.

Monitor: Hb and Hct values, reticulocyte count, serum Fe levels, TIBC, ferritin levels.

■ **Epoetin Alfa**   (Epogen; Amgen. Procrit; Ortho Biotech)

How Supplied:
Parenteral:
    2000, 3000, 4000, 10,000 U/ml, 1 ml single-dose vial.
    10,000 U/ml 2 ml multiple-dose vial.

Administration:
    IV or subcutaneous.

Mechanism of Action: Recombinant human erythropoietin: stimulates erythropoiesis in anemic patients with low endogenous erthropoietin levels (<500 mU/ml).

Dose: Initially 50–150 U/kg 3 times/wk. Rise in Hct occurs after 2–6 wk. Reduce dose as Hct approaches 36% or rises by >4 points in a 2-wk period. Maintenance dose averages 75 U/kg 3 times/wk (range 12.5–525). In cases of inadequate response, rule

Table 19-2
FAT-SOLUBLE VITAMINS

Vitamin	RDA (Female-Male)	Deficiency States	Signs of Toxicity
A: Retinol	4000–5000 U	Night blindness, keratomalacia; follicular hyperkeratosis; epithelial keratinization; urinary calculi	Pruritic, desquamating skin; fissures; headache; papilledema; increased intracranial pressure
D: Cholecalciferol Caliciferol	400 U	Rickets; osteomalacia	Hypercalcemia
E: Tocopherol	8–10 mg	Neuropathy, myopathy, anemia	Unknown
K: Phytonadione Maraquinone	1 μg/kg (newborn: 0.5–1 mg immediately after delivery)	Deficiency of vit K–dependent clotting factors (II, VII, IX, X)	Usually nontoxic

out underlying iron deficiency, infection, malignancy, hematologic disease (e.g., thalassemia), vitamin deficiency; occult blood loss; hemolysis.

Indication: Treatment of anemia of chronic renal failure, HIV patients on zidovudine, and cancer patients (nonmyeloid malignancy) on anemia-causing chemotherapy.

Contraindications: Uncontrolled HTN (especially chronic renal failure patients). Use with caution if history of seizures, underlying hematologic disease, (e.g., sickle cell anemia, myelodysplastic syndromes, hypercoagulable disorders), porphyria; lactation.

Adverse Effects/Toxicity: In chronic renal failure: HTN; seizures; thrombosis of vascular access; diarrhea. In zidovudine-treated HIV patients and cancer chemotherapy patients: pyrexia, headache, GI complaints, rash, URTI. Baseline and periodic iron status to determine need for iron supplementation (required by most patients); transferrin saturation = Fe/TIBC (should be > 20%) and serum ferritin (should be > 100 ng/ml).

Monitor: Erythropoietin levels in HIV patients on zidovudine; BP, periodic Hct, if on heparin and dialysis.

■ Dihydrotachysterol   (DHT; Roxane)

How Supplied:
PO: 0.125, 0.2, 0.4 mg tablets.
   0.2 mg/ml 30 ml solution.

Administration: *PO.*

Mechanism of Action: Vit D analog; increases serum calcium by stimulating intestinal calcium absorption and mobilizing bone calcium in the absence of PTH and functioning renal tissue; also increases renal phosphate excretion.

Dose: Initially 0.8–2.4 mg/day × 1–2 wk, then 0.2–1.0 mg/day to maintain serum calcium at 9–10 mg/100 ml; supplement with 10–15 gm/day calcium lactate or gluconate.

Indications: Treatment of acute, chronic and latent forms of postoperative tetany, idiopathic tetany and hypoparathyroidism.

Contraindications: Hypercalcemia: hypovitaminosis D. Use with caution in patients with renal osteodystrophy and hyperphosphatemia (need to maintain serum phosphate in normal range to avoid metastic calcification); patients with renal stones; pregnancy; lactation.

Adverse Effects/Toxicity: Symptoms of hypocalcemia/hypervitaminosis D, weakness, headache, anorexia, GI distress, vertigo, ataxia, depression, disorientation, hallucinations, syncope, coma.

Monitor: Serum calcium, phosphate levels.

Interactions: Thiazides increase risk of hypercalcemia.

IRON, VIT; & MIN.

■ Calcitriol   (Calcijex; Abbott)

How Supplied:
Parenteral: 1 µg/ml and 2 µg/ml ampules.

Administration:
IV bolus.

Mechanism of Action: Active form of vit D_3 (cholecalciferol); stimulates intestinal calcium transport, renal tubular calcium reabsorption, and with PTH, calcium reabsorption from bone. Also directly suppresses PTH secretion and synthesis.

Dose: 0.5 µg (0.01 µg/kg) 3 times/wk; increase by 0.25–0.5 µg q2–4 wk to average dose 0.5–3.0 µg (0.01–0.05 µg/kg). Ensure proper calcium dietary intake or supplementation (800–1500 mg/day); use a non-aluminum phosphate binding compound to control serum phosphorus in patients on dialysis.

Indications: To treat hypocalcemia and reduce PTH levels in patients on chronic renal dialysis; also improves renal osteodystrophy.

Table 19-3
WATER-SOLUBLE VITAMINS

Vitamin	RDA (Female–Male)*	Physiologic Function	Deficiency States
B₁: Thiamine	1.0–1.5 mg	Coenzyme in carbohydrate metabolism	Beriberi (neuritis, cardiomyopathy), Wernicke's encephalopathy, Korsakoff's syndrome, alcoholic polyneuropathy
B₂: Riboflavin	1.2–1.7 mg	Coenzyme	Stomatitis, glossitis, dermatitis; anemia; neuropathy
B₃: Niacin	13–19 mg	Coenzyme for oxidation-reduction reactions essential for tissue respiration	Pellagra (dermatitis, diarrhea, and dementia)
B₆: Pyridoxine	1.6–2.0 mg	Coenzyme in amino acid metabolism	Dermatitis, glossitis, stomatitis; peripheral neuritis; anemia
B₁₂: Cyanocobalamin	3 μg (4 μg for pregnancy and lactation)	Coenzyme essential for cell growth and replication	Megaloblastic anemia, irreversible demyelinating neuropathy

Table 19-3
WATER-SOLUBLE VITAMINS

Vitamin	RDA (Female–Male)*	Physiologic Function	Deficiency States
C: Ascorbic acid	60 mg (pregnant, 70; smokers, 100)	Osteoid formation; collagen synthesis; vascular function; iron absorption	Scurvy (poor wound healing, loosening of teeth, gingivitis, petechiae, subperiosteal bone hemorrhage (infants)
Folate: Pteroylglutamic acid	160–200 µg (preconception and pregnant 400)	Coenzyme in amino acid + RBC metabolism	Megaloblastic anemia
Pantothenic acid	4–7	Coenzyme for metabolism of carbohydrates, glyconeogenesis, degradation of fatty acids, steroid synthesis	Neuromuscular degeneration (paresthesias, impaired coordination), adrenocortical insufficiency

*Requirements for pregnant and lactating women approximately the same as for adult men.

Contraindication: Hypercalcemia, hypervitaminosis D. Use with caution in patients on digitalis (hypercalcemia may precipitate cardiac dysrhythmia).

Adverse Effects: Weakness, headache, GI distress, muscle and bone pain.

Toxicity: Polyuria, polydipsia; weight loss; calcific conjunctivitis; pancreatitis; hyperthermia; ectopic calcification; elevated BUN, SGOT, SGPT; HTN; cardiac dysrythmias; psychosis.

Monitor: Baseline and periodic serum calcium, phosphorus, magnesium, alkaline phosphatase; 24 hr urinary calcium and phosphorus.

Interaction: Use with magnesium-containing antacids may cause hypermagnesemia.

■ **Etidronate Disodium** (Didronel; Procter & Gamble. Didronel IV Infusion; MGI Pharma)

How Supplied:
PO: 200, 400 mg tablets.
Parenteral: 300 mg/6ml ampule.

Administration:
PO: avoid food (especially dairy products) or metal-containing antacids (calcium, iron, magnesium, aluminum) within 2 hr of dosing.
IV: diluted in > 250 ml NS, slow infusion; maintain adequate hydration with saline and give with loop or high-ceiling diuretic for optimal response.

Mechanism of Action: Disodium salt of (1-hydroxyethylidene) diphosphonic acid: Slows the formation and dissolution of hydroxyapatite crystals, thus slowing accelerated bone turnover and protecting against calcification of soft tissues.

Dose:
PO: Initially 5 mg/kg/day × 6 mo; or up to 10–20 mg/kg/day × 3
  mo, followed by drug-free interval of at least 3 mo.
IV: 7.5 mg/kg/day × 3 days.

Elimination: Excreted unmetabolized by kidney; decrease
dose in renal insufficiency.

Indications:
PO: Symptomatic Paget's disease of the bone, to reduce pain and
  improve mobility; heterotopic ossification (myositis ossifi-
  cans) after total hip replacement or spinal cord injury.
IV: Hypercalcemia of malignancy not responding to dietary
  changes and/or oral hydration.

Contraindications:
PO: Overt osteomalacia.
IV: Higher renal functional impairment (creatinine >5 mg/dl).

Adverse Effects: GI distress (lessen by dividing dose); arthralgias; rash; osteomalacia; confusion; hallucinations; paresthesias,
agranulocytosis; pancytopenia.

Toxicity: Nephrotic syndrome; fracture; ECG changes.

Monitor: CBC, creatinine, BUN, calcium and phosphate levels.

Interactions: Concomitant NSAIDs and over-aggressive
diuretic therapy may precipitate renal failure with IV drug.

Table 19-4

MINERALS: RDA

	Adult Female	Adult Male	Pregnancy	Lactation
Calcium (mg)				
11–24 y.o.	1200–1500	1000	1200–1500	1200–1500
24–50	1000		1200–1500	1200–1500
50–65	1000*			
>65	1500			
Copper (mg)	2	3	3	3
Phosphorus (mg)	800	800	1200	1200
Magnesium (mg)	280	350	320	350
Iron (mg)	15	10	45–75	45–75
Zinc (mg)	12	15	15	17
Iodine (µg)	150	150	175	200
Selenium (µg)	55	70	65	75

*1500 if not on hormone replacement therapy.

Table 19-5
PRENATAL VITAMINS

Vitamin (Co.)	Vit A (IU)	B₁ (mg)	B₂ (mg)	B₃* (mg)	B₆ (mg)	B₁₂ (μg)	C (mg)	D (IU)	E (IU)	Folate (mg)	Calcium (mg)	Iron (mg)	Zinc (mg)	Copper (mg)
Materna (Lederle)	5000	3	3.4	20	10	12	100	400	30	1	250	60	25	2
Mission Prenatal Rx (Mission)	8000	4	2	20	20	8	240	400	—	1	175	60	15	2
Nestabs (Fielding)	5000	3	3	20	3	8	120	400	30	1	200	36	15	—
Niferex (PN Forte)	5000	3	3.4	20	4	12	80	400	30	1	250	60	25	2
Pramilet FA (Ross)	4000	3	2	10	3	3	60	400	—	1	250	40	0.085	0.15
PreCare (Northampton Medical)	—	—	—	—	2	—	50	240	3.5	1	250	40	15	2
Prenate 90† (Bock)	4000	3	3.4	20	20	12	120	400	30	1	250	90	25	2
Stuart Prenatal (Stuart)	4000	1.84	1.7	18	2.6	4	100	400	11	0.8	200	60	25	—
Stuart Natal Plus (Stuart)	4000	1.84	3	20	10	12	120	400	11	1	200	65	25	2
Zenate (Reid-Rowell)	4000	1.5	1.6	17	2.2	2.2	70	—	10	—	200	—	15	—

*As niacinamide.
†Also contains 50 mg docusate sodium (stool softener).

351

Table 19-6

COMMON MULTIVITAMIN AND MINERAL PREPARATIONS

Preparation (Co.)	A (IU)	B$_1$ (mg)	B$_2$ (mg)	B$_3$* (mg)	B$_6$ (mg)	B$_{12}$ (μg)	C (mg)	D (IU)	E (IU)
Berocca (Roche)	—	15	15	100	4	5	500	—	—
Berocca Plus (Roche)	5000	20	20	100	25	50	500	—	30
Centrum (Lederle Consumer)	5000	1.5	1.7	20	2	6	60	400	30
Gerimed	5000	3	3	25	2	6	120	400	30
Megadose (Arco)	5000	80	80	80	80	80	250	1000	100
One-A-Day Maximum Formula (Miles)	5000	1.5	1.7	20	2	6	60	400	30
55 Plus (Miles)	6000	4.5	3.4	20	6	25	120	400	60
Sigtab-M (Roberts)	6000	5	5	25	3	18	100	400	45
Stresstabs (Lederle)	—	10	10	100	5	12	500	—	30
Stresstabs + Iron (Lederle)	—	10	10	100	5	12	500	—	30
Stresstabs + Zinc (Lederle)	—	10	10	100	5	12	500	—	30
Theragran (Bristol Myers)	5000	3	3.4	20	3	9	90	400	30
Theragran Antioxidant (Bristol Myers)	5000	—	—	—	—	—	250	—	200
Theragran-M (Bristol Myers)	5000	3	3.4	20	3	9	90	400	30
Zymacap (Roberts)	5000	2.25	2.6	30	3	9	90	400	15

*As niacinamide.

Folate (mg)	Calcium (mg)	Iron (mg)	Zinc (mg)	Copper (mg)	Magnesium (mg)	Calcium Pantothenate
0.5	—	—	—	—	—	18
0.8	—	—	22.5	3	50	25
0.4	162	18	15	2	100	10
—	370	—	15	—	—	—
0.4	50	—	25	0.5	7	80
0.4	130	18	15	2	100	10
0.4	220	—	15	2	100	20
0.4	200	18	15	2	100	15
0.4	—	—	—	—	—	20
0.4	—	18	—	—	—	20
0.4	—	—	23.9	3	—	20
0.4	—	—	—	—	—	10
—	—	—	7.5	1	100	20
0.4	40	27	15	2	—	10
0.4	—	—	—	—	—	15

Table 19-7
COMMON CALCIUM PREPARATIONS*

Preparation (Co.)	Calcium Form - Mg =	Elemental Calcium (mg)	Vit. D. (mg)	Iron (mg)
Calcet (Mission)	Lactate 240			—
	Gluconate 240	152.8	100	—
	Carbonate 240			—
Calci-Chew (Purdue Frederick)	Carbonate 1250	500	—	—
Caltrate 600 (Lederle)	Carbonate 1500	600	—	—
Caltrate 600 + Vit D (Lederle)	Carbonate 1500	600	125	00
Caltrate 600 + Iron + Vit D (Lederle)	Carbonate 1500	600	125	18†
Centrum Singles-Calcium (Lederle)	Carbonate 500		—	—
Citracal (Mission)	Citrate 950	200	—	—
Os-Cal 250 + D (Smith-Kline Beecham)	Carbonate 625	250	125	—
Os-Cal 500 (Smith-Kline Beecham)	Carbonate 1250	500	—	—
Os-Cal 500+ D (Smith-Kline Beecham)	Carbonate 1250	500	125	—
Rolaids (Warner Lambert)	Carbonate 550	220	—	—
Tums (Smith-Kline Beecham)	Carbonate 500	200	—	—

*Also see Table 16-1: Tums, Rolaids.
†Elemental iron mg (approximately 55 mg ferrous fumarate).

354

CHAPTER 20

INTRAVENOUS FLUIDS AND ELECTROLYTES

Common intravenous fluids are listed in Table 20-1.

GENERAL PRINCIPLES

1. *Total body water* = 50% (obese) to 70% (lean) of body weight = extracellular fluid (ECF) + intracellular fluid (ICF).
2. *ECF* = interstitial compartment ($\frac{3}{4}$) + intravascular compartment ($\frac{1}{4}$) (i.e., plasma volume).
   a. Sodium (Na^+): Major cation + osmotic component determining size of compartment.
      (1) Elevated Na^+ = H_2O lack (1 L H_2O deficit/3 mEq Na^+ above normal).
      (2) Low Na^+ = H_2O excess.
   b. Chloride (Cl^-) + bicarbonate (HCO_3^-): Major anions.
3. *ICF:*
   a. Potassium (K^+): Major cation + osmotic gradient.
   b. Magnesium (Mg^{2+}): Accessory cation.
   c. Phosphates, sulfates, proteins: Major anions.
4. *Osmolality (osm):* Normal serum range = 285–295.
   a. Maintained by adjustments in ADH and thirst-mediated H_2O intake.
   b. $Osm_{ECF} = Osm_{ICF}$, since H_2O moves freely across cell membranes.
5. *Acid-base balance:*
   a. Normal.

	pH	P_{CO_2}(mm Hg)	HCO_3^-(mEq/L)
(1) Arterial blood	7.37–7.43	33–44	22–26
(2) Venous blood	7.32–7.38	42–50	23–27

   b. Essential equation: $CO_2 + H_2O \leftrightarrows H_2CO_3 \leftrightarrows H^+ + HCO_3^-$

$$pH = 6.1 + \log\left[\frac{HCO_3^-}{CO_2}\left(\frac{Kidney}{Lung}\right)\right]$$

Table 20-1
IV SOLUTIONS

	NaCl	Na Lactate*	KCL (mEq/L)	CaCl₂	Glu (gm/L)	Cal (kcal/L)	mOsm/L
D₅W	—	—	—	—	50	85	126
D₁₀W	—	—	—	—	100	340	505
D₅₀W	—	—	—	—	500	1700	2525
0.45 NS	77	—	—	—	—	—	154
0.9 NS	154	—	—	—	—	—	308
D₅/0.2 NS	34	—	—	—	50	170	321
D₅/0.45 NS	77	—	—	—	50	170	407
D₅/0.9 NS	154	—	—	—	50	170	561
D₁₀/0.225 NS	38	—	—	—	100	340	581
D₁₀/0.45 NS	77	—	—	—	100	340	659
D₁₀/0.9 NS	154	—	—	—	100	340	868
Lactated Ringer's (LR)	103	27	4	4	—	—	274
D₅/LR	103	27	4	4	50	170	527

Modified from Costrini NV, Thomson WM, editors: *Manual of Medical Therapeutics*, Boston, 1977, Little Brown; Benwitz WE, Taltro DS: *Pediatric Drug Handbook*, ed 2, St Louis, 1988 Mosby.

*HCO₃⁻ precursor.

356

   c. Compensatory mechanisms:
     (1) Renal: Reabsorb filtered HCO_3^-, excrete 50–100 mEq H^+/day.
     (2) Lung: Eliminate $CO_2 + H_2O$ formed from $HCO_3^- + H^+$.
6. *Average daily maintenance:*

	Amount/Day
(a) Water	1500–2000 ml (500–1000 ml urine, 500–1000 ml insensible loss 100–200 ml in stool)
(b) Na + (NaCl)	70 mEq (4 gm)
(c) K^+	40–60 mEq
(d) Carbohydrate	150–200 gm

7. *Additional losses/24 hr:*

	Max Vol (ml)	Na^+	K^+	H^+	Cl^-	HCO_3^-
a. *Normal:*						
(1) Gastric secretions	Variable	40–60	10	80–100	100–400	—
(2) Bile	1500	140	10	—	100	30
(3) Pancreatic secretions	1000	140	10	—	50–75	90
(4) Succus entericus	3500	100–130	10–20	—	110	25
b. *Abnormal:*						
(1) Fever: 38.4° C– 39.4° C	500	50	5	—	55	—
> 39.5° C	1000	50	5	—	55	—
(2) Diarrhea	1000–4000	50–60	30	—	40	45
(3) New ileostomy	500–2000	130	20	—	110	—
(4) Adapted ileostomy	400	50	10	—	60	—
(5) New cecostomy	400	50	10	—	40	—
(6) Colostomy (transverse loop)	300	50	10	—	45	—

8. *Replacement guidelines:*
   a. In general: Replace one half of deficit in first 8 hr, remainder over next 16 hr.

9. Exceptions:
   a. Shock: Replace isotonic fluid at appropriate rate to avoid cardiovascular compromise.
   b. Hypertonic dehydration: Replace Na^+ + H_2O deficit over 48 hr; too rapid correction may cause cerebral edema.
   c. K^+: Replace over 72 hr; too rapid replacement can lead to hyperkalemia.
10. Monitor electrolytes serially for best guideline to ongoing losses and adequate replacement.

COMMON ACID-BASE DISORDERS*

Physiologic features of acid-base disorders are given in Table 20-2.

Metabolic Acidosis

1. Organic or fixed acid excess (associated with high anion gap):
   a. Diabetic ketoacidosis.
   b. Lactic acidosis: sepsis, shock, starvation, hypoperfusion (e.g., vasopressor, prolonged peripheral anoxia in major vessel surgery).
   c. Intoxication with salicylates, paraldehyde, methanol (formate anion), ethylene glycol, NH_4Cl.
   d. Hyperalimentation (relative excess acidic amino acids).
2. Impaired renal excretory mechanism:
   a. Acute oliguric renal failure.
   b. Chronic azotemic renal failure (phosphate anion excess; associated with high anion gap).
   c. Renal tubular acidosis:
      (a) Congenital, hereditary, familial.
      (b) Acquired: pyelonephritis, drug or toxin ingestion (outdated tetracycline, amphotericin B, gentamicin, toluene [glue or paint sniffing], phenacetin, lithium, acetazolamide, streptozotocin, cadmium, lead), hyperglobulinemias, cirrhosis.
3. Abnormal bicarbonate loss:
   a. Diarrhea, small bowel suction or fistula, pancreatic fistula.

*Data in this section is from Condon RE, Nyhus LM, editors: *Manual of surgical therapeutics,* Boston, 1982, Little Brown; Papper S, Williams GR, editors: Manual of medical care of the surgical patient, Boston, 1981, Little Brown.

b. Cholestyramine.
c. Ureterosigmoidostomy.
d. Acetazolamide (Diamox) therapy.

Metabolic Alkalosis

1. Increased GI H^+ losses:
   a. Vomiting.
   b. Nasogastric suction.
   c. Intestinal fistula.
   d. Congenital chloridorrhea.
2. Renal H^+ losses:
   a. Mineralocorticoid excess: Cushing's syndrome, steroid therapy.
   b. Hypoparathyroidism.
3. Hypokalemia:
   a. Diuretics
4. HCO_3^- retention:
   a. $NaHCO_3$ administration.
   b. Massive blood transfusion.
   c. Milk-alkali syndrome.
   d. Contraction alkalosis.

Respiratory Acidosis

1. Inhibited respiratory drive:
   a. Drugs, opiates, anesthetics.
   b. CNS lesions.
   c. O_2 administration in chronic hypercapnia.
   d. Cardiac arrest.
2. Respiratory muscle/chest wall derangement:
   a. Muscle weakness: Myasthenia, poliomyelitis, multiple sclerosis, aminoglycoside Rx (with anesthetics).
   b. Morbid obesity.
   c. Thoracic trauma: Flail chest.
3. Impaired gas exchange:
   a. Chronic obstructive pulmonary disease: Asthma, emphysema.
   b. Increase in nonventilated lung areas: Pulmonary edema, pneumonia.
   c. Hamman-Rich syndrome.

Respiratory Alkalosis

1. Hypoxemia: Pulmonary disease (e.g., embolus), high altitude, congenital heart disease with right-to-left shunt, congestive heart failure.

Table 20-2

PHYSIOLOGY OF ACID-BASE DISORDERS*

Abnormality	Mechanism		Associated Metabolic Abnormality	Physiologic Response	Therapy
Metabolic acidosis	Added H+ or fixed acid Loss of HCO_3^-	$\downarrow$ pH + $\downarrow$ HCO_3^-	Anorexia, nausea, lethargy, somnolence Kussmaul's respirations Venoconstriction $\downarrow$ Myocardial contractility	$\uparrow$ RR $\rightarrow$ $\downarrow$ P_{CO_2}	$\downarrow$ Protein intake (20–40 gm/day) $\rightarrow$ $\downarrow$ acid production $\uparrow$ Caloric intake carbohydrates and fat (800–2000 kcal/day) to decrease protein tissue breakdown Administer base: PO: $NaHCO_3$, 6–8 gm/day (12 mEq Na^+ + 12 mEq HCO_3^-/gm) IV: Na HCO_3^-, 1–2 ampule/L dextrose + H_2O (44 mEq/amp) Shohl's solution: 15 ml bid–qid (1 mEq HCO_3^- + 1 mEq Na + 1 mEq K+/ml) Diuretics (e.g., furosemide 20–2000 mg/day) to aid salt + H_2O excretion

Table 20-2

PHYSIOLOGY OF ACID-BASE DISORDERS*—Cont'd

Abnormality	Mechanism	Associated Metabolic Abnormality	Physiologic Response	Therapy
Metabolic alkalosis	Loss of H⁺ } ↑ pH + ↑ HCO₃⁻ Excess HCO₃⁻ }	Hypocalcemia → tetany, seizures, dysrhythmias Paradoxical aciduria (impaired HCO₃⁻ excretion)	↓ RR → ↓ PCO_2	Fluid + K⁺ replacement Management of underlying cause
Respiratory acidosis	Retained CO_2 } ↓ pH } pCO_2 > 40 mm Hg	Hypoxia; respiratory depression CNS changes: Stupor, coma Cerebral vasodilation and ↑ pressure	↑ Renal tubular HCO₃⁻ reabsorption + Cl⁻ excretion → ↑ plasma HCO₃⁻	Respiratory support: Positive pressure ventilation Lower PCO_2 gradually to avoid metabolic alkalosis from renal compensatory mechanisms Cl⁻ (e.g. NaCl) unless hypervolemic
Respiratory alkalosis	↑ RR → ↑ PCO_2 + total CO_2 → ↑ pH	Perioral, peripheral paresthesias Lightheadedness Tetany Hypophosphatemia	↑ renal HCO₃⁻ → ↓ Plasma HCO₃⁻	Treat underlying cause Rebreathe exhaled air

Modified from Condon RE, Nyhus LM, editors: *Manual of Surgical Therapeutics*, Boston, 1981, Little Brown; Papper S, Williams GR, editors: *Manual of Medical Care of the Surgical Patient*, Boston, 1981, Little Brown.

*See Table 20-2 for common etiologies.

INTRAVENOUS

2. CNS disease (e.g., subarachnoid hemorrhage).
3. Psychogenic hyperventilation (e.g., anxiety states).
4. Salicylate intoxication.
5. Hypermetabolic states (e.g., fever, septic shock, thyrotoxicosis, exercise).
6. Liver failure.
7. Assisted ventilation.

HYPERALIMENTATION: TOTAL PARENTERAL NUTRITION (TPN)

General Principles

1. Definition: Method of delivering large quantity of hypertonic protein dextrose solution (Table 20-3) into a large central vein (i.e., superior vena cava via a subclavian line).
2. Delivery into a large vein allows for rapid adjustment of osmolality by dilution.
3. Rigid surgical sterile technique essential; catheter infection is life-threatening in these patients.

Indications:

Patients in negative nitrogen balance because of bowel disease (e.g., malabsorption, fistula), inability to ingest food (CNS trauma), or increased metabolic requirements (cancer, burns, trauma, sepsis, renal failure) where oral feeding is not feasible in the near future or is otherwise contraindicated.

Contraindications:

1. Terminal states where inevitable dying would thus be prolonged (e.g., irreversible decerebration).
2. Cardiovascular decompensation or severe metabolic derangement requiring stabilization before hypertonic IV feeding is attempted.
3. Gastrointestinal tract intake feasible (in general this is still the preferred method of nutritional support).

Fluid Preparation: Anticipating Requirements

1. Basic fluid composition: 500 ml $D_{50}W$ + 500 ml amino acid solution (8% most commonly used preparation; see Table 20-3); 3.5% amino acid solutions may be given peripherally.
2. Thus, final amino acid mix approximately 4%; 25% glucose; calorie/nitrogen (N) ratio 150–200 cal/gm N.

3. Electrolytes, vitamins, and minerals added to meet specific patient requirements (Tables 20-4 to 20-6).
4. Total number of calories required by average adult: 2000 (nl)–4000 (hypermetabolic states, e.g., burns).
5. Follow BUN to determine N utilization: e.g., excess amino acids result in increased BUN; adjust glucose–amino acid ratio accordingly.
6. Start infusion rate at 50–100 ml/hr, depending on CV and renal status.
7. Increase daily amount of TPN solution administered (and thus number of calories) slowly; i.e., by 20–50 ml/hr every 2–3 days to allow time for adaptive mechanisms (e.g., endogenous insulin release) to adjust and utilize new nutrition most effectively: 1 L/day initially, up to 3 L/day by end of first week.
8. *Intralipid* (Kabi Vitrum) 10% or 20%: fat emulsion derived from soybean oil.
   a. Usual recommended fat dosage 1–2 gm/kg body weight/day.
   b. Usual recommended fat-carbohydrate ratio 40%:60%.
   c. Since it is isotonic, preferred administration is peripheral vein (may be piggybacked into central line but should not be infused via filter or with glucose–amino acid solution; it will cause emulsion breakdown).
   d. Infuse at 1 ml/min for first 30 min; if no adverse effects, complete in not less than 4 hr.
   e. Provides 9 kcal/gm energy and thus more calories at smaller fluid volume.
   f. Twenty percent emulsion indicated only when high caloric intake and severe fluid restriction are essential.
   g. Dose: Usually 500 ml 10% solution, 2 × weekly; max 500 ml/8 hr (or 60% calorie intake).
   h. Specific complications: Allergic reactions, acute febrile response, hyperlipidemia, hypercoagulability, hepatosplenomegaly with cholestasis.

Monitor

1. Baseline: CBC, platelets, SMA-20, (i.e., Ca, PO_4, Fe, TIBC, uric acid, total protein, albumin, AST [SGOT], alkaline phosphatase), Mg, fasting blood glucose, PT, urinalysis, chest x-ray film, ECG.

Text continued on p. 368.

Table 20-3

COMMONLY USED AMINO ACID SOLUTIONS

	Travasol 8.5% (500 ml)	FeAmine II 8.5% (500 ml)	Aminosyn 3.5% (680 ml)	Nephramine 5.1%* (250 ml)
PROTEIN†				
Grams (100% utilizable)	42.5 gm	39 gm	33.3 gm	5.1 gm
AMINO ACIDS (mg/100 ml)				
Leucine	526	770	313	880
Phenylalanine	526	480	174	880
Methionine	492	450	133	880
Lysine	492	620	240	640
Isoleucine	406	590	240	560
Valine	390	560	267	650
Threonine	356	340	173	400
Tryptophan	152	130	53	200
Histidine	372	240	100	—
Arginine	880	310	327	—
Nonessential AAs	+	+	+	—

Table 20-3

COMMONLY USED AMINO ACID SOLUTION—Cont'd

NITROGEN				
Grams (100% utilizable)	7.15	6.25	5.34	1.46
ELECTROLYTES (mEq/L)				
Na	—	10	—	6
K	—	—	3.6	—
Cl	17	—	—	—
MgPO₄	—	20	—	—
Acetate	2.6	—	20	—

*Designed for use in high metabolic stress states (e.g., renal failure).
†Derived from soybean oil.

Table 20-4
COMMON CATION AND ANION PARENTERAL ADDITIVES

Solution	Concentration	Indication, Dose, and Route
Calcium Chloride		
10% injection (Astra)	14 mEq/10 ml; 100 mg/ml	Cardiac arrest: 2.4 mg/kg or 2.5–5 ml q10 min via central venous catheter
Calcium Gluconate		
10% injection (Elkins-Sinn, Warner-Chilcott, Astra)	14 mEq/10 ml; 100 mg/ml	Cardiac arrest (asystole or electromechanical dissociation): 500–800 mg/dose IV q10 min
		Hypocalcemia: 2 gm IV bolus, then 3–4 gm IV over 3–12 hr via D_5W or NS mainline
Magnesium Sulfate		
10% injection (Astra)	0.8 mEq/ml; 100 mg/ml	Hypomagnesemia or refractory hypocalcemia 25–50 mg/kg IM or IV q4–6 hrs × 3–4 doses
50% injection	4 mEq/ml; 500 mg/ml	
Potassium Chloride		
14.9% injection	2 mEq/ml	Based on ongoing losses
Sodium Bicarbonate		
7.5% injection (Astra)	0.9 mEq/ml; 75 mg/ml	Cardiac arrest: 1 mEq/kg/dose × 1 if adequate ongoing CPR; maintenance 0.5 mEq/kg q10 min or prn as per ABGs
8.4% injection (Astra)	1 mEq/ml; 84 mg/ml	

Table 20-5
TPN: BASIC REQUIREMENTS/24 HOURS*

	Amount	Comment
Water	2500–3500 ml	
Calories	2500–3500	
Protein	100–150 gm	
Nitrogen	16–25 gm	
Carbohydrate	525–750 gm	
Sodium	100–200 mEq	As NaCl, NaPO$_4$ or NaHCO$_3$
Potassium	50–160 mEq (varies)	As KPO$_4$ or KCl
Magnesium	10–30 mEq	As MgSO$_4$
Calcium	5–25 mEq	As Ca gluconate (add last to avoid insoluble calcium phosphate precipitation)
Phosphate	20 – 25 mEq/1000 kcal	

*Total as divided into 3 liters of fluid, administered entirely via TPN line or with peripheral line supplementation.

Table 20-6
TPN: BASIC REQUIREMENTS

Vitamin/ Mineral	Requirements/ 24 Hr*	Comment
Multivitamin infusion	1 vial/day	
Folate	1 mg/day	Add to different liter than multivitamin infusion
Vitamin K	10 mg/wk	IM or IV
Vitamin B$_{12}$	1000 µg/mo	IM
Insulin	Variable	Add to IV solution or administer subcutaneously prn
Vitamin C	500 mg/day	
Zinc	12 mg/day	
Copper	1.5 mg/day	
Manganese	0.25–2 mg/day	
Chromium	2–15 µg/day	
Intralipid 10%	2 × wk (minimum)	To prevent folic acid deficiency
Intralipid 10% or 20%	500 ml/8 hr	As caloric supplement

*Total as divided into 3 liters of fluid, administered entirely via TPN line or with peripheral line supplementation.

2. Daily during stabilization (5–7 days): urine glucose qid (with blood glucose during first 24–48 hr to establish renal threshold for glucosuria), SMA–6, intake and output (I/O), body weight.
3. Routine after stabilization:
   a. Daily: I/O, weight, urine glucose.
   b. 3 × weekly: SMA–6.
   c. Every wk: CBC, platelets, PT, SMA-20 (includes triglycerides, cholesterol, liver function tests).

Complications

1. Metabolic:
   a. Hyperglycemia with or without hyperosmolar nonketotic hyperglycemic coma. Most common if infusion rate increased too rapidly.
   b. Rebound hypoglycemia, if TPN discontinued too abruptly.
   c. Hyperchloremic metabolic acidosis: Excessive Cl^- salt administration or HCl from metabolism of arginine and lysine (avoid by giving part of Na^+ + K^+ as lactate salts rather than as chlorides).
   d. Prolonged prothrombin time: Relative vitamin K deficiency.
   e. Hyperammonemia, elevated AST (SGOT), ALT (SGPT), bilirubin, alkaline phosphatase values because of the inability of the liver to handle excess nitrogen.
   f. Prerenal azotemia with elevated BUN value because of excessive amino acid infusion.
   g. Essential fatty acid deficiency if no Intralipid supplied.
   h. Specific electrolyte deficiencies: Hypophosphatemia, hypocalcemia, hypercalcemia.
2. Infectious:
   a. Infected catheter most common event; majority of these septicemias are fungal.
   b. Fever workup in patient receiving TPN:
      (1) Remove TPN bottle and administration set and culture.
      (2) Keep line open with $D_{10}W$.
      (3) Take blood cultures from peripheral vein.
      (4) Search for other cause of fever (will be noncatheter related in 75%).
      (5) If no other source found and fever persists more

than 24 hr, draw blood culture from catheter, remove catheter, and culture tip.

3. Catheter related, noninfectious:
   a. Pneumothorax, hemothorax, hydrothorax.
   b. Injury to brachial plexus, subclavian or carotid artery.
   c. Catheter embolus.
   d. Tracheal perforation.
   e. Subclavian, internal jugular vein thrombosis.
   f. Arteriovenous fistula.
   g. Air embolus.
   h. Cardiac perforation or tamponade.

CHAPTER 21

LIPID–LOWERING AGENTS

■ **Lovastatin**   (Mevacor; Merck)

How Supplied:
PO: 10, 20, 40 mg tablets.

Administration:
PO: Well absorbed.

Mechanism of Action: Inhibits HMG-COA reductase, rate-limiting step in cholesterol synthesis in the liver. Reduces VLDL cholesterol concentration, LDL synthesis and apolipoprotein B and TG levels; also may increase LDL catabolism and HDL levels.

Dose: Initially 20 mg/day, single dose with evening meal; titrate q4 wk to max 80 mg/day, single dose or divided. Lower dose in patients on immunosuppressives and with renal insufficiency (creatinine clearance 30 ml/min).

Elimination: Extensive first-pass extraction in the liver; metabolites excreted in bile.

Indications: To reduce elevated total and LDL cholesterol levels in patients with primary hypercholesterolemia (Types IIa & IIb) when dieting restrictions alone prove inadequate. (Table 21-1 on p. 373).

Contraindications: Active liver disease; unexplained elevated serum transaminases; pregnancy; lactation. Use with caution in patients with severe renal insufficiency or renal transplant, especially if on immunosuppressives, other lipid-lowering drugs, or with other increased risk for renal failure caused by rhabdomyolysis; e.g., severe infection, hypotension, major surgery, uncontrolled seizures; also in patients with high alcohol consumption or past history of liver disease.

Adverse Effects: GI distress; myalgia; rash; elevated serum transaminases and CPK.

Toxicity: Rhabdomyolysis with renal failure; optic nerve degeneration.

Monitor: Cholesterol, CPK, SGOT, SGPT.

Interaction: Cyclosporine increases lovastatin levels and risk of rhabdomyolysis; gemfibrozil and systemic azole antifungals given concurrently may also increase rhabdomyolysis risk. Additive cholesterol-lowering effects with other hypolipidemics.

■ Fluvastatin   (Lescol; Sandoz)

How Supplied:
PO: 20, 40 mg capsules.

Administration:
PO: Well and rapidly absorbed.

Mechanism of Action: See Lovastatin on p. 370.

Dose: 20–40 mg qhs or divided bid (40 divided bid maximizes LDL response).

Elimination: Biliary excretion.

Indications: See Lovastatin on p. 370 and Table 21-1.

Contraindications: See Lovastatin on p. 370.

Adverse Effects: GI distress, hypersensitivity reaction; elevated liver enzymes.

Toxicity: Theoretical risk of rhabdomyolysis; myopathy.

LIPID LOWERING

Monitor: Lipid profile, SGOT, SGPT, CPK, digoxin levels.

Drug Interaction: Additive hypolipidemic effect when combined with a bile-acid binding resin (e.g., cholestyramine) or niacin (take fluvastatin >2 hr after resin to avoid drug binding).

■ **Pravastatin**   (Pravachol; Bristol-Myers Squibb)

How Supplied:
PO: 10, 20, 40 mg tablets.

Administration:
PO: Rapidly absorbed.

Mechanism of Action: See Lovastatin on p. 370.

Dose: 10–40 mg qhs; lower dose in patients with significant renal/hepatic dysfunction, the elderly, or if on immunosuppressive drugs (e.g., cyclosporine).

Elimination: Extensive first-pass hepatic metabolism; 70% excreted in feces.

Indications: See Lovastatin on p. 370 and Table 21-1.

Contraindications: See Lovastatin on p. 370. Also avoid concurrent use of fibrates and gemfibrozil.

Adverse Effects: Rash, malaise, headache.

Toxicity: Rhabdomyolysis with acute renal failure caused by myoglobinuria.

Monitor: Baseline and periodic lipid profile, SGOT, SGPT, CPK.

Interactions: Concomitant erythromycin, cyclosporine, niacin, and fibrates increase risk of rhabdomyolysis.

Table 21-1

PRIMARY HYPERLIPOPROTEINEMIAS*

Type	Disorder	Biochemical Defect	Plasma Lipoprotein Elevation	Drug Therapy First Choice	Other
I.	Familial lipoprotein lipase deficiency (hyperchylomicronemia)	Deficiency of lipoprotein lipase	Chylomicrons	None	None
IIa.	Familial hypercholesterolemia	Deficiency of LDL receptor	LDL	Lovastatin and bile acid-binding resin	Probucol or nicotinic acid and bile acid resin
IIb.	Multiple lipoprotein-type hyperlipidemia (familial combined hyperlipidemia)	Unknown	LDL + VLDL (rarely chylomicrons)	Nicotinic acid; gemfibrozil	Clofibrate; bile-acid resin; lovastatin; probucol
III.	Familial type-III hyperlipoproteinemia (dysbetalipoproteinemia)	Abnormal apo E (of VLDL)	Chylomicron remnants and IDL	Gemfibrozil; clofibrate	Nicotinic acid
IV.	Familial hypertriglyceridemia	Unknown	VLDL (rarely chylomicrons)	Gemfibrozil; nicotinic acid	Clofibrate
V.	Familial apoprotein CII deficiency	Deficiency of apoprotein CII	Chylomicrons and VLDL	None	Nicotinic acid†

*Adapted from Wilson JD, Braunwald E, Isselbacher KJ et al (eds), *Harrison's principles of internal medicine*, ed 12, McGraw-Hill, 1991, New York. *Goodman & Gilman's The pharmacologic basis of therapeutics*, ed 8, McGraw-Hill, 1993, New York.

†If at risk of pancreatitis.

■ Simvastatin (Zocor; Merck)

How Supplied:
PO: 5, 10, 20, 40 mg tablets.

Administration: *PO.*

Mechanism of Action: See Lovastatin on p. 370.

Dose: Initially 5–10 mg qhs; titrate q4 wk to max of 40 mg/day. Individualize according to baseline LDL and patient's response. Decrease dose in severe renal insufficiency.

Elimination: See Lovastatin on p. 370.

Indications: See Lovastatin on p. 370 and Table 21-1.

Contraindications: See Lovastatin on p. 370.

Adverse Effects: Constipation, elevated serum transaminases and CPK.

Toxicity: See Pravastatin on p. 372.

Monitor: See Pravastatin on p. 372.

Interaction: Increased risk of rhabdomyolysis in cardiac transplant patients on cyclosporine, nontransplant patients on gemfibrozil or lipid-lowering doses of nicotic acid, or seriously ill patients on erythromycin or systemic azole derivative antifungals.

■ Gemfibrozil (Lopid; Parke Davis)

How Supplied:
PO: 600 mg tablets.

Administration:
PO: Rapidly and completely absorbed, especially with food.

Dose: 600 mg bid, 30 min before AM and PM meal.

Mechanism of Action: Increases lipoprotein lipase activity, thus promoting catabolism of TG-rich lipoproteins, VLDL, and IDL. May also decrease hepatic synthesis and secretion of VLDL, and indirectly raise HDL.

Elimination: Enterohepatic circulation; final excretion via kidneys, mostly as glucuronide.

Indications: Treatment of high serum TGs (types IV and V hyperlipidemia) who are at risk of pancreatitis and have not responded to diet alone: e.g., increased TGs, VLDL and chylomicrons (see Table 21-1).

To reduce risk of CHD in type IIb patients that have not responded to weight loss, diet and exercise and other agents such as nicotinic acid and bile acid-binding resins, with low HDL, high LDL, and TGs.

Contraindications: Severe renal or hepatic dysfunction, including primary biliary cirrhosis; preexisting gallbladder disease or gallstones developing on therapy; pregnancy; lactation. Use with caution in patients with severe renal insufficiency.

Adverse Effects/Toxicity: Mild GI distress, skin rash, alopecia, blurred vision, weight gain, leukopenia, anemia, flulike syndrome with severe muscle cramps. Cholelithiasis may occur caused by increased cholesterol excretion into the bile. Increased LFTs, bilirubin, CPK, alkaline phosphatase.

Monitor: Lipid profile, LFTs, bilirubin, alkaline phosphatase; creatinine; CBC; PT if on anticoagulants.

Interaction: Prolonged PT if on anticoagulants; rarely, rhabdomyolysis if on HMG-CoA reductase inhibitor.

■ **Clofibrate** (Atromid-S; Wyeth-Ayerst)

How Supplied:
PO: 500 mg capsule

Administration: See Gemfibrozil on p. 374.

LIPID LOWERING

Mechanism of Action: Inhibits hepatic release of lipoproteins, especially VLDL; potentiates lipoprotein lipase activity. Lowers triglyceride-rich VLDL, and also serum cholesterol (if elevation is because of IDL as in type III hyperlipoproteinemia). Reduces risk of fatal and nonfatal myocardial infarction.

Dose: 2 gm/day, divided bid–qid.

Elimination: See Gemfibrozil on p. 375.

Indications: To treat high VLDL and IDL, such as in type III primary dysbetalipoproteinemia (type III hyperlipidemia) not responding to diet; and to lower TGs in type IV and V hyperlipidemia at risk for pancreatitis where other measures have failed (see Table 21-1).

Contraindications: See Gemfibrozil on p. 375.

Adverse Effects/Toxicity: See Gemfibrozil on p. 375. Clofibrate has relatively greater risk cholelithiasis; rhabdomyolysis with hyperkalemia (if severe preexisting renal insufficiency); atrial and ventricular dysrrhythmias.

Monitor: See Gemfibrozil on p. 375.

Interactions: Potentiates concurrent anticoagulants (reduce dose by 50% and monitor PT); theoretically increases levels of phenytoin and tolbutamide (by displacement from binding sites).

BILE ACID BINDING AGENTS
■ **Cholestyramine** (Questran; Bristol-Myers Squibb)

How Supplied:
PO: 1 gm tablets.
   5, 9 gm powder packets (containing 4 gm drug) for oral suspension.

Administration: *PO,* not absorbed. To be taken 1 hr after or 4–6 hr before any other drugs.

Mechanism of Action: Chloride salt of an anion-exchange resin. Binds bile acids in the intestine, thus increasing their fecal excretion, and resulting in increased conversion of cholesterol to bile acids. A compensatory increase in hepatic LDL receptors leads to increased uptake of LDL from plasma and lower circulatory LDL by 20% in 2 wk (by 50% if administered with HMG CoA reductase inhibitor) and cholesterol levels. Continued therapy lowers rates of CHD and nonfatal MI. In patients with biliary obstruction, lower serum bile acid levels reduces bile acids deposited in dermal tissue and decreased pruritus.

Dose: 10–40 mg qhs; lower dose in renal/hepatic dysfunction, the elderly and on immunosuppressives (max 20 mg/day).

Elimination: Excreted in feces.

Indications: To reduce elevated LDL in patients with primary hypercholesterolemia with inadequate response to diet; relieves pruritus caused by partial biliary obstruction.

Contraindications: Complete biliary obstruction; phenylketonuria; hypoprothombinemia not on vitamin K supplementation; chronic constipation. Inadequate data on use in pregnancy and lactation.

Adverse Effects/Toxicity: Constipation (common); GI distress; fecal impaction; aggravation of hemorrhoids; hyperchloremic acidosis; steatorrhea; hypoprothrombinemia caused by absorption of fat-soluble vitamins (counteract with water-soluble vitamin supplementation or parenteral vitamin K); elevated serum transaminases and alkaline phosphatase; transient increase in serum triglycerides.

Monitor: Periodic and baseline lipid profile; PT; phenobarbital, digitalis and thyroid drug levels.

Interaction: Enhanced hypolipidemic effect with HMG-CoA reductase inhibitors and nicotinic acid; reduces absorption of phenylbutazone, warfarin, chlorothiazide, propranolol, tetracycline, PCN G, phenobarbital, thyroid and thyroxine preparations and digitalis.

LIPID LOWERING

■ Colestipol Hydrochloride (Colestid; Upjohn)

How Supplied:
PO: 5 gm packets for oral suspension.
  300, 500 gm bottles.

Administration: See Cholestyramine on p. 376.

Mechanism of Action: See Cholestyramine on p. 377.

Dose: 5–30 gm/day, single or divided dose. Increase dose cautiously in patients with chronic constipation (see Table 21-1).

Indications: As an adjunct to diet for reduction of elevated total and LDL-cholesterol in primary hypercholesterolemia.

Contraindication: See Cholestyramine on p. 377.

Adverse Effects/Toxicity: See Cholestyramine on p. 377.

Monitor: See Cholestyramine on p. 377.

Interactions: See Cholestyramine on p. 377. Also decreases absorption of furosemide and gemfibrozil, but does not appear to change warfarin levels.

NICOTINIC ACID
■ Niacin (Nicobid, Nicolar; Rhone-Poulenc Rorer)

How Supplied:
PO: 125, 250 mg sustained-release capsule.
  500 mg immediate-release tablet.

Administration: *PO;* rapidly absorbed. Timed-release capsule and immediate-release tablet form not interchangeable.

Mechanism of Action: Lowers VLDL and daughter particle LDL by inhibition of lipolysis in adipose tissue, decreased hepatic esterification of TGs and increased lipoprotein lipase activity.

Dose:
Timed-release capsule: 125–500 mg/day, single dose or divided bid.
Tablet: 1–2 gm bid–tid.

Indications: Used with a bile-acid binding resin or alone to lower LDL and total cholesterol in patients with primary hypercholesterolemia (types IIa and IIb), when response to diet alone is inadequate. Also as adjunctive therapy to lower triglycerides in patients with type IV and V hyperlipidemia at risk for pancreatitis (see Table 21-1).

Contraindications: Hepatobiliary dysfunction; active peptic ulcer disease; arterial bleeding; heart disease (especially with angina or recent heart attack); gout; glaucoma; diabetes; pregnancy.

Adverse Effects: Cutaneous flushing and pruritus (prevent with aspirin or NSAID 30 min before dose); GI distress and peptic ulceration; hyperpigmentation, acanthosis nigricans. Hyperglycemia may occur in nondiabetic patients; elevated uric acid; postural hypotension if on antihypertensives. Rarely, toxic amblyopia and cystic macular degeneration.

Toxicity: Fulminant hepatic necrosis if sustained-release capsules are substituted for immediate-release tablets.

Interactions: Rhabdomyolysis reported (rarely) with HMG-CoA reductase inhibitors; postural hypotension if used with ganglionic blockers and vasoactive drugs.

Monitor: Lipid profile; SMA-20; CPK.

MISCELLANEOUS AGENTS
■ **Probucol** (Lorelco; Marion Merrell Dow)

How Supplied:
PO: 250, 500 mg tablets.

Administration: *PO:* Less than 10% absorbed (slightly better with food).

Mechanism of Action: Lowers total LDL cholesterol by increasing LDL catabolism; increasing fecal bile acid excretion; inhibiting early stages of cholesterol biosynthesis and slightly lowering absorption of dietary cholesterol.

Dose: 500 mg bid, pc.

Elimination: Via bile and feces.

Indications: To reduce cholesterol in patients with primary hypercholesterolemia (type IIa and IIb hyperlipoproteinemia) after inadequate response to diet and DM control (see Table 21-1).

Contraindication: Recent/progressive myocardial damage; ventricular dysrhythmia; syncope; prolonged QT interval on ECG (use with caution in patients on other drugs that may prolong QT interval such as tricyclic antidepressants, class I & III antiarrhythmias, phenothiazines, beta blockers; digitalis); pregnancy; lactation.

Adverse Effects: GI distress; paresthesias; angioneurotic edema; eosinphilia; prolonged QT interval.

Monitor: Baseline and periodic lipid profile; ECG; CBC.

Interactions: See contraindication, above. Also, clofibrate may cause lowering of HDL.

CHAPTER 22

NEWBORN DRUGS

■ **Naloxone HCl** (Narcan; Du Pont)

How Supplied:

Parenteral:

0.4 mg/ml, 1 ml ampule, 1 ml prefilled syringe, 10 ml vial.

1.0 mg/ml, 1, 2 ml prefilled syringe, 2 ml ampule, 10 ml vial.

Administration:

IM, IV, SC: Undiluted. IV onset of action almost immediate and recommended for emergencies.

Dose:

1. Narcotic-induced depression: 0.01 mg/kg IM, IV, SC; repeat q2–3min prn; excessive dose may increase BP.
2. Postoperative narcotic depression: 0.1–0.2 mg/kg IV q2–3 min prn; excessive or too rapid reversal may also reverse analgesia, increase BP, or result in nausea, vomiting, or circulatory stress.

Mechanism of Action: Antagonizes opioid effects by competing for same receptor sites. Increases respiratory rate within 1–2 min in patients with respiratory depression, reverses sedative effects, and returns BP level to normal.

Elimination: Conjugated with glucuronic acid in liver; excreted in urine; half-life 1 hr in adults, 3 hr in neonates.

Indications: Reversal of narcotic depression, including respiratory depression, induced by opioids (natural and synthetic); diagnosis of acute suspected opioid overdosage; and neonatal respiratory depression casued by maternal opioid administration or use.

Contraindications: Known drug hypersensitivity. Use with caution in patients with cardiovascular disease; may see hypotension, hypertension, ventricular tachycardia and fibrillation, pulmonary edema.

Toxicity: Abrupt narcotic reversal in newborns of opioid-dependent mothers may precipitate acute abstinence syndrome with vomiting, sweating, increased BP and HR, tremors, seizures, and cardiac arrest.

■ Naltrexone Hydrochloride (Trexan; DuPont Pharma)

How Supplied:
PO: 50 mg tablets.

Administration:
PO, well absorbed. Patient must be confirmed to be opioid-free × 7–10 days.

Mechanism of Action: Pure opioid antagonist; reversibly blocks subjective effects of IV opioids (e.g., morphine, butorphanol, pentazocine).

Dose: Narcan Challenge Test:
  IV: 0.2 mg; another 0.6 mg after 30 sec if no signs of withdrawal (sweating, vomiting, piloerection). See Opioids in Chapter 29).
  SC: 0.8 mg.
  If no withdrawal signs in 20 (for IV) or 45 min (for SC), 25 mg, then another 25 mg in 1 hr; 50 mg/day (or 350 mg/wk, divided q 2–3 days) thereafter.

Elimination: Metabolized in liver; primarily renal excretion.

Indications: To block pharmacologic effects of exogenous opioids as an aid to maintenance of an opioid-free state in detoxified exaddicts.

Contraindications: Patients receiving opioid analgesics; opioid-dependent patients; patients in acute opioid withdrawal; positive opioid urine screen; acute hepatitis or liver failure. Use with caution in patients with recent liver disease; pregnancy; lactation.

Adverse Effects: Hepatocellular injury; anxiety; GI distress; vomiting; joint and muscle pain; headache; abnormal liver function; increased WBCs.

Toxicity: Severe opioid withdrawal symptoms precipitated by accidental ingestion of naltrexone while opioid-dependent: confusion, somnolence, hallucinations, vomiting, diarrhea.

Monitor: LFTs; CBC; urine opioid screens.

Interactions: See Toxicity, above.

BLEEDING PROPHYLAXIS
Vitamin K
See Chapter 19.

EYE PROPHYLAXIS
■ **Erythromycin** (Ilotycin Ointment; Dista)
As directed.

LUNG SURFACTANTS
■ **Colfosceril Palmitate** (Exosurf Neonatal; Burroughs Wellcome)

How Supplied:
Parenteral: 10 ml vial for suspension with 10 ml sterile H_2O.

Administration: *Endotracheal*, after appropriate reconstitution.

Mechanism of Action: Synthetic lung surfactant. Stabilizes alveoli by reducing surface tension, thus improving V/P and gas exchange; also increases elasticity and dynamic compliance to lessen risk of mechanical ventilator complications (e.g., pneumothorax).

Dose: 5 ml/kg q12 hr.

Indications: Prophylactic RDS prevention in infants at risk < 1350 gm, infants >1350 gm with pulmonary immaturity, and treatment of RDS at any weight.

Adverse Effects: Slightly increased risk of pulmonary hemorrhage, apnea.

Monitor: Ventilator parameters.

■ Beractant   (Survanta; Ross)

How Supplied:
Parenteral: 200 mg phospholipids/8 ml in 0.9% NS; single-dose vial.

Administration:
Endotracheal, with infant positioned appropriately to ensure homogenous distribution.

Mechanism of Action: See Colfosceril Palmitate on p. 383.

Dose   4 ml/kg, divided over several minutes (see *PDR*); then q6h.

Indications: Preventon and treatment of RDS in premature infants to reduce mortality and air leak complications.

Contraindications: None known, but controlled data lacking in patients <600 or >1750 gm birth weight.

Adverse Effects: Usually associated with dosing procedure: Transient bradycardia, oxygen desaturation, rales.

Monitor: Ventilator parameters.

NEONATAL RESUSCITATION

Agents used for resuscitation in newborn infants are listed in Table 22-1.

Table 22-1

NEONATAL RESUSCITATION

Agent/Dose	Indications	Goals	Complications
O_2:			
Facemask: 100% at 10 l/min. flow	Respiratory depression	Improve HR and color	PaO_2 over 110 mm Hg not desirable
ET tube: 60–80% O_2 with peak pressure 20–25 cm H_2O, 10 l/min flow	Inadequate improvement via facemask	Improve HR and color	
Sodium bicarbonate: Diluted to 0.5 mEq/ml, infused at 1 mEq/kg/min; total dose 2–3 mEq/kg	pH 7.25, not corrected by adequate ventilation; base deficit more than 15–20 mEq/l	Correct acidosis	If CO_2 retention persists, bicarb metabolized to CO_2 may exacerbate respiratory acidosis Associated with intracranial hemorrhage in prematures
5% Albumin: 10 ml/kg	Hypovolemia with poor peripheral perfusion	Improve peripheral circulation and correct hypotension	Volume overload, if e.g. unable to measure aortic (central) BP versus peripheral
Epinephrine (1:10,000): 0.1 mg/kg IV or through ET tube	Cardiac arrest	Increase HR	
Atropine: 0.01 mg/kg/IV	Severe bradycardia	Increase HR	
Isuprel: 4 mg/250 ml $D_{20}N$	Heart block	Cardiac stimulant; bronchodilator	

385

CHAPTER 23

OBESITY CONTROL: ANORECTICS

Most anorexigenic drugs are chemically similar to amphetamines and decrease appetite by stimulating the hypothalamus to release catecholamines. In addition, these drugs increase physical activity and have various metabolic effects on lipogenesis, lipolysis, and carbohydrate metabolism.

Anorexigenic drugs should be used only in conjunction with caloric restriction, exercise, and other weight reduction programs. Because of tolerance, these drugs should not be used for more than 4 to 6 wk unless significant weight loss has occurred.

The amphetamines are no longer recommended for the treatment of obesity because of the high risk of drug dependence (controlled substances class II). Available drugs in class III or IV or OTC are not so effective in weight loss but have reduced CNS stimulation and low risks of drug dependence.

All anorectics are contraindicated in pregnancy; teratogenesis has been reported. Neonatal withdrawal symptoms can occur. Most anorexigenic drugs are secreted in breast milk and can cause side effects in the newborn.

Table 23-1 lists various anorexigenic agents.

INDICATIONS

Use only in the management of exogenous obesity as a short-term adjunct in a regimen of weight reduction based on caloric restriction.

CONTRAINDICATIONS

- Hyperthyroidism.
- Arteriosclerosis.
- Severe hypertension.

Table 23-1

ANOREXIGENIC AGENTS

Generic Name	Brand Name	Dose	How Supplied	Manufacturer
CONTROLLED SUBSTANCES CLASS				
Schedule IV				
Fenfluramine HCL	Pondimin	20 mg tid	20 mg tab	Robins
Mazindol	Mazanor	1 mg tid	1 mg tab	Wyeth-Ayerst
	Sanorex		1, 2 mg tab	Sandoz
Phentermine HCL	Adipex-P	37.5 mg daily	37.5 mg tab/cap	Teva
	Fastin	30 mg daily	30 mg caps	SKB
Schedule III				
Benzphetamine HCL	Didrex	25–50 mg daily/tid	25,50 mg tab	Upjohn
Phendimetrazine tartrate	Plegine	35 mg bid or tid	35 mg tab	Wyeth-Ayerst
	Prelu-2	1 cap daily	105 mg caps	Boehringer Ingelheim
Schedule II				
Dextroamphetamine sulfate	Dexedrine	5–10 mg daily/bid	5 mg tab	SKB
Methamphetamine HCL	Desoxyn	5 mg daily/bid	5, 10, 15 mg spans	Abbott
Phenmetrazine HCL	Preludin	75 mg daily	5, 10, 15 mg tab	Boehringer Ingelheim
			75 mg Endurets	

387

- Glaucoma.
- Hypersensitivity.
- History of drug abuse.
- Concomitant MAO inhibitor administration.

ADVERSE EFFECTS

1. Cardiovascular: Palpitations, tachycardia, elevation of blood pressure.
2. CNS: Dizziness, overstimulation, insomnia, headache, tremor.
3. GI: Dryness of mouth, diarrhea or constipation.
4. Endocrine: Changes in libido, impotence.
5. Skin: Allergic manifestations.

CHAPTER 24

OVER-THE-COUNTER PREPARATIONS

STANDARD COMPONENTS

Sympathomimetic Amines: Nasal Decongestants

1. Phenylpropanolamine:
   a. Sympathomimetic amine.
   b. Pharmacologic action and potency similar to ephedrine except less CNS stimulation.
   c. Often combined with H_1 antagonist for oral relief of nasal or sinus congestion.
2. Pseudoephedrine:
   a. Sympathomimetic amine.
   b. Stereoisomer of ephedrine.
   c. For oral relief of nasal congestion.
3. Phenylephrine:
   a. Powerful α-sympathomimetic amine.
   b. Forms: PO, nasal, ophthalmic.
   c. Uses: Nasal decongestant, mydriatic.

Antihistamines: Antiallergic

1. Chlorpheniramine:
   a. Alkylamine type of potent H_1–blocker with anticholinergic (drying) secondary effects.
   b. Side effects: Drowsiness less common but CNS stimulation more common.
2. Brompheniramine: Similar to chlorpheniramine.
3. Diphenhydramine:
   a. Ethanolamine type of potent H_1–blocker.
   b. Significant antimuscarinic effects.
   c. Side effects: Sedation frequent, GI distress rare.

Antitussives

1. Dextromethorphan:
   a. D-Isomer of codeine analog of levorphanol but without the analgesic or addictive properties.
   b. Acts centrally to raise cough threshold.
   c. Fewer subjective and GI side effects.

MISCELLANEOUS OTC PREPARATIONS

Tables 24-1 to 24-7 list various analgesics, antacids, appetite suppressants, stimulants, respiratory infection remedies, and sleep aids.

Table 24-1
ANALGESICS

Agent (Co.)	Formula (mg)	Form	Usual Dose (Max/24 hr)*
I. ACETAMINOPHEN CLASS			
Arthritis Foundation	Acetaminophen 500	Caplet	TT q4-6h (8)
Aspirin Free (McNeil Consumer)			
Panadol (Smith-Kline Beecham)	Acetaminophen 500	Tablet, caplet	TT q4h (8)
Tylenol, Regular Strength (McNeil)	Acetaminophen 325	Tablet, caplet	T–TT tid-qid
Tylenol, Extra Strength (McNeil)	Acetaminophen 500	Tablet, caplet, gelcap	TT tid-qid
		Liquid (500 mg/15 ml)	30 ml q4-6h (120 ml)
II. ACETAMINOPHEN COMBINATIONS			
Maximum Strength Arthritis Foundation	Acetaminophen 500	Caplet	TT hs
Night Time (McNeil)	Diphenhydramine 25		
Bayer Select Maximum Strength	Acetaminophen 500 + caffeine 65	Caplet	TT q4-6h (8)
Headache (Miles)			
Bayer Select Maximum Strength	Acetaminophen 500 +	Caplet	TT q4-6 (8)
Menstrual (Miles)	pamabrom 75		
Bayer Select Night Time Pain	Acetaminophen 500 +	Caplet	TT qhs
Relief (Miles)	diphenhydramine 25		
Teen Multi-Symptom Formula	Acetaminophen 400 +	Caplet	TT q4-6h (8)
Midol (Miles)	pamabrom 25		
Maximum Strength Multi-Symptom	Acetaminophen 500 + caffeine 60	Caplet, gelcap	TT q4-6h (8)
Formula Midol (Miles)	Pyrilamine maleate 15		

*T, 1 tablet; TT, 2 tablets; TTT, 3 tablets.

Continued.

391

Table 24-1			
ANALGESICS—Cont'd			
III. ASPIRIN CLASS			
Arthritis Foundation Safety-Coated Aspirin (McNeil)	Aspirin 500	Tablet	TT q6h (8)
Genuine Bayer Aspirin (Miles)	Aspirin 325	Tablet, caplet	T–TT q4h (12)
Maximum Bayer Aspirin (Miles)	Aspirin 500	Tablet, caplet	T–TT q4h (8)
Empirin Aspirin (Warner Wellcome)	Aspirin 325	Tablet	T–TT q4h (12)
IV. ASPIRIN COMBINATIONS			
Anacin (Whitehall)	Aspirin 400 + caffeine 32	Tablet, caplet	TT q4h (10)
Ascriptin (CIBA)	Aspirin 325 + maalox	Tablet	TT q4h (12)
Maximum Strength Anacin (Whitehall)	Aspirin 500 + caffeine 32	Tablet	TT tid–qid (8)
Arthritis Pain Formula (Whitehall)	Aspirin 500 + aluminum hydroxide 27 + magnesium hydroxide 100	Tablet, caplet	TT tid–qid
Ecotrin (Smith-Kline Beecham)	Aspirin 325, enteric coated	Tablet, caplet	TT q4h or TTT q6h
	Aspirin 500, enteric coated	Tablet, caplet	TT q6h
Excedrin (Bristol-Myers)	Aspirin 250 + acetaminophen 250 + caffeine 65	Tablet, caplet	TT q4h (8)
Extra Strength Bayer PM Aspirin (Miles)	Aspirin 500 + diphenhydramine 25	Caplet	TT qhs
Vanquish (Miles)	Aspirin 227 + acetaminophen 194 + caffeine 33 + aluminum hydroxide 25 + magnesium hydroxide 50	Caplet	TT q4h (12)

Table 24-1
ANALGESICS—Cont'd

V. NSAIAs

Advil (Whitehall)	Ibuprofen 200	Tablet, caplet	T–TT q4–6h (6)
Aleve (Procter & Gamble)	Naproxen sodium 200	Tablet	T q8–12h (3)
Arthritis Foundation OTL (McNeil)	Ibuprofen 200	Tablet	T–TT q4–6h (6)
Bayer Select Ibuprofen (Miles)	Ibuprofen 200	Caplet	T q4–6h (6)
Medipren (McNeil)	Ibuprofen 200	Tablet, caplet	T–TT q4–6h (6)
Motrin IB (Upjohn)	Ibuprofen 200	Tablet, caplet	T–TT q4–6h (6)
Nuprin (Bristol-Myers)	Ibuprofen 200	Tablet	T–TT q4–6h (6)

Table 24-2

ANTACIDS

Preparation (Mfr)	Formula	Form	ANC[1]/Tab or 5 ml (mEq)	Usual Dose (Max/24 hr)
Alka-Seltzer (Miles)	Aspirin 325 + $NaHCO_3^-$ 1916 + citric acid 1000	Effervescent tablet	17.2	TT/6 oz H_2O q4h (8)
Amphojel (Wyeth-Ayerst)	AL $(OH)_3$ 320/5 ml AL $(OH)_3$ 300, 600	PO suspension 0.3, 0.6 gm tablet		10 ml 5-6 ×/day (60 ml) TT (0.3) or T (0.6) 5-6 ×/day (12; 6)
Maalox (CIBA-Geigy)	AL $(OH)_3$ 225 + Mg $(OH)_2$ 200 AL $(OH)_3$ 200 + Mg $(OH)_2$ 200	Suspension Tablet	13.3 9.7	10–20 ml qid (80) TT–IV qid (16)
Extra Strength Maalox (CIBA-Geigy)	AL $(OH)_3$ 400 + Mg $(OH)_2$ 400	Tablet	23.4	T–TT qid (8)
Extra Strength Maalox Plus (CIBA-Geigy)	AL $(OH)_3$ 500 + Mg $(OH)_2$ 450 + simethicone 40	Suspension Tablet	29 11.4	10–20 ml qid (60) T–IV qid (16)
Phillips Milk of Magnesia (Miles)	MG $(OH)_2$ 405 Mg $(OH)_2$ 311	Suspension Tablet		5–15 ml qid (60) TT–IV qid (16)
Rolaids (Warner-Lambert)	A1 $(OH)_3$/$NaHCO_3$ 334	Tablet	8	T–TT qhr prn (24)

Table 24-2
ANTACIDS—Cont'd

Preparation (Mfr)	Formula	Form	ANC¹/Tab or 5 ml (mEq)	Usual Dose (Max/24 hr)
Extra Strength Rolaids (Warner-Lambert)	$CaCO_3$ 1000	Tablet		T–TT qhr prn (8)
Tums (Smith-Kline Beecham)	$CaCO_3$ 500	Tablet	10	T–TT qhr prn (16)
Tums E-X (Smith-Kline Beecham)	$CaCO_3$ 750	Tablet		T–TT qhr prn (10)
Tums Liquid Extra Strength (Smith-Kline Beecham)	$CaCO_3$ 1000	Suspension	20	5–10 ml qhr prn (40)
Tums Liquid Extra Strength + Simethicone (Smith-Kline Beecham)	$CaCO_3$ 1000 + simethicone – 30	Suspension	20	5–10 ml qhr prn (40)

$NaHCO_3$, sodium bicarbonate; $AL(OH)_3$, aluminum hydroxide; $Mg (OH)_3$, magnesium hydroxide; ANC, acid neutralizing capacity; $A1(OH)_3/NaHCO_3$, trihydroxy aluminum calcium carbonate; $CaCO_3$, calcium carbonate; $NaHCO_3$, sodium carbonate.

Table 24-3
APPETITE SUPPRESSANTS

Preparation (Co.)	Active Ingredient (mg)	Usual Dose
Acutrim 16 Hour (CIBA)	Phenylpropanolamine HCL* 75	T qAM
Acutrim Maximum Strength (CIBA)	Phenylpropanolamine HCL 75	T qAM
Acutrim Late Day (CIBA)	Phenylpropanolamine HCL 75	T qAM
Dexatrim Maximum Strength (Thompson)	Phenylpropanolamine HCL 75	T qAM
Dexatrim Maximum Strength Plus Vitamin C (CIBA)	Phenylpropanolamine HCL 75 plus Vitamin C 180	T qAM

*Phenylpropanolamine: Sympathomimetic amine; pharmacologic action and potency similar to ephedrine but less CNS stimulation.

Table 24-4
STIMULANTS

Preparation (Co.)	Active Ingredient (mg/tab)	Usual Dose
No Doz (Bristol-Myers)	Caffeine 100	T–TT q3–4h

Table 24-5

RESPIRATORY INFECTION REMEDIES: ANTIHISTAMINES, DECONGESTANTS, AND COMBINATIONS

Brand (Co.)	Formula mg/tab or 5 ml	Form	Usual Dose (Max/24 hr)
Actifed (Warner Wellcome)	Pseudoephedrine 60/triprolidine 2.5	Capsule, tablet	T q4–6h (4)
Actifed Plus (Warner Wellcome)	Acetaminophen 500/pseudoephedrine 30/ triprolidine 1.25	Caplet, tablet	TT q6h (8)
Actifed Syrup (Warner Wellcome)	Pseudoephedrine 30/triprolidine 1.25	Syrup	10 ml q4–6h (40)
Alka-Seltzer Plus (Miles)	Phenylpropanolamine 24/chlorpheniramine 2/ aspirin 325	Effervescent tablet	TT + 6 oz H₂O q4h (8)
Alka-Seltzer Plus Night-Time (Miles)	Phenylpropanolamine 24/diphenhydramine 38.3/ aspirin 325	Effervescent tablet	TT + 6 oz H₂O q4–6h (8)
Allerest (CIBA)	Phenylpropanolamine 18.7/chlorpheniramine 2	Tablet	TT q4h (8)
Allerest Sinus Pain Formula (CIBA)	Phenylpropanolamine 18.7/chlorpheniramine 2/ acetaminophen 500	Tablet	TT q6h (8)
Chlor-Trimeton Allergy (Schering)	Chlorpheniramine 4	Tablet Syrup	T q4–6h (6) 10 ml q4–6h (60)
Chlor-Trimeton Decongestant (Schering)	Chlorpheniramine 4/pseudoephedrine 60	Tablet	T q4–6h (4)
Comtrex (Bristol-Myers)	Chlorpheniramine 2/pseudoephedrine 30/ acetaminophen 325/dextromethorphan 10	Tablet; caplet	TT q4h (8)
Contac (Smith-Kline Beecham)	Phenylpropanolamine 75/chlorpheniramine 8	Capsule	T q12h (2)
Contac Sinus Non-Drowsy (Smith-Kline Beecham)	Pseudoephedrine 30/acetaminophen 500	Tablet; caplet	TT q6h (8)
Contac Severe Cold (Smith-Kline Beecham)	Phenylpropanolamine 12.5/chlorpheniramine 2/ acetaminophen 500/dextromethorphan 15	Caplet	TT q6h (8)

Continued.

OVER THE COUNTER

Table 24-5

RESPIRATORY INFECTION REMEDIES: ANTIHISTAMINES, DECONGESTANTS, AND COMBINATIONS—Cont'd

Brand (Co.)	Formula mg/tab or 5 ml	Form	Usual Dose (Max/24 hr)
Coricidin (Schering)	Chlorpheniramine 2/acetaminophen 325	Tablet	TT q4h (12)
Coricidin-D (Schering)	Chlorpheniramine 2/acetaminophen 325/ phenylpropanolamine 12.5	Tablet	TT q4h (12)
Dimetapp (Robins)	Brompheniramine 4/phenylpropanolamine 25	Tablet	T q4h (6)
Dimetapp Plus (Robins)	Brompheniramine 2/phenylpropanolamine 12.5/ acetaminophen 500	Caplet	TT q6h (8)
Drixoral (Schering)	Pseudoephedrine 120/dexbrompheniramine 6	Tablet	T q12h (2)
	Pseudoephedrine 30/brompheniramine 2	Syrup	10 ml q4–6h (40)
Sine-Off Maximum Strength (Smith-Kline Beecham)	Pseudoephedrine-30/chlorpheniramine 2/ acetaminophen 500	Caplet	TT q6h (8)
Sine-Off Aspirin Formula (Smith-Kline Beecham)	Phenylpropanolamine 12.5/chlorpheniramine 2/ aspirin 325	Tablet	TT q4h (8)
Sinutab Allergy (Warner Wellcome)	Pseudoephedrine 120/dexbrompheniramine 6	Tablet	T q12h (8)
Sinutab Maximum Strength (Warner Wellcome)	Pseudoephedrine 30/chlorpheniramine 2/ acetaminophen 500	Tablet, caplet	TT q6h (8)
Triaminic (Sandoz)	Phenylpropanolamine 12.5/ chlorpheniramine 2	Tablet Syrup	TT q4h (12) 20ml q4h
Tylenol Cold Medication (McNeil)	Pseudoephedrine-30/ chlorpheniramine 2/ dextromethorphan 15 acetaminophen 325	Tablet, caplet Syrup	TT q6h (8) 30 ml q6h (120)
Tylenol Allergy Sinus (McNeil)	Pseudoephedrine 30/ chlorpheniramine 2/ acetaminophen 500	Caplet	TT q6h (8)
Tylenol Sinus (McNeil)	Pseudoephedrine 30/acetaminophen 500	Tablet, caplet	TT q4–6h (8)

Table 24-6
RESPIRATORY INFECTION REMEDIES: ANTITUSSIVES, EXPECTORANTS, AND COMBINATIONS

Brand (Co.)	Formula (mg per 5 ml)	Alcohol Content (%)	Usual Dose (Max/24 hr)
Benylin (Warner Wellcome)	Diphenhydramine 12.5	5	10 ml q5h (60)
Benylin-DM (Warner Wellcome)	Dextromethorphan 10	5	5–10 ml q4h or 15 q6–8h (60)
Benylin Decongestant (Warner Wellcome)	Diphenhydramine 12.5/pseudoephedrine 30	5	10 ml q4h (40)
Benylin Expectorant (Warner Wellcome)	Dextromethorphan 20/guaifenesin 400	5	10–20 ml q4h (120)
Contact Cough Formula (Smith-Kline Beecham)	Dextromethorphan 30/guaifenesin 200*	–	15 ml q6–8h (60)
Contact Nighttime Cold Medicine (Smith-Kline Beecham)	Dextromethorphan 30/doxylamine succinate* 7.5/ pseudoephedrine 60/acetaminophen 100	25	30 ml qhs or q6h (120)
Robitussin (Robins)	Guaifenesin 100	3.5	10–20 ml q4h (120)
Robitussin-CF (Robins)	Guaifenesin 100/phenylpropanolamine 12.5/ dextromethorphan 10	4.75	10 ml q4h (60)
Robitussin-DM (Robins)	Guaifenesin 100/dextromethorphan 15	1.4	10 ml q6–8h (40)
Robitussin-PE (Robins)	Guaifenesin 100/pseudoephedrine 30	1.4	10 ml q4h (40)
Triaminic Expectorant (Sandoz)	Guaifenesin 100/phenylpropanolamine 12.5	5	10 ml q4h (60)
Triaminic-DM (Sandoz)	Dextromethorphan 10/phenylpropanolamine 12.5	–	10 ml q4h (60)
Triaminic Multi-Symptom Relief (Sandoz)	Dextromethorphan 10/phenylpropanolamine 12.5/ chlorpheniramine 2	–	10 ml q4h (60)

*Antihistamine with some hypnotic effects.

Table 24-7
SLEEP AIDS

Brand (Co.)	Formula (mg per 5 ml)	Form	Usual Dose
Excedrin P.M. (Bristol-Myers)	Diphenhydramine 38/acetaminophen 500	Tablet; caplet	ṪṪ qhs
Nytol (Block)	Diphenhydramine 25	Caplet	ṪṪ qhs
Sleepinol (Thompson)	Diphenhydramine 50	Capsule, softgel	Ṫ qhs
Unisom (Pfizer)	Doxylamine 25	Tablet	Ṫ qhs
Unisom with Pain Relief (Pfizer)	Diphenhydramine 50/acetaminophen 650	Tablet	Ṫ qhs

CHAPTER 25

OVULATION STIMULATION AND FERTILITY-PROMOTING AGENTS

■ Clomiphene Citrate   (Serophene; Serono)

Nonsteroidal compound with estrogenic activity, which may induce ovulation in anovulatory women. The apparent mechanism of action is the drug-induced release of pituitary gonadotropin hormones.

How Supplied: 50 mg tablet.

Dose: Starting about the fifth day of cycle, give 50 mg/day for 5 days. If ovulation does not occur, a second course of 100 mg/day may be given. Treatment beyond three courses usually is not recommended.

Indication: Treatment of ovulatory failure.

Contraindications:
1. Pregnancy.
2. Liver disease.
3. Abnormal uterine bleeding.
4. Ovarian cyst of undetermined origin.

Warning: Careful evaluation of patient must be done before clomiphene therapy is begun, including liver function, determination of endogenous estrogen production, and evaluation of husband's fertility.

Adverse Effects:
1. Ovarian hyperstimulation syndrome (see Urofollitropin).
2. Multiple gestations.
3. Vasomotor symptoms.
4. Ovarian enlargement and abdominal pain.
5. Breast tenderness.
6. Visual symptoms.
7. Other symptoms, usually minor.
8. Various congenital anomalies reported in 2.5% of pregnancies, which does not exceed the rate in general population.

■ Urofollitropin   (Metrodin; Serono)

Preparation of gonadotropins extracted from urine of postmenopausal women containing 75 IU FSH and less than 1 IU LH. Mechanism of action is to stimulate ovarian follicular activity and maturation. To effect ovulation, in the absence of endogenous LH surge, give hCG at the appropriate time.

How Supplied: 1 ampule containing 75 IU urofollitropin as sterile lyophilized powder and 1 ampule (2 ml) NaCl injection.

Dose: Individualize starting with 75 IU/day IM for 7–12 days, followed by 5000 to 10,000 units hCG 1 day after last dose of urofollitropin. As guide to therapy, ultrasound and serum or urinary estrogen levels are essential. If ovaries are abnormally enlarged on last day, no hCG should be administered. If there is evidence of ovulation and no pregnancy occurs, the cycle of drug therapy may be repeated for at least two more cycles, increasing urofollitropin to 150 IU/day.

Indications:
1. Combined with hCG, used for induction of ovulation in women with polycystic ovary disease and other pituitary-ovarian disorders.
2. Stimulate development of multiple oocytes in assisted reproduction methods.

Contraindications:
1. Primary ovarian failure (high FSH level).
2. Pituitary tumor.
3. Abnormal uncontrolled thyroid or adrenal dysfunction.

4. Ovarian cysts not caused by polycystic ovary disease.
5. Pregnancy.
6. Abnormal uterine bleeding of undetermined origin.

Warning:
1. Ovarian hyperstimulation may occur, causing increased vascular permeability, leading to rapid accumulations of fluid in all body cavities and to serious life-threatening cardiovascular and pulmonary changes.
2. Multiple gestations can occur, including quintuplets.
3. Metrodin should be used by physicians experienced with treatment of infertility.

Adverse Reactions:
1. Ovarian hyperstimulation syndrome.
2. Ovarian enlargement, usually cystic.
3. Abdominal pain and GI symptoms.
4. Breast enlargement and tenderness.
5. Rash, swelling, pain at injection site.

■ **Menotropins** (Pergonal; Serono. Humegon; Organon)

Preparation of gonadotropins extracted from urine of postmenopausal women containing 75 or 150 IU FSH and 75 or 150 IU LH.

How Supplied:
1. 1 ampule containing 75 IU FSH and 75 IU LH with 1 ampule (2 ml) NaCl for injection.
2. 1 ampule containing 150 IU FSH and 150 IU LH with 1 ampule (2 ml) NaCl for injection.

Indications:
1. Menotropins are used to stimulate ovarian follicular development and maturation. To effect ovulation, give hCG after the administration of menotropins.
2. In infertile men, menotropins are used in combination with hCG to stimulate spermatogenesis.

OVULATION

Contraindications, Warnings, Adverse Effects:
See Urofollitropin on p. 402.

■ Human Chorionic Gonadotropin (Profasi; Serono. Pregnyl; Organon)

Product derived from human pregnancy urine containing 5000 or 10,000 USP units/ampule. The mechanism of action is to stimulate production of gonadal steroid hormones, primarily testosterone in the men and progesterone in the women.

How Supplied: 10 ml multidose vial containing 5000 or 10,000 USP units/vial in lyophilized powder, to be combined with sterile water for injection. When reconstituted and refrigerated will last for 60 days.

Dose: 5000 to 10,000 USP units administered 1 day after last dose of human menotropins.

Indications:
Women: hCG is used to induce ovulation after appropriate treatment with menotropins or urofollitropin.
Men: hCG is used to treat hypogonadotropism, infertility, and prepubertal cryptorchidism not resulting from anatomic defect.

Contraindications:
1. Precocious puberty.
2. Androgen-dependent neoplasm.
3. Previous hypersensitivity to hCG.

Warning:
1. hCG has not been demonstrated to be of use in the treatment of obesity.
2. hCG should be used only by physicians experienced with treatment of infertility.

Adverse Effects: See urofollitropin.

■ Leuprolide Acetate (Lupron; TAP)

A synthetic nonpeptide analog of GnRH possessing greater potency than the natural hormone. Acting as an LHRH agonist, the compound paradoxically is a potent inhibitor of gonadotropin secretion, initially stimulating ovarian and testicular steroidogenesis but with continued administration suppressing ovulation and spermatogenesis. The effect is completely reversible when the drug is discontinued.

In premenopausal women, an initial increase in FSH and LH levels leads to a transient increase in ovarian production of estrone and estradiol. In men, transient increases are noted in testosterone and dihydrotestosterone levels.

How Supplied:
Injection only: 2.8 ml multidose vial; each 0.2 ml contains 1 mg leuprolide acetate.
Lupron Depot: Single-dose vial contains 7.5 mg leuprolide acetate.

Dose:
SC: 1 mg (0.2 ml) daily injection.
IM Depot: 7.5 mg injection monthly.

Indications:
1. Palliative treatment of advanced prostatic cancer.
2. Endometriosis.
3. Uterine leiomyomata tumors.

Contraindications: Pregnancy must be excluded.

Precautions: In women, suppression of ovarian steroidogenesis causes menopausal symptoms and signs (flashes, sweats, osteoporosis, many other changes). Allergic skin reactions.

■ Goserelin Acetate Implant (Zoladex; Zeneca)
Synthetic decapeptide analog of luteinizing hormone-releasing hormone (LHRH). In women and men, down-regulation of the pituitary gland occurs, leading to suppression of gonadotropin secretion and decrease in estradiol production in the ovary and decrease in testosterone production in the testes.

How Supplied/Dose: Disposable syringe containing 3.6 mg to be administered subcutaneously q28 days into the abdominal wall. See manufacturer's instructions.

OVULATION

Indications: Endometriosis: Treat for 6 months. Prostatic carcinoma: individualize.

Contraindications: Pregnancy must be excluded.

■ Gonadorelin Acetate (Lutrepulse; Ortho. Factrel; Wyeth-Ayerst)

Synthetic preparation of gonadotrophin-releasing hormone (GnrH) for pulsatile intravenous injection. Use approximates the natural hormonal secretary pattern of the hypothalamus; the primary effect is the synthesis and release of luteinizing hormone (LH) in the pituitary gland.

Indication: Diagnosis and treatment of primary hypothalamic amenorrhea.

Contraindication:
If pregnancy is contraindicted.
Presence of certain types of ovarian cysts.

Adverse Effects: See Urofollitropin section.

Dose and Administration: See manufacturer's instructions.

■ Nafarelin Acetate (Synarel; Syntex)
See Chapter 28.

■ Bromocriptine Mesylate (Parlodel; Sandoz)

How Supplied: *PO:*
2.5 mg tablet (Snap tabs)
5 mg capsule

Administration:
PO: Fractional systemic bioavailability because of limited (30%) and extensive first-pass metabolism.

Dose:
1. Hyperprolactinemia: Initially 1.25 mg hs or bid if side effects tolerated; increase by 2.5 mg/day q1–4 wk. Usual therapeutic dose 5–7.5 mg/day (range 2.5–25 mg/day).
2. Acromegaly: Initially 1.25–2.5 mg hs; increase by 1.25–2.5 mg/day q3–7 days until optimally effective. Usual therapeutic dose 20-30 mg/day; max 100 mg/day.
3. Parkinson's disease: Initially 1.25–2.5 mg pc bid; increase 2.5 mg/day q1–2 wk. Adjust concurrent levodopa dosage.

Mechanism of Action: Lysergic acid derivative and potent dopaminergic agonist. Action on postsynaptic dopamine (DA) receptors in the tuberoinfundibular process releases prolactin-inhibiting factor (= DA) to reduce prolactin levels in patients with hyperprolactinemia, both pathologic and physiologic (lactation). Also lowers growth hormone levels in acromegaly; reinstitutes ovulatory menstrual cycle in 75% of patients with amenorrhea-galactorrhea syndrome. Antiparkinson effect results from direct stimulation of DA receptors in the corpus striatum.

Elimination: Metabolized in liver; excreted in feces and bile.

Indication:
1. Hyperprolactinemia: Amenorrhea with or without galactorrhea, infertility, hypogonadism, prolactinoma.
2. Acromegaly: Alone or with radiation, surgery.
3. Parkinson's disease.

Contraindications: Uncontrolled hypertension (HTN); risk of seizures, pregnancy-induced HTN; ergot alkaloid sensitivity; pregnancy; children younger than 15 yr. Use with caution in patients with renal or liver disease.

Toxicity:
1. Initially: Nausea (49%), headache, dizziness, GI distress, nasal congestion, hypotension.
2. Long-term treatment: Constipation, dyskinesia, erythromelalgia, psychiatric symptoms, alcohol intolerance, digital vasospasm.

OVULATION

CHAPTER 26

PSYCHO-PHARMACOLOGIC DRUGS

ANTIANXIETY DRUGS

Anxiety is a normal response of the autonomic nervous system that results from the anticipation of danger, either internal or external. Abnormal function of the individual may occur when the anxiety is disproportionate to the stimulus. Anxiety disorders are classified as primary or situational. The causes of the latter may be medical conditions such as substance abuse, psychiatric disorders, hyperthyroidism, or psychosocial stresses.

Psychopharmacologic therapy in the form of anxiolytic medication can be extremely useful in alleviating the myriad emotional and physical complaints of the patient. Specific disorders that are amenable to drug therapy include anxiety neuroses (e.g., panic disorders), obsessive-compulsive disorders, posttraumatic stress disorder, sleep disorders, and phobic disorders.

BENZODIAZEPINES

The benzodiazepines are usually the drugs of choice for anxiety syndromes. Their sedative and hypnotic actions are useful in a variety of conditions. Compared with other drugs, benzodiazepines offer distinct advantages regarding adverse effects, tolerance, abuse, and toxicity (Table 26-1).

Indications

1. Management of anxiety disorders.
2. Symptomatic relief in acute anxiety attacks.
3. Alcoholic withdrawal symptoms.

Table 26-1
BENZODIAZEPINES

Name Generic	Brand	(Mfr)	Equivalent Dose (mg)	Half-life (hr)	Onset of Action	Usual Dose*	How Supplied
LONG-ACTING							
Chlordiazepoxide	Librium	(Roche)	10	20	Intermediate	5 or 10 mg tid	5, 10, 25 mg tab
Chlorazepate	Tranxene	(Abbott)	7.5	60	Rapid	15–30 mg OD	3.75, 7.5, 15 mg tab 11.25, 22.5 mg single-dose tab
Diazepam	Valium	(Roche)	5	40	Rapid	2–10 mg bid/tid	2, 5, 10 mg tab
Flurazepam	Dalmane	(Roche)	15	80	Rapid	15–30 mg hs	15, 30 mg tab
SHORT-ACTING							
Alprazolam	Xanax	(Upjohn)	0.5	11	Intermediate	0.25–0.5 mg tid	0.25, 0.5, 1.0 mg tab
Lorazepam	Ativan	(Wyeth-Ayerst)	1	14	Intermediate	2–6 mg OD	0.5, 1, 2 mg tab
Oxazepam	Serax	(Wyeth-Ayerst)	15	8	Slow	10–15 mg tid	10, 15, 30 mg tab
Temazepam	Restoril	(Sandoz)	15	12	Intermediate	15–30 mg hs	15, 30 mg Tab
Triazolam	Halcion	(Upjohn)	0.125	3	Rapid	0.25 mg hs	0.125, 0.25 mg tab

*The dosage will vary depending on the clinical condition treated and the individual requirements.

PSYCHOPHARMACOLOGIC

409

4. Preoperative for relief of anxiety.
5. Seizures.
6. Skeletal muscle spasm.

Contraindications

Known hypersensitivity to the drug.

Adverse Effects:

1. Drowsiness, mental confusion, ataxia: These drugs may impair mental and physical performance and could be hazardous when one is driving or operating machinery. The concomitant use of alcohol or other CNS depressants may have an additive effect. In older women the dosage should be kept very low to preclude ataxia or oversedation. Drug interactions may occur and should be considered when adverse symptoms develop.
2. Allergic manifestations.
3. Extrapyramidal symptoms.
4. Increased or decreased libido.
5. Jaundice, blood dyscrasias.
6. Drug abuse and dependence; withdrawal symptoms.
7. Use in pregnancy: There are reports of congenital malformations when these drugs were taken during the first trimester of pregnancy; therefore these drugs should not be prescribed during early pregnancy. In the case of unsuspected pregnancy and drug administration, the patient should be counseled regarding the risks of fetal abnormalities.

ANTIDEPRESSANTS

Affective disorders (depression) may be ameliorated and controlled with drug therapy. Various agents, including the heterocyclic antidepressants, monoamine oxidase inhibitors, and lithium, are used. Anxiety often accompanies depression but is usually relieved by one of these agents. However, if an anxiolytic is indicated, the benzodiazepines are the drugs of choice.

Indications

These agents are used to treat symptoms of acute depression and to prevent relapse. Use of these drugs elevates mood, increases mental alertness, improves sleep patterns, and reduces morbid preoccupation. Table 26-2 lists antidepressants used in gynecology.

Table 26-2

SOME ANTIDEPRESSANTS USED IN GYNECOLOGY

Type-Generic Name	Brand Name (Mfg.)	Anticholinergic Effects	Sedative/Agitation Effects	Usual Daily Dose (mg)	How Supplied
TRICYCLIC TERTIARY AMINES					
Amitriptyline	Elavil (Stuart)	High	High	75–150	10, 25, 50, 75, 100, 150 mg tab
	Endep (Roche)				
Doxepin	Sinequan (Roerig)	High	High	75–100	10, 25, 50, 75, 100, 150 mg tab
Imipramine	Tofranil (Geigy)	High	High-moderate	75–100	75, 100, 125, 150 mg cap
Trimipramine	Surmontil (Wyeth-Ayerst)	High	High	75–150	25, 50, 100 mg cap
TRICYCLIC SECONDARY AMINES					
Amoxapine	Asendin (Lederle)	Low-moderate	Low-moderate	75–200	25, 50, 100, 150 mg tab
Desipramine	Norpramin (Merrell Dow)	Low	Low	75–100	10, 25, 50, 75, 100, 150 mg tab
Nortriptyline	Pamelor (Sandoz)	Moderate	Low-Moderate	20–100	10, 25, mg cap
					10 mg/5 ml liquid
Protriptyline	Vivactil (Merck)	Moderate-high	None-low	15–40	5, 10 mg tab

Continued.

411

Table 26-2

SOME ANTIDEPRESSANTS USED IN GYNECOLOGY-Cont'd

MONOAMINE OXIDASE INHIBITORS				
Phenelzine	Nardil (Parke-Davis)	Hypertensive crisis	45–90	15 mg tab
Tranylcypromine	Parnate (SKB)	Hypertensive crisis	20–40	10 mg tab
SEROTONIN REUPTAKE INHIBITORS				
Fluoxetine	Prozac (Dista)	None	20	10, 20 mg pulvules; 20 mg/5 ml liquid
Nefazodone	Serzone (BMS)	None	200	100, 150, 200, 250 mg tab
Paroxetine	Paxil (SKB)	None	20	20, 30 mg tab
Sertraline	Zoloft (Roerig)	None	50	50, 100 mg tab

Adverse Reactions

1. Anticholinergic and ß-adrenergic effects (diaphoresis, flushes, blurred vision, constipation, hypotension, tachycardia).
2. Aggravation of angle-closure glaucoma.
3. Urinary retention.
4. Adynamic ileus.
5. Excessive sedation, insomnia.
6. Overeating.
7. Seizures.
8. Cardiac toxicity (with overdosage).
9. Hypertensive crisis (with MAO inhibitors) secondary to interactions with certain foods or drugs.

BARBITURATES (TABLE 26-3)

Barbituric acid derivatives have hypnotic and anticonvulsant activity because of their nonselective depression of the CNS. All levels of CNS mood alteration can occur, from excitation to deep coma, depending on the drug and dosage. These drugs cross the placenta and are excreted in breast milk, which may cause fetal

Table 26-3
BARBITURATES

Generic	Brand (Mfg.)	How Supplied
Amobarbital	Amytal sodium (Lilly)	15, 30, 50, 100 mg tab 65, 200 mg cap 250, 500 mg in powder for injection
Butabarbital	Butisol (Wallace)	15, 30, 50, 100 mg tab 30 mg/5 ml elixir
Mephobarbital	Mebaral (Winthrop)	32, 50, 100 mg tab
Pentobarbital	Nembutal (Abbott)	50, 100 mg cap 100 mg/2 ml amp injection 30, 60, 120, 200 mg suppository
Phenobarbital	Generic (Lilly)	15, 30, 60 mg tab 20 mg/5 ml elixir 30, 65, 130 mg/ml injection
Secobarbital	Seconal (Lilly)	50, 100 mg tabs/cap 120, 200 mg suppository 50 mg/ml vial injection

PSYCHOPHARMACOLOGIC

abnormalities, respiratory depression of the newborn, coagulation defects in the neonate, and drug dependance in the nursing infant.

Dosage

The dosage must be individualized, based on the condition treated, the age and weight of the patient, and the particular barbiturate prescribed. These drugs are classified according to their onset and duration of action.

1. Long acting: Onset of action in about 60 min; duration about 10 hr.
   a. Mephobarbital (Mebaral)
   b. Phenobarbital
2. Intermediate acting: Onset of action in 45–60 min; duration 6–8 hr.
   a. Amobarbital (Amytal) sodium
   b. Butabarbital (Butisol) sodium
3. Short acting: Onset of action in 10–15 min; duration 3–4 hr.
   a. Pentobarbital sodium (Nembutal)
   b. Secobarbital (Seconal) sodium

Indications

1. Treatment of insomnia.
2. Sedation.
3. Preanesthetic anxiety relief.
4. Epilepsy.
5. Seizures.

Contraindications

1. Hypersensitivity to barbiturates.
2. First trimester of pregnancy.
3. Cautionary use throughout pregnancy and lactation.

Adverse Effects

1. Respiratory depression, apnea, laryngospasm.
2. Hypersensitivity effects; exfoliative dermatitis.
3. Barbiturate dependence.
4. CNS symptoms (e.g., drowsiness, confusion, slurred speech).

HYPNOTICS AND SEDATIVES: NONBENZODIAZEPINES-NONBARBITURATES

■ Buspirone HCl   (Buspar; BMS)

How Supplied: 5, 10 mg tablet.

Dose: 5 mg tid.
   Sedation or ataxia uncommon; low incidence of extrapyramidal side effects; little potential for abuse or withdrawal syndrome. Not listed as controlled substance.

Chloral Hydrate

How Supplied:
   200, 500 mg capsule.
   250, 500 mg/5 ml syrup.
   500 mg suppository.

Dose:
   250 mg tid pc.
   500 mg hs.

■ Ethchlorvynol   (Placidyl; Abbott)

How Supplied: 200, 500, 750 mg capsule.

Dose: 500–1000 mg hs.

■ Hydroxyzine HCl   (Atarax; Roerig)

How Supplied:
   10, 25, 50, 100 mg tablet.
   10 mg/5 ml syrup.

Dose: 50–100 mg qid.

■ Hydroxyzine HCl (Vistaril; Roerig)

How Supplied:
    50 mg/ml,
    100 mg/2 ml IM solution.

Dose: 25–100 mg IM.

■ Hydroxyzine Pamoate (Vistaril; Pfizer)

How Supplied:
    25, 50, 200 mg capsule.
    25 mg/5 ml suspension.

Dose: 50–100 mg qid.

Meprobamate
Equanil (Wyeth-Ayerst)

How Supplied: 200, 400 mg tablet.

Dose: 200, 400 mg tablet.
Equagesic (Wyeth-Ayerst)

How Supplied: Meprobamate 200 mg + aspirin 325 mg.

Dose: 1–2 tablets tid–qid.
Miltown (Wallace)

How Supplied:
    200, 400, 600 mg tablet.
    400 mg sustained-release caps (Meprospan).

Dose: 1200–1600 mg in 3–4 divided doses.

■ Zolpidem Tartrate (Ambien; Searle)

How Supplied: 5, 10 mg tablets.

Dose: 10 mg tabs qhs.

RESPIRATORY SYSTEM AGENTS

SYMPATHOMIMETICS (TABLE 27-1)

■ **Epinephrine** (EpiPen; Center. Sus-Phrine; Forest. Bronkaid Mist; Miles. Primatene; Whitehall)

How Supplied:
Aerosol: 0.16, 0.2 mg/inhalation.
Parenteral:
For injection 1:1000 (1 mg/ml), 1 mg ampule, 30 ml vial.
Suspension for SC injection: 1:200 (5 mg/ml), 0.3 ml ampule, 5 ml vial.

Administration:
Inhalation: Shake dispenser; exhale. Inhale deeply with lips firmly around nozzle and hold in as long as possible before exhaling slowly.
SC: 1:1000 injection for rapid effect; 1:200 for sustained effect; give via tuberculin syringe and 26-gauge 1/2-in needle.
IV, intracardiac: Severe emergencies only (see Chapter 12).

Dose:
1. *Inhalation:* 1 inhalation; repeat after 1 min if no relief; repeat q3–4h prn.

Table 27-1

COMBINATION AGENTS

Antiasthmatics	Components (Pharmaceutical Company)
Bronkaid Tablets	Ephedrine sulfate 24 mg, guaifenesin 100 mg, theophylline 100 mg (Miles)
Marax Tablets	Ephedrine sulfate 25 mg, theophylline 130 mg, hydroxyzine 10 mg (Roerig)
Marax Syrup	Each 5 ml ephedrine sulfate 6.25 mg, theophylline 32.5 mg, hydroxyzine 2.5 mg, alcohol 5% (Roerig)
Mudrane-GG-Tablets	Potassium iodide 195 mg, anhydrous aminophylline 130 mg, phenobarbital 8 mg, ephedrine 16 mg (ECR)
Mudrane GG-2 Tablets	Guaifenesin 100 mg, anhydrous aminophylline 130 mg, phenobarbital 8 mg, ephedrine 16 mg (ECR)
Mudrane GG Elixir	Guaifenesin 100 mg, anhydrous aminophylline 13 mg (ECR)
Primatene Tablets	Each 5 ml: guaifenesin 26 mg, theophylline 20 mg, phenobarbital 2.5 mg, ephedrine 4 mg, alcohol 20% (ECR)
Primatene Dual Action Formula	Anhydrous theophylline 130 mg, ephedrine 24 mg (Whitehall)
	Theophylline anhydrous 60 mg, ephedrine 12.5 mg, guaifenesin 100 mg (Whitehall)
Quadrinal Tablets	Theophylline 65 mg, ephedrine 24 mg, phenobarbital 24 mg, potassium iodide 320 mg (Knoll)
Quibron Capsules	Each capsule 150 mg anhydrous theophylline, 90 mg guaifenesin (Roberts)
Slo-Phyllin GG Capsules and Syrup	Each capsule or 15 ml syrup: theophylline anhydrous 150 mg, guaifenesin 90 mg (Rhone-Poulenc Rorer)

Continued.

Table 27-1
COMBINATION AGENTS—Cont'd

Mucolytics

Congess SR Capsules	Guaifenesin 250 mg, pseudoephedrine 120 mg (Fleming)
Congess JR Capsules	Guaifenesin 125 mg, pseudoephedrine 60 mg (Fleming)
Entex Capsules	Phenylephrine 5 mg, phenylpropanolamine 45 mg, guaifenesin 200 mg (Procter & Gamble)
Entex LA Tablets	Phenylpropanolamine 75 mg, guaifenesin 400 mg (Procter & Gamble)
Entex Liquid	Each 5 ml/phenylephrine 5 mg, phenylpropanolamine 20 mg, guaifenesin 100 mg, alcohol 5% (Procter & Gamble)
Humibid LA Tablets	Guaifenesin 600 mg (Adams)
Humibid DM Tablets	Guaifenesin 600 mg, dextromethorphan hydrobromide 30 mg (Adams)

2. *SC:*
   a. 1:1000 injection: 0.3–0.5 ml (= mg)/dose q15–30 min ×
      3–4 doses or q4h prn. (Terbutaline may be preferred.)
   b. 1:200 injection suspension: 0.1–0.3 ml q6h.

Mechanism of Action: β-Stimulation bronchodilates by relaxing bronchial muscle; α-stimulation relieves bronchial mucosal
congestion and constricts pulmonary vessels, thus increasing
vital capacity.

Elimination: Metabolized by catechol-O-methyltransferase
(COMT) and monoamine oxidase (MAO); excreted in urine.

Indications: Bronchial asthma, bronchospasm seen in chronic
bronchitis and emphysema; hypersensitivity reactions to drugs
and allergens.

Contraindications: Narrow-angle glaucoma, shock (may
accentuate), and cerebral arteriosclerosis (may induce angina).
Not for use in patients with organic heart disease during general
anesthesia with halogenated hydrocarbons or cyclopropane (may
provoke ventricular fibrillation). Not for use with local anesthesia in distal extremities (may induce tissue sloughing from vasoconstriction). Not for use in labor; may delay second stage. Use
with caution in the elderly, diabetic patients (α-stimulation
inhibits insulin secretion), patients with hypertension or hyperthyroidism (anxiety, tremor, palpitations more likely), or psychoneurosis (baseline symptoms increased). See Interactions
below.

Toxicity:
1. Major: Accidental rapid IV injection may cause sharp rise in
   BP with cerebral hemorrhage. Ventricular dysrhythmias may
   result after use with certain anesthetics (discussed earlier)
   and in patients with organic heart disease. Peripheral vasoconstriction and cardiac stimulation may result in pulmonary
   edema, sometimes fatal. Rarely, shock and central retinal
   artery occlusion may be seen.
2. Minor: Anxiety, restlessness, headache, tremor, respiratory
   distress, palpitations; more often in patients with hyperthyroidism and hypertension.

Antidote: Counteract marked pressor response with rapidly acting vasodilators (nitrites, α-blocking agents); treat cardiac dysrhythmias with appropriate antidisrrhythmic or β-blocker.

Interactions: See contraindications, p.420. Also, digitalis or mercurial diuretics promote potential for dysrhythmias. Epinephrine's effects potentiated by additional sympathomimetics, tricyclic antidepressants, L-thyroxine, and certain antihistamines (e.g., diphenhydramine, tripelennamine, chlorpheniramine).

■ **Isoproterenol** (Isuprel; Sanofi Winthrop. Norisodrine; Abbott. Duo Medihaler Aerosol; 3M)

How Supplied:
Aerosol: 0.25%; 10, 15 ml controlled-dose nebulizer.
Inhalation solution:
    1:100 (1%; 10 mg/ml) 10 ml bottle.
    1:200 (0.5%; 5 mg/ml) 10, 60 ml bottle.
Parenteral: 1:5000 (0.2 mg/ml) 1, 5 ml ampule.

Administration:
    Inhalation: See Epinephrine, p. 417, for aerosol dispenser technique. May also be given by hand-bulb nebulizer, compressed air- or oxygen-operated nebulizer (to deliver more dilute form of mist over longer period and achieve deeper penetration and better dilatation in finer bronchioles) or IPPB devices.
    IV infusion: Dilute with D_5W.

Dose:
  1. Aerosol: 1–2 dispenser doses; max 5 times/day.
  2. Hand-bulb nebulizer:
      a. 1×200 solution: 5–15 deep inhalation q4h.
      b. 1:100 solution: 3–7 deep inhalations; may repeat after 5–10 min in severe bronchospasm; maximum 5 times/day.
  3. Compressed air or O_2 nebulizer; IPPB: Dilute in 1:100 or 1:200 solution with H_2O or 0.9 NS to 1:800 or 1:1000; regulate flow to deliver diluted solution over 10–20 min; max 5 times/day.

4. IV:
    a. Shock, hypoperfusion states: Initial infusion 0.1 µg/kg/min increased incrementally to 0.5–5 µg/kg/min, depending on ventilatory status + vital signs.
    b. Bronchospasm during anesthesia: 0.01–0.02 mg bolus, repeat prn.

Mechanism of Action: Primarily β-receptor stimulation; relieves bronchoconstriction and eases pulmonary secretion expectoration. Positive inotropic and chronotropic effects bring about an increase in HR and ejection velocity without changing stroke volume. Systemic and pulmonary vascular resistance are reduced, with a fall in diastolic BP, and improved venous return and tissue perfusion.

Elimination: Readily absorbed parenterally and by aerosol; metabolized primarily by hepatic COMT. Duration of action brief but longer than epinephrine.

Indications:
 1. Bronchoconstriction in acute and chronic asthma; reversible bronchospasm in chronic bronchitis and emphysema, or during anesthesia. (β$_2$-specific agents; e.g., terbutaline, may be preferred.)
 2. CV: Mild cardiac stimulant in transient heart block not requiring electroshock or pacemaker; serious heart block and Adams-Stokes attacks (except ventricular tachycardia or fibrillation); cardiogenic shock after MI; septicemic shock.

Contraindications: May aggravate tachydysrhythmias, tachycardia, or heart block because of digitalis intoxication, ventricular dysrhythmias requiring inotropic therapy, or angina. Avoid repeated excessive inhalant use; may develop severe paradoxical airway resistance. Use with caution in patients with coronary insufficiency, diabetes, hyperthyroidism. Other agents preferred in pregnancy (peripheral vasodilation may decrease uterine blood flow and shunt blood away from fetus).

Adverse Effects/Toxicity: Overall, less common than with epinephrine: palpitations, tachycardia, headache; uncommonly, angina, nausea, tremor; rarely, cardiac dysrhythmias, Adams-Stokes seizures.

Interactions: Do not give simultaneously with epinephrine because additive cardiac stimulation may evoke dysrhythmias (but may give alternately at proper intervals). Potent inhalation anesthetics (e.g., halothane) may sensitize myocardium to sympathomimetics.

SELECTIVE β_2-ADRENERGIC STIMULANTS

■ **Metaproterenol Sulfate** (Alupent; Boehringer Ingelheim. Metaprel; Sandoz)

How Supplied:
Aerosol: 0.65 mg/dose (15 mg/ml), 150 mg/10 ml dispenser and refill.
Inhalation solution:
    5%; 10, 30 ml bottle.
    0.4%, 0.6%; 2.5 ml/vial.
Syrup: 10 mg/5 ml, 16 oz bottle.
PO: 10, 20 mg tablet.

Administration:
PO aerosol: See Epinephrine on p. 417.
Inhalation solution: Undiluted for handheld nebulizer; diluted with 0.9 NS via IPPB device.
PO: 40% absorbed.

Dose:
Aerosol: 2–3 inhalations, repeated q3–4h. Maximum 12 inhalations/day.
Inhalation solution:
    Hand-held nebulizer: 5–15 inhalations, tid–qid.
    IPPB: 0.2–0.3 ml (after dilution with 2.5 ml 0.9 NS), tid– qid.
Syrup: 10 ml tid–qid.
Tablet: 20 mg tid–qid.

Mechanism of Action: Activates adenyl cyclase, thus increasing local cAMP (bronchodilator). Primarily β_2-adrenergic agonist, thus has little effect on β_1-cardiac receptors. Lessens bronchospasm and dyspnea by increasing 1-sec forced expiratory volume (FEV_1), maximum and peak expiratory flow rate, forced vital capacity, and decreasing airway resistance.

Elimination: Excreted in urine as glucuronic acid conjugates; longer duration than other β-sympathomimetics since not metabolized by COMT.

Indications: Bronchodilator in asthma; relieves reversible bronchospasm in bronchitis and emphysema. In pregnancy, may use aerosol to treat mild, infrequent bronchospasm and oral form in asthmatics still symptomatic on maximum theophylline therapy.

Contraindications: Tachydysrhythmias. Use with caution in patients potentially sensitive to sympathomimetics (e.g., coronary artery disease, CHF, hypertension, cardiac dysrhythmias, hyperthyroidism diabetes, and convulsive disorders).

Toxicity: Nervousness, tremor, nausea, tachycardia, hypertension, angina.

Interactions: Additive effects with other β–adrenergic aerosol bronchodilators; sympathomimetic effects also potentiated by MAOIs and tricyclic antidepressants.

■ **Terbutaline Sulfate** (Brethaire, Brethine; Geigy. Bricanyl; Marion Merrell Dow)

How Supplied:
Aerosol: 0.2 mg/dose; 75 mg/75 ml dispenser and refill.
PO: 2.5, 5 mg tablets.
Parenteral: 1 mg/ml ampule.

Administration:
Oral inhalation: See Epinephrine, p. 417. More rapid onset of action with SC form than PO tablet (5 min vs. 1 hr) and shorter duration (4 vs. 7 hr).

Dose:
Aerosol: 2 inhalations separated by 1 min, repeated q4–6h.
Tablet: 2.5–5 mg tid.
SC: 0.25 mg; may repeat in 15–30 min.
Consider alternate therapy if no response in another 15–30 min. Maximum total dose 0.5 mg/4 hr.

Tocolysis (NOTE: Not FDA approved for this purpose.): 0.25 mg SC q6h; once preterm labor arrested, switch to 2.5–7.5 mg PO q6h until 36–37 wk gestation.

Mechanism of Action: Selective β_2-adrenergic agonist; improves pulmonary function via decreased airway and pulmonary resistance and bronchodilatation.

Elimination: Partially metabolized in liver to sulfur conjugate excreted in urine, 60% unchanged.

Indications: Bronchodilator in asthma, relieves reversible bronchospasm in bronchitis and emphysema. Use oral form in pregnancy for asthmatic patients still symptomatic on maximum terbutaline therapy. Not FDA approved for tocolysis, but oral and SC forms have been widely used with some success and relative safety.

Contraindications: Known drug hypersensitivity; age < 12 yr. Use with caution in patients with diabetes (may precipitate ketoacidosis), hypertension, hyperthyroidism, history of seizures, and cardiac disease (may provoke dysrhythmias). Usual contraindications to tocolysis (see Chapter 31).

Toxicity: Nervousness, tremor, headache, nausea, tachycardia, and palpitations. Maternal side effects in labor include transient hyperglycemia, hypokalemia, and pulmonary edema; also, fetal tachycardia and neonatal hypoglycemia.

Indications: May potentiate deleterious cardiovascular effects of other sympathomimetic amines.

■ **Albuterol** (Aicet; Adams. Proventil; Schering. Ventolin; Allen and Hanburys)

How Supplied:
Aerosol: 90 µg/dose; 17 gm dispenser and refill.
PO:
    2, 4 mg tablet.
    4 mg sustained-release tablet.
    2 mg/5 ml syrup.

Inhalation solution:
    0.5%, 20 ml bottle.
    0.083%, 2.5 mg/3 ml bottle.
    2 mg/5 ml, 16 oz bottle.
Syrup: 2 mg/5 ml, 16 oz bottle.

Administration:
Aerosol inhaler: See Epinephrine on p. 417.
    Inhalation solution: Dilute 0.5% with NS or give 0.83% undiluted, by nebulizer. Gradually absorbed from bronchial mucosa; rapidly absorbed orally.

Dose:
    Inhaler: 2 inhalations q4–6h or 2 inhalations 15 min before exercise for prophylaxis.
    Nebulizer: 2.5 mg tid–qid.
    Syrup: 2–4 mg (5–10 ml) tid; max 8 mg qid (use lower dosage ranges in elderly and those sensitive to β-adrenergic stimulants).
    Tablets: 2–4 mg tid–qid; increase cautiously to max 8 mg qid (use lower dosage range in elderly and sensitive patients).

Mechanism of Action: Selective β_2-adrenergic agonist; adenyl cyclase stimulation increases local cAMP with resultant bronchial smooth muscle relaxation and inhibition of release of mediators of immediate hypersensitivity from cells (e.g., mast cells). Fewer cardiovascular effects than isoproterenol because of β_2-selectivity; longer duration of action since not metabolized by COMT.

Elimination: Excreted in urine partially metabolized. Half life 3–4 hr.

Indications: Relief of bronchospasm in reversible obstructive airway disease; prevention of exercise-induced bronchospasm.

Contraindications: Known drug hypersensitivity. Use with caution in patients with cardiac disease (especially coronary insufficiency, dysrhythmias), hypertension, convulsive disorders, hyperthyroidism, diabetes (may precipitate ketoacidosis), and in patients sensitive to effects of sympathomimetic amines. Not approved for tocolysis; inadequate data for use in lactation.

Toxicity: Tachycardia, tremor, headache, dizziness. Rarely, immediate hypersensitivity reactions, with urticarial rash, angioedema, bronchospasm, and anaphylaxis. Use in labor can induce maternal tachycardia, hypotension, acute CHF, pulmonary edema and death; also, fetal tachycardia and neonatal hypoglycemia.

Interactions: Effects potentiated by MAOIs, tricyclic antidepressants, and other sympathomimetic amines. β-Receptor blocking agents and albuterol counteract each other.

■ **Isoetharine** (Isoetharine Inhalation Solution; Roxane. Bronkometer, Bronkosol; Sanofi Winthrop)

How Supplied:
Aerosol: 0.34 mg/dose; 10, 15 ml unit vial and refill.
Inhalation solution:
    0.062%, 2.5 mg/4 ml vial.
    0.125%, 5 mg/4 ml vial.
    0.167%, 5 mg/3 ml vial.
    0.2%, 5 mg/2.5 ml vial.
    0.25%, 5 mg/2 ml vial.
    0.1%; 10, 30 ml bottle.

Administration:
Aerosol dispenser: See Epinephrine on p. 417.
    Inhalation solution: Undiluted via hand nebulizer, or diluted 1:3 with NS via O_2 aerosolization, or IPPB.

Dose:
Aerosol dispenser: 1–2 inhalations, repeat after 1 min prn, then q4h prn.
Hand nebulizer: 3–7 inhalations undiluted.
    Oxygen aerosolization: 1/4–1/2 ml with O_2 4–6 L/min over 15–20 min q4h prn.
    IPPB: 1/4–1 ml at appropriate flow rate and cycling pressure, q4h prn.

Mechanism of Action: β-Selective sympathetic agonist, primarily β_2. Relieves bronchospasm and improves vital capacity by effect on bronchial and arteriolar smooth muscle.

Elimination: Metabolized by COMT.

Indications: Bronchodilator in asthma; reversible bronchospasm in bronchitis and emphysema.

Contraindications: Known drug hypersensitivity. Inadequate data on use in pregnancy.

Toxicity: Nausea, headache, tachycardia, palpitations, severe paradoxical airway resistance.

Interactions: Other sympathomimetic amines may potentiate certain effects (e.g., tachycardia).

■ Salmeterol Xinafoate   (Serevent; Allen and Hanburys)

How Supplied: Aerosol 21 µg/inhalation; 6.5, 13 gm canister.

Administration: Oral inhalation daily.

Mechanism of Action: Long-active selective β_2 agonist. See Metaproterenol p. 423.

Dose: 2 inhalations bid or 30–60 min before exercise.

Indications: See Metaproterenol on p. 423. Also for prevention of exercise-induced bronchospasm.

Contraindications: See Metaproterenol on p. 423.

Adverse Effects/Toxicity: See Metaproterenol on p. 423.

Interactions: See Metaproterenol on p. 423.

ANTICHOLINERGICS

Atropine
   See Chapter 12.

■ Ipratropium Bromide   (Atrovent; Boehringer Ingelheim)

How Supplied: Aerosol: 18 µg/inhalation; 14 gm vial dispenser.
   Inhalation solution: 0.02%; 2.5 ml vial.

Administration: Local, site-specific effect; not well absorbed systemically.

Dose: Aerosol: Two inhalations (36 µg) qid; max 12 inhalations/24 hr.

Inhalation solution: 500 µg tid–qid.

Mechanism of Action: Synthetic quaternary ammonium compound. Anticholinergic (congener of methyl-atropine) bronchodilator, producing significant increase in FEV without affecting viscosity or volume of sputum.

Elimination: Serum half-life 2 hr.

Indications: Maintenance treatment of bronchospasm in COPD, including chronic bronchitis and emphysema.

Contraindications: Hypersensitivity to atropine-like drugs.

Toxicity: Cough, nervousness, nausea, palpitations, worsening of narrow-angle glaucoma.

METHYLXANTHINES
■ Aminophylline   (Barre-National; Roxane)

How Supplied:
PO: 100, 200 mg tablet.
Solution: 150 mg/5 ml, 210 mg/10 ml, 315 mg/15 ml.

Administration: *PO*. Lactating women should nurse just before dose to decrease amount of drug passed to neonate.

Dose:
600–1600 mg/day divided tid or qid.

Do not exceed maximum 24-hr dose unless inadequate serum levels documented.

Mechanism of Action: Direct relaxation of smooth muscle of bronchial airways and pulmonary vasculature. Secondary xanthine effects include coronary vasodilator, diuretic, and cardiac, cerebral, and skeletal muscle stimulant.

Elimination: Hepatic metabolism, accelerated by smoking and other liver enzyme inducers and slowed in hepatic cirrhosis and acute pulmonary edema.

Indications: Relief and prevention of asthma symptoms and reversible bronchospasm of chronic bronchitis and emphysema. Also for status asthmaticus refractory to adrenergic agonist inhalation. Drug of choice for asthma during pregnancy.

Contraindications: Active peptic ulcer disease (may increase volume and acidity of gastric secretions); known drug hypersensitivity. Use with caution in patients with severe heart disease, acute myocardial injury, CHF (prolonged drug serum levels), hypertension, hyperthyroidism, cor pulmonale, severe hypoxemia, liver dysfunction, alcoholism, and in the elderly (especially men).

Adverse Effects: At therapeutic drug levels: nausea, vomiting, headache, nervousness, palpitation, tachycardia, increased respirations (children may be more sensitive). Contains sodium sulfite with potential for allergic and anaphylactic reactions.

Toxicity: Seen with overdosage: In addition to the above, diarrhea, convulsions (treat with diazepam or short-acting barbiturates), hypotension, circulatory failure; cardiac dysrhythmia and sudden death after too rapid IV infusion.

Monitor: Therapeutic serum levels:
    Bronchial asthma: 10–20 µg/ml.
    Status asthmaticus: 16–20 µg/ml.

Interactions: Toxic synergism possible with sympathomimetic bronchodilators (e.g., ephedrine). Halothane anesthesia may provoke sinus tachycardia or ventricular dysrhythmias. Phenobarbital and phenytoin (Dilantin) may increase theophylline clearance and lower seizure threshold. Excretion of lithium carbonate is increased. Elevated theophylline levels occur with concomitant use of cimetidine, troleandomycin, erythromycin, allopurinol, or oral contraceptives. May antagonize propranolol's effect.

■ **Theophylline** (T-Phyl; Purdue Frederick. Theo-24; Whitby. Theox; Carrnick. Theo-Dur; Key. Theolair; 3M Pharmaceuticals. Uniphyl; Purdue Frederick)

How Supplied:
PO:
    200 mg tablet.
    50, 75, 100, 125, 200, 250, 300, 400, 450, 500 mg sustained-release tablet.
    300 mg divided-dose tablet.
    100, 125, 200, 300, 400 mg capsule.
    50, 75, 125, 200 mg sustained-action capsule.
Syrup: 80 mg/15 ml, 16 oz bottle.

Administration: PO: Well absorbed; food decreases GI distress and slows but does not reduce absorption.

Dosage:
1. Acute bronchospasm with need to attain therapeutic levels quickly.
    a. Not currently taking theophylline: Loading dose 5 mg/kg, then:
        (1) Normal adults: 3 mg/kg q8h maintenance.
        (2) Smokers: 3 mg/kg q6h maintenance.
        (3) Elderly or those with cor pulmonale: 2 mg/kg q8h maintenance.
        (4) CHF: 1–2 mg/kg q12h.
    b. Currently taking theophylline:
        (1) If serum level known: 0.5 mg/kg loading dose for each desired 1.0 µg/ml increase in level.

      (2) If serum level not known: Estimate loading dose (based on time and amount of drug last taken) by assuming 2.5 mg/kg loading dose will raise serum level 5 µg/ml.

2. Long-term therapy:
    a. Initially 16 mg/kg/24 hr or 400 mg/24 hr (whichever is less), divided tid–qid.
    b. Increase by 25% q3d as long as tolerated or until maximum dose is reached (900 mg/day or 13 mg/kg/day, whichever is less).

Mechanism of Action: See Aminophylline on p. 429,

Elimination: Metabolized in liver. Mean half-life 3–5 hr in children, 8 hr in nonsmoking adults. Elimination variable and slower in liver disease (e.g., cirrhosis), CHF, and acute pulmonary edema and when taken concurrently with certain other drugs (see later discussion).

Indications: Relief/prevention of asthma symptoms and reversible bronchospasm in chronic bronchitis and emphysema. Drug of choice for asthma in pregnancy.

Contraindications: See Aminophylline on p. 429.

Adverse Effects/Toxicity: See Aminophylline on p. 429. Serious toxicity not always preceded by lesser side effects.

Monitor/Interactions: See Aminophylline on p. 429.

■ **Oxtriphylline** (Choledyl, Choledyl S.A.; Parke-Davis)

How Supplied:
PO: 100, 200 mg tablet.
    400, 600 mg sustained-action tablet (equivalent to 254, 382 mg anhydrous theophylline).

Administration: See Theophylline on p. 431.

Dose: Initially 25 mg/kg/day or 625 mg/day divided tid–qid. Increase by 25% q2–3d to max dose of 20 mg/kg/day or 1400 mg/day, whichever is less. Optimally, monitor serum levels to determine appropriate maintenance dosage, usually 1 sustained-action tablet (400 or 600 mg) bid.

Mechanism of Action/Elimination/Indications/Contraindications: See Theophylline on p. 431.

Toxicity: See Theophylline on p. 431. Film-coated tablets cause less GI irritation.

Monitor/Interactions: See Theophylline on p. 431.

MISCELLANEOUS ANTIASTHMATICS

■ Beclomethasone Dipropionate (Beclovent, Beconase; Allen and Hanburys. Vancenase, Vanceril; Schering)

How Supplied:
Aerosol: 42 µg/inhalation, 6.7 gm, 16.8 gm canister refill.
Nasal spray: 0.042%, 25 gm bottle.

Administration: After nasal inhalation, deposited primarily in nasal passages and partly swallowed, with rapid absorption. Therapeutic effects may not be obvious for several days. Vasoconstrictor therapy may aid delivery during first 2–3 days, especially with excessive secretions or mucosal edema.

Dose:
Aerosol:
    Adults: One inhalation in each nostril bid–qid.
    Children (6–12 yr): One inhalation in each nostril tid.
    Nasal spray: 1–2 inhalations in each nostril bid.

Mechanism of Action: Antiinflammatory synthetic halogenated steroid with potent glucocorticoid and weak mineralocorticoid activity.

Elimination: Primarily in feces.

Indications: Symptom relief in seasonal and perennial rhinitis unresponsive to conventional therapy; prevention of nasal polyp recurrence after removal. Not for use in acute asthmatic attack; bronchospasm may prevent distribution to more distal airways.

Contraindications: Hypersensitivity to drug or its propellant (trichlorofluoromethane and dichlorofluoromethane). Inadequate data on use in pregnancy and lactation.

Toxicity: Hoarseness, nasal irritation, oral candidiasis, hypersensitivity reactions with urticaria, rash, angioedema. Also, rebound bronchospasm if discontinued abruptly.

■ Cromolyn Sodium (Gastrocrom, Intal, Nasalcrom; Fisons)

How Supplied:
PO: 100 mg capsules.
Aerosol inhaler: 800 µg/spray; 8.1, 14.2 gm controlled-dose turboinhaler.
Nasal solution: 400 mg/ml; 13, 26 ml bottle.

Administration: Poorly absorbed orally, thus given by turboinhaler (for asthma) to dispense finely powdered drug; 10% penetrates deep into lungs and is absorbed. In allergic perennial rhinitis, effects may not be obvious for 2–4 wk; may also require concomitant antihistamine or decongestant.

Dose:
Inhaler: 2 metered sprays qid.
    Nasal solution: 1 spray in each nostril tid–qid.
PO: 200 mg qid 30 min before meals and hs; reduce dose with severe hepatorenal dysfunction.

Mechanism of Action: Inhibits mast cell degranulation (histamine and leukotriene release) by indirectly blocking calcium entry into mast cells. Prevents immediate and nonimmediate bronchoconstrictive reaction during allergic responses mediated by IgE, including bronchospasm caused by exercise, toluene diisocyanate, aspirin, cold air, sulfur dioxide, and environmental pollutants. No intrinsic bronchodilator, antihistamine, or anti-inflammatory actions. Also blocks release of histamine and leukotrienes from mast cells.

Elimination: Excreted equally in urine and bile, unchanged.

Indications:
Aerosol inhaler: Prophylactic treatment of bronchial asthma, but must be administered before antigen exposure. Not for acute asthmatic attacks; may aggravate bronchial irritation.
Nasal solution: Prevention and treatment of allergic rhinitis.
PO: Mastocytosis, to reduce diarrhea, abdominal pain, flushing, urticaria.

Contraindications: Known drug hypersensitivity. Exercise caution in patients with severe renal or hepatic dysfunction. Apparently well tolerated in pregnancy, although extensive data are lacking.

Toxicity: Most commonly related to direct irritant effect (e.g., bronchospasm, wheezing, cough, nasal congestion, ocular stinging). Rarely, dizziness, nausea, headache, or hypersensitivity reaction with laryngeal and angioedema, urticaria, and anaphylaxis.

■ Flunisolide   (AeroBid; Forest)

How Supplied: Aerosol: 250 μg/inhalation, 100 controlled-dose canister.

Administration: See Beclomethasone dipropionate on p. 433. Rinse mouth after inhalation.

Dose: Two inhalations bid; max 4 inhalations bid.

Mechanism of Action: Antiinflammatory and antiallergic corticosteroid; allows for decrease in concomitant systemic steroid dosage.

Elimination: Rapid hepatic metabolism to water–soluble conjugates.

Indications: Bronchial asthma requiring chronic steroid therapy. Not indicated in status asthmaticus or nonasthmatic bronchitis.

Contraindications: Known drug hypersensitivity; age < 6 yr. Inadequate data on use in pregnancy and lactation.

Toxicity: Symptoms of adrenal insufficiency if concomitant systemic steroids reduced too rapidly, especially when exposed to trauma, surgery, or infections (e.g., gastroenteritis); arthralgias, myalgias, depression, hypotension, weight loss, and death. Other side effects include GI distress, diarrhea, sore throat, oropharyngeal fungal overgrowth, and palpitations.

Monitor: Early morning resting cortisol level.

ANTISECRETORIES

Atropine

See Chapter 12.

■ Glycopyrrolate   (Robinul; Robins)

How Supplied:
PO: 1, 2, mg tablet.
Parenteral: 0.2 mg/ml; 1, 2, 5, 20 ml vial.

Administration: PO absorption variable. Inject IM or IV undiluted.

Dose:
PO: 1–2 mg bid–tid.
Parenteral:

    Preanesthetic medication: 0.002 mg (0.01 ml)/lb IM, 30–60 min before induction.

    Intraoperative: 0.1 mg (0.5 ml) IV q2–3 min prn.

    Neuromuscular blockade reversal: 0.2 mg (1.0 ml) IV for each 1 mg neostigmine or 5 mg pyridostigmine.

Peptic ulcer: 0.1 mg (0.5 ml) tid–qid IM or IV.

Mechanism of Action: Anticholinergic; inhibits acetylcholine effects on postganglionic cholinergic nerves and autonomic effector cells of smooth muscle, cardiac muscle, sinoatrial node, atrioventricular node, exocrine glands, and autonomic ganglia. Decreases volume and free acidity of gastric secretions; controls excess respiratory tract secretions. Also antagonizes other muscarinic symptoms (e.g., bradycardia, intestinal hypermotility) induced by cholinergic drugs.

Indications: Preoperatively to reduce oropharyngeal, tracheobronchial, and gastric secretions and to block cardiac vagal inhibitory reflexes during anesthetic induction and intubation. Intraoperatively can counteract drug-induced or vagal inhibitory reflexes and/or dysrhythmias. Serves similar purpose when administered with neostigmine and pyridostigmine for neuromuscular blockade reversal. Adjunctive therapy in peptic ulcer disease for rapid anticholinergic effect or when patient is intolerant to oral medication.

Contraindications: Know drug hypersensitivity. Exercise caution in patients with glaucoma or asthma or during prolonged therapy in patients with obstructive uropathy. Obstructive GI tract disease, paralytic ileus, intestinal atony (elderly or debilitated patient), unstable cardiovascular status in acute hemorrhage, severe ulcerative colitis, toxic megacolon, myasthenia gravis, hypertension, hyperthroidism, severe asthma. Inadequate data on use in pregnancy and lactation.

Toxicity: Drowsiness, blurred vision, urinary retention, increased intraocular pressure, dysrhythmias, impotence, decreased lactation.

Antidote:
For peripheral anticholinergic effects: quaternary ammonium anticholinesterase (e.g., neostigmine methylsulfate).
For CNS symptoms (convulsions, psychosis): physostigmine (crosses blood-brain barrier).

Interactions: IV use in conjunction with cyclopropane anesthesia can induce ventricular dysrhythmias.

■ MUCOLYTICS

■ **Acetylcysteine** (Mucosil; Dey Bristol-Myers)
See Table 27-1.

How Supplied:
Solution:
   10% (100 mg/ml); 4, 10, 30 ml vial.
   20% (200 mg/ml); 4, 10, 30 ml vial.

Administration:
   Pulmonary: Inhalation via nebulizer or direct instillation via endotracheal tube or catheter.
   Catheter: Dilute with cola, juice, or water to 5%.

Dose:
   Inhalation: 1–10 ml 20% solution or 2–20 ml 10% solution q2–6h.
   Instillation: 1–2 ml 10% or 20% solution q1–4h.
   PO: Loading dose 140 mg/kg, then 70 mg/kg q4h × 17 doses.

Mechanism of Action: Free sulfhydryl group acts directly on mucoproteins to open disulfide bonds and thus liquefy mucus and DNA (component in pus that accounts for its viscosity). It has no effect on fibrin, blood clots, or living tissue. In acetaminophen poisoning, it replenishes hepatic glutathione stores.

Indications: Adjunct therapy in patients with abnormal, viscid, or inspissated mucous secretions. Reduces hepatotoxicity when given within 24 hr of acetaminophen overdose.

Contraindications: Use with caution in patients with severe asthma. No data on use in pregnancy and lactation.

Toxicity: Bronchospasm, stomatitis, bronchorrhea, rhinorrhea, nausea, vomiting, and hemoptysis with prolonged use.

■ COUGH SUPPRESSANTS

Dextromethorphan

   Various preparations available; see Chapter 24 and Table 27-1.

Administration:
PO: capsule, tablet, lozenge, syrup.

Dose: 60–120 mg/day divided bid–qid.

Mechanism of Action: D-Isomer of codeine analog of levorphanol but without analgesic or addictive effects. Acts centrally to elevate coughing threshold, without codeine's subjective or GI side effects. Does not inhibit ciliary action.

Elimination: Hepatic metabolism; renal excretion.

Indications: Temporary relief of cough from minor throat and bronchial irritation (e.g., common cold, inhaled irritants).

Contraindications: Known drug hypersensitivity.

Toxicity: Rarely, extremely high doses may produce nausea, vomiting, and visual and CNS disturbances.

■ **Guaifenesin** (Various Combination Agents; see Table 27-1)

How Supplied:
PO:
　　300 mg sustained-release capsule.
　　600 mg sustained-release tablet.
Syrup: Various other preparations.

Administration: PO; rapidly absorbed.

Dose: 600–1200 mg bid.

Mechanism of Action: Expectorant: increases respiratory tract fluid secretions; reduces viscosity of secretions, thus loosening phlegm and improving cough reflex efficiency and ciliary action.

Elimination: Rapidly metabolized and excreted in urine; half-life 1 hr.

Indications: Temporary relief of cough caused by respiratory tract infections (including sinusitis, pharyngitis, bronchitis) and asthma when complicated by tenacious mucus, mucous plugs, and congestion.

Contraindications: Known drug hypersensitivity. Inadequate data on usage in pregnancy and lactation.

CHAPTER 28

STEROID HORMONES

ANDROGENS

Dosage: Dosage varies depending on the preparation and disease being treated; check the *PDR* for appropriate dosage. Table 28-1 lists androgens available for clinical use.

Action:
1. Stimulates RNA synthesis and other proteins in target tissues.
2. Suppresses GnRH, causing decreased FSH and LH levels.
3. Stimulates erythropoietic factors.

Indications:
1. Replacement therapy in male patients with hormone deficiency states.
2. Restoration of libido in postmenopausal syndrome.
3. Postpartum breast engorgement.
4. Endometriosis.
5. Breast carcinoma.
6. Fibrocystic disease of breast.
7. Lichen sclerosis.
8. Osteoporosis.
9. Hereditary angioedema.
10. Refractory anemia.
11. Protein anabolism.

Contraindications:
1. Known hypersensitivity to drug.
2. Suspected pregnancy.
3. Serious hepatic, cardiac, or renal disease.

Table 28-1

ANDROGENS AVAILABLE FOR CLINICAL USE

Type	Generic Name	Brand Name (Mfg)	How Supplied
Oral	Fluoxymesterone	Halotestin (Upjohn)	2, 5, 10 mg tab
	Methyltestosterone	Android (ICN)	10, 25 mg tab
		Oreton Methyl	10 mg cap
	Oxymethalone	Anadrol (Syntex)	50 mg tab
	Stanozolol	Winstrol (Sanofi/Winthrop)	2 mg tab
Injectable	Testolactone	Teslac (BMS)	50 mg tab
	Testosterone Cypionate	Depo-Testosterone (Upjohn)	100, 200 mg/ml
	Testosterone Enanthate	Delatestryl (BTG)	100, 200 mg/ml
Transdermal	Testosterone	Testoderm (Alza)	4 mg/6 mg patch

Adverse Reactions:
1. Virilism in women, including hirsutism (facial hair), voice deepening, oily skin, alopecia, acne, clitoral enlargement, increased libido, and menstrual irregularities.
2. Liver dysfunction, including jaundice and increased liver enzymes.
3. Benign and malignant liver tumors.
4. Hypercalcemia.
5. Salt and fluid retention.
6. Increased fibrinolysis.
7. Induce premature epiphyseal closure.

ANDROGEN-ESTROGEN MIXTURES

Useful in restoring libido in postmenopausal women, suppressing lactation, arresting osteoporosis. Table 28-2 lists androgen-estrogen mixtures.

■ Impeded Androgen (Danazol, Danocrine; Sanofi/Winthrop)
Synthetic derivative of 17 α-ethynyltestosterone.

Dose:
1. Endometriosis:
    a. Moderate to severe: 800 mg/day in two doses.
    b. Mild: 200–400 mg/day.
    c. Therapy should continue for 3–9 mo.
    d. Start therapy with menses to avoid treating unsuspected pregnancy.

Table 28-2
ANDROGEN-ESTROGEN MIXTURES

Brand Name (Mfg)	Ingredients	How Supplied
Estratest (Solvay)	Esterified estrogens 1.25 mg Methyltestosterone 2.5 mg	Oral tab
Estratest H.S. (Solvay)	Esterified estrogens 0.625 mg Methyltestosterone 1.25 mg	Oral tab
Premarin with Methyltestosterone (Wyeth-Ayerst)	Conjugated estrogens 0.625/1.25 mg Methyltestosterone 5/10 mg	Oral tab

2. Fibrocystic breast disease:
   a. 100–400 mg/day in two doses.
   b. Nonhormonal contraception is required; low dosage may not prevent ovulation.

Action:
1. Suppresses pituitary-ovarian axis by inhibiting FSH and LH release from the pituitary, resulting in amenorrhea and anovulation.
2. Direct inhibitory effect at gonadal sites.
3. Weak androgenic activity.
4. No estrogenic or progestational activity.

Indications:
1. Endometriosis.
2. Fibrocystic breast disease.
3. Hereditory angioedema.

Adverse Effects:
1. Fluid retention, edema.
2. Weight gain.
3. Androgenic effects, including oily skin, decreased breast size, hirsutism.
4. Hypoestrogenic symptoms, including hot flashes, sweating, vaginal dryness, nervousness, emotional lability.
5. Abnormal liver function.
6. Many other adverse effects reported.

ESTROGENS

Dose: Varies depending on the patient disorder, but the lowest dose possible should be used. See *PDR* for recommended estrogen dose and type of drug. Table 28-3 lists various estrogens and estrogenic preparations available for clinical use.

Action:
1. Increases synthesis of DNA, RNA, and other proteins in estrogen-sensitive cells.
2. Suppresses GnRH release, reducing pituitary FSH and LH secretion.

Table 28-3

ESTROGENS AVAILABLE FOR CLINICAL USE

Brand Name (Mfg)	Generic Name	How Supplied (mg)
ORAL		
Premarin (Wyeth-Ayerst)	Conjugated equine estrogens-estrone, equilin, 17-alpha dihydroequilin, 17-alpha-estradiol, equilenin	0.3, 0.625, 0.9, 1.25, 2.5
	17-beta estradiol-micronized	1, 2
Estrace (BMS)	Esterified estrogens	0.3, 0.625, 1.25, 2.5
Estratab (Solvay)	Esterified estrogens	0.3, 0.625, 1.25, 2.5
Menest (SKB)	Piperazine estrone sulfate (Estropipate)	0.625
Ogen (Upjohn)	Estropipate USP	0.75, 1.5
Ortho-Est (Ortho)		
NONSTEROIDAL ESTROGENS		
Diethylstilbestrol, USP (Lilly)	Diethylstilbestrol	1, 5
INJECTABLE		
Estradurin (Wyeth-Ayerst)	Polyestradiol phosphate	40 mg/2ml
Premarin IV (Wyeth-Ayerst)	Conjugated equine estrogens	25 mg/ml
	Estradiol benzoate (Generic)	0.5 mg/ml
	Estradiol valerate (Generic)	10, 20, 40 mg/ml
	Estradiol cypionate (Generic)	5 mg/ml

Continued.

445

Table 28-3
ESTROGENS AVAILABLE FOR CLINICAL USE—Cont'd

Brand Name (Mfg)	Generic Name	How Supplied (mg)
TOPICAL-VAGINAL		
Estrace (BMS)	17-beta estradiol	0.1 mg/gm 42.5 gm tube
Ogen (Upjohn)	Piperazine estrone sulfate	1.5 mg/gm 42.5 gm tube
Premarin (Wyeth-Ayerst)	Conjugated equine estrogens	0.625 mg/gm 42.5 gm tube
TRANSDERMAL		
Climara (Wyeth-Ayerst)	17-beta estradiol	0.05 mg/day; 0.10 mg/day
Estraderm (CIBA)	17-beta estradiol	0.05 mg; 0.10 mg/day
MIXTURES		
Premphase (Wyeth-Ayerst)	Conjugated equine estrogens	0.625 mg tabs
	Medroxyprogesterone acetate	5.0 mg tabs
Prempro (Wyeth-Ayerst)	Conjugated equine estrogens	0.625 mg tabs
	Medroxyprogesterone acetate	2.5 mg tabs
PMB-200/400 (Wyeth-Ayerst)	Conjugated equine estrogens	0.45
	Meprobamate	200 and 400

STEROID HORMONES

Indications:
 1. Estrogen deficiency states.
 2. Menstrual cycle abnormalities.
 3. Contraception (combined with progestin).
 4. Postcoital contraception.
 5. Menopausal syndrome.
 6. Osteoporosis prevention.
 7. Female hypogonadism.
 8. Female castration.
 9. Primary ovarian failure.
10. Hirsutism.
11. Postmenopausal atherosclerosis.
12. Breast cancer (palliation only).
13. Prostatic cancer (metastatic).

Contraindications:
 1. Pregnancy, suspected pregnancy.
 2. Known or suspected breast cancer (except as palliation therapy in metastatic disease).
 3. Known or suspected estrogen-dependent neoplasia.
 4. Undiagnosed genital bleeding.
 5. Active thrombophlebitis or thromboembolic disorder.
 6. Past history of thrombosis, thrombophlebitis, and related disorders.
 7. Acute liver disease.
 8. Chronic hepatic dysfunction.

Adverse Effects:
 1. Fluid retention.
 2. Abnormal uterine bleeding.
 3. Mastodynia.
 4. Increased risk of endometrial hyperplasia.
 5. Induction of endometrial carcinoma.
 6. Increase size of leiomyoma.
 7. Increased risk of gallbladder disease.
 8. Increased risk of thromboembolic disease, including thrombophlebitis, thrombotic stroke, myocardial infarction (thrombosis), pulmonary embolism.
 9. Induction of hepatic adenoma.
10. Increase blood pressure.
11. Hypercalcemia.
12. Gastrointestinal effects (nausea and vomiting, cholestatic jaundice).

13. Chloasma.
14. Skin eruptions (erythema multiforme, erythema nodosum).
15. Corneal curvature changes.
16. Headache, dizziness, other CNS effects.
17. Reduced carbohydrate tolerance.
18. Libido changes.
19. Aggravation of porphyria.
20. Vaginal candidiasis.
21. Increased risk of fetal abnormalities.
22. Alterations in lab values and tests (see Table 14-4).

PROGESTINS

Progestins are a group of chemically similar compounds having varying degrees of progestational, androgenic, estrogenic, and antiestrogenic activity.

Dose: Varies depending on the patient disorder, but the lowest dose possible should be used. See *PDR* for recommended progestin type and dosage. Table 28-4 lists progestins available for clinical use. Progestins used in contraceptive formulations are discussed in Chapter 14.

Action:
1. Increase synthesis of RNA in target-susceptible tissues.
2. Suppress gonadotropin synthesis and release.
3. Suppress ovulation.
4. Increase cervical mucous viscosity.

Indications:
1. Menstrual cycle irregularities.
2. Contraception (usually in conjunction with estrogen).
3. Postmenopausal syndrome.
4. Endometrial hyperplasia.
5. Endometrial carcinoma.
6. Endometriosis.
7. Polycystic ovary syndrome.
8. Precocious puberty.
9. Premenstrual syndrome.
10. Renal carcinoma (metastatic).
11. Breast carcinoma (metastatic).

Table 28-4
PROGESTINS AVAILABLE FOR CLINICAL USE*

Generic Name	Brand Name (Mfg)	How Supplied
Medroxyprogesterone acetate	Provera (Upjohn)	2.5, 5, 10 mg tabs
	Depo-Provera Contraceptive (Upjohn)	150 mg/ml injection
	Depo-Provera (Upjohn)	400 mg/ml injection
	Curretab (Solvay)	10 mg tab
	Cycrin (ESI)	10 mg tab
	Amen (Carrick)	10 mg tab
Megesterol acetate	Megace (BMS)	20, 40 mg tab
		40 mg/ml suspension
Norethindrone acetate	Aygestin (ESI)	5 mg tab
Progesterone		25, 50, 100 mg/ml IM
		25, 50 mg suppository
		100 mg micronized suspension

*For progestins used in contraceptive preparations, see Chapter 14.

Contraindications:
1. Presence or history of thrombophlebitis, cerebral stroke, thromboembolic disorder.
2. Severe liver dysfunction.
3. Carcinoma of breast (nonmetastatic).
4. Undiagnosed uterine bleeding.
5. Missed or threatened abortion.
6. Diagnostic test for pregnancy.

Adverse Effects:
1. May be associated with vascular clot formation.
2. May be associated with breast carcinoma.
3. Masculinization of female fetus.
4. Decreased breast milk production.
5. May decrease glucose tolerance.
6. May adversely affect lipids and lipoproteins.
7. Breast tenderness.

8. Galactorrhea.
9. Fluid retention.
10. Acne, oily skin, hirsutism.
11. Gingivitis.
12. Irregular uterine bleeding or spotting.

GONADOTROPIN-RELEASING HORMONE AGONISTS

■ Nafarelin Acetate   (Synarel; Syntex)

Potent agonistic analog of GnRH, which initially stimulates FSH-LH release, causing increased steroidogenesis; continued administration causes decreased steroidogenesis, leading to ovulation suppression in women and azoospermia in men.

How Supplied/Dose: Spray pump for nasal administration delivers 200 µg/spray. Recommended daily dose is 400 µg in alternating nostrils.

Indication: Endometriosis.

Contraindications:
1. Hypersensitivity.
2. Undiagnosed vaginal bleeding.
3. Pregnancy or potential pregnancy while on therapy.
4. Breast feeding.

Warning: Safe use of nafarelin acetate during pregnancy not established; patients should use nonhormonal contraception.

Adverse Effects: Hypoestrogenism, including decreased bone density, hot flashes, and sweats.

■ GOSERELIN ACETATE IMPLANT   (Zoladex; Zeneca)

See Chapter 25.

CHAPTER 29

SUBSTANCE ABUSE CHEMICALS

GENERAL PRINCIPLES

1. Tolerance: Repetitive use results in need for increasingly larger drug doses to reproduce original pharmacologic effect. May occur secondary to more rapid drug metabolism or decrease in receptor cell sensitivity.
2. Cross-tolerance: Tolerance to one drug accompanied by tolerance to other drugs in same class.
3. Physical dependence (neuroadaptation): State of altered cellular physiology, seen after repeated drug use, that results in need for continued drug administration to avoid withdrawal syndrome.
4. Psychologic dependence: Profound psychoemotional need for continued drug use.
5. Addiction: Behavioral pattern manifested by overwhelming compulsion to use drug purposive activity to secure its supply and the tendency to relapse after withdrawal.
6. Withdrawal (abstinence) syndrome: Stereotypical syndrome based on signs of physical dependence that appear after drug is withdrawn.

OPIATES

How Supplied: Various tablets, powders, liquids, PO solutions, resins, depending on member of class (see individual agents in Chapter 1):

1. Natural alkaloids of opium derived from resin of opium poppy: opium, morphine, codeine.
2. Semisynthetic morphine derivatives: diacetylmorphine (hero-

in), hydromorphone (Dilaudid), oxycodone (Percodan).

3. Purely synthetic opiates, not derived from morphine: meperidine (Demerol), methadone (Dolophine), propoxyphene (Darvon).

4. Opiate-containing preparations, such as elixir of terpin hydrate with codeine and paregoric.

Administration: Readily absorbed from GI tract, nasal mucosa, and lung; parenteral administration elevates blood levels more rapidly. Heroin IV is rapidly hydrolyzed to morphine by liver with peak levels in 30 min; thereafter rapidly leaves blood and is concentrated in body tissues, including brain (crosses blood-brain barrier since highly lipid soluble).

Dose: Varies depending on route, degree of tolerance, and drug purity (i.e., pharmaceutical company vs. "street" drug); e.g., some addicts may self-administer 2 gm morphine IV over 2.5 hr or 3–4 gm meperidine/day without significant respiratory depression.

Mechanism of Action (Table 29-1): Same as morphine (see Chapter 1) (in vivo conversion product; i.e., descending CNS depression).

Miscellaneous Effect:
1. "Rush," "kick": Warm flushing of skin and orgasmic pulsations in lower abdomen, felt shortly after IV administration and lasting about 45 sec. With chronic intake, insomnia, decreased sexual function, excessive sweating.

2. In the neonate: Lethargy, disturbed thermoregulation, hypertonia, poor sucking reflex.

Overdose:
1. May occur because of clinical overdosage, accidental overdosage in addicts (fluctuation in purity of illicit heroin; combining with other CNS depressants, e.g., alcohol), suicide attempts.

2. Lethal dose depends on degree of tolerance and drug. In non-tolerant individual, toxicity is rare unless dose of methadone is >40–60 mg PO, morphine 120 mg PO or 30 mg parenterally.

3. Signs and symptoms: Classic triad of coma, pinpoint pupils, respiratory depression (RR may be 2–4/min). Hypotension leads to cyanosis, possible shock (severe hypoxia may cause dilated pupils), convulsions.

Table 29-1
OPIATE EFFECTS

Symptom/Sign	Mechanism	Tolerance Develops
Euphoria	Cross BBB* (high lipid solubility) and bind to specific opiate receptors in brain	+
Analgesia	Increases pain threshold or magnitude of stimulus required to evoke pain	+
Respiratory depression (decreased volume and slower rate)	Inhibition of brainstem respiratory center	+
Nausea/vomiting	Brainstem CTZ† stimulation	+
Orthostatic hypotension	Peripheral vasodilatation	
Constipation	Decreased GI secretions (stomach, biliary tract, pancreas); inhibition of smooth muscle contractility	
Urinary hesitancy	Decreased smooth muscle tone in ureters and bladder	+
Miosis	Inhibition of smooth muscle of iris	

*BBB: Blood-brain barrier.
†CTZ: Chemoreceptor trigger zone.

SUBSTANCE ABUSE

Complications of Illicit Opiate Use
1. Because of shared needles, unhygenic procedures: Infection, (e.g., septicemia, endocarditis, hepatitis, AIDS, tetanus), abscesses of lung, brain, and subcutaneous tissue.
2. Because of foreign body and contaminant injection: Emboli, granulomas, pulmonary edema.
3. In obstetric patients: Preterm labor, toxemia, abruptio placentae, retained placenta, postpartum hemorrhage, ruptured marginal sinus.
4. In fetus or neonate of addicted mother: Prematurity, low birth weight, intraventricular hemorrhage, histiocytosis.

Withdrawal Symptoms
1. Early (e.g., 8–12 hr after last heroin or morphine dose): Lacrimation, rhinorrhea, yawning, sweating; then tossing, restless sleep ("yen").

2. Later (after 24 hr): Dilated pupils, anorexia, gooseflesh from increased pilomotor activity ("going cold turkey"), irritability, tremor.

3. Late (after 72 hr): Exaggerated level of items in 1 and 2, with diarrhea, abdominal cramps, elevated HR and BP, signs of CNS hyperexcitability (ejaculation in men, orgasm in women), dehydration, ketosis, possible CV collapse.

4. In the neonate (onset variable depending on type of drug and analgesics used intrapartum, within first 24–48 hr with heroin or day 4–12 with methadone): Hyperactivity, irritability, tremors, disturbed sleep, frantic sucking, vomiting, fever, seizures, poor weight gain.

Treatment of Withdrawal in Labor: 5–20 mg methadone IM, with low dose of short-acting narcotic IV (morphine, meperidine, hydromorphone HCl) if symptoms severe and treatment needed until IM dose is effective.

In newborn: Paregoric, 0.2 ml PO q3–4h if no simultaneous alcohol or other sedative use. Pentazocine (Talwin) contraindicated since it also acts as narcotic antagonist and can exaggerate withdrawal symptoms.

■ **Methadone** (Methadone HCl; Lilly, Roxane. Dolophine HCl; Lilly)

How Supplied:
PO:
    5, 10 mg tablet.
    40 mg dispersible tablet.
    1, 2, 10 mg/ml solution.
Parenteral: 10 mg/ml ampule and 20 ml vial.

Administration: Well absorbed PO, SC, IM.

Dose:
1. Pain relief: 2.5–10 mg q3–4h.
2. Maintenance in pregnancy: Use lowest possible dose (e.g., 5–40 mg/day).
3. Detoxification:
    a. Initially 15–20 mg to suppress acute withdrawal symptoms.

    b. Stabilization: 40 mg/day divided, × 2–3 days.
    c. Cure: Decrease dose by 20% q2d as tolerated over next
       2 ½ wk.

Mechanism of Action: Synthetic narcotic analgesic, actions similar to morphine. Advantages include effective analgesia, oral efficacy, extended duration of action in suppressing withdrawal symptoms in physically dependent patients, and persistent pharmacologic effects even with chronic intake.

Elimination: Metabolized in liver; half-life 1–1.5 days.

Indications: Severe pain relief; maintenance and detoxification treatment of narcotic addiction.

Contraindications: Use with caution in patients with head injury and increased intracranial pressure (may aggravate ICP); acute asthma attack, COPD, cor pulmonale or decreased respiratory reserve (may further decrease respiratory drive and increase airway resistance to point of apnea); hypotension (may exacerbate). Discourage breast feeding.

Toxicity: See Opioids (Chapter 1).

Antidote (for overdose):   Naloxone; repeated doses may be required because of shorter duration of action (1–3 hr) compared with methadone (36–48 hr).

Interaction: Rifampin and phenytoin accelerate metabolism and may precipitate withdrawal symptoms. Potentiates effects of other CNS depressants (narcotics, general anaesthetics, phenothiazines, tranquilizers, sedative-hypnotics, tricyclic antidepressants, alcohol) with possible respiratory depression, hypotension, and coma.

SUBSTANCE ABUSE

COCAINE

How Supplied: Powder, often diluted with procaine, for intranasal administration. "Free-base": Prepared by alkalinization and extraction of hydrochloride salt with organic solvents (volatilized at 90° C); for smoking. "Crack": Highly purified free alkaloid form. Coca paste: 60%–80% cocaine sulfate; smoked.

Administration: Intranasal ("snorting"), IV, PO, smoking the free alkaloid form (free-basing). Onset of action rapid (a few seconds) when free-base is smoked or used IV.

Dose: Varies depending on route of administration, degree of tolerance, drug purity. Average "line" contains 25 mg; one "rock" of crack contains 100–300 mg. Typical intranasal dose contains 100 mg; addicts may smoke 4 gm/day.

Mechanism of Action: Local anesthetic derived from leaves of the *Erythroxylon coca* tree (indigenous to Peru and Bolivia). Blocks presynaptic sympathetic neurotransmitter uptake (epinephrine, norepinephrine, dopamine), thus allowing for excess transmitter at postsynaptic receptor. Potentiation of norepinephrine manifests in CV system as massive adrenergic stimulation with hypertension, tachycardia, acute rise in arterial BP, and intense vasoconstriction (accounts for at least some of toxic fetal effects). Potentiation of dopamine in CNS engenders euphoria and reinforces addictive properties; subsequent dopamine depletion leads to "lows" after use.

Elimination: Degraded by plasma and hepatic cholinesterases to water-soluble metabolites, ecgonine methyl ester and benzoylecgonine (the latter detectable in urine in toxicology screens 24–48 hr after last dose). Elimination half-life 4–5 hr.

Toxicity:
1. Psychiatric: Anxiety, agitation, paranoia, tactile hallucinations.
2. Metabolic: Hyperthermia from increased muscle activity and seizures plus poor heat loss from vasoconstriction.
3. Neurologic: Seizures.
4. CV: Coronary artery constriction with ischemia or acute MI (even without underlying coronary artery disease), dysrhythmias, rupture of ascending aorta, CVA, subarachnoid hemorrhage, coma, cardiorespiratory arrest.
5. Obstetric: Spontaneous abortion, preterm births (≤25%), SGA infants (≤20%), abruptio placentae, neurobehavioral abnormalities (e.g. irritability, low threshold for overstimula-

tion). Congenital anomalies (e.g., intestinal atresia, genitourinary abnormalities) may be explained by cocaine-mediated vasoconstriction with infarction and interrupted blood flow, leading to disrupted morphogenesis.

Antidote: Chlorpromazine, propanolol (in acute intoxication).

METHAMPHETAMINE

How Supplied: Clear crystalline formation (also known as "Ice" or "Crystal").

Administration: Usually burned in a pipe and then smoke is inhaled; the parent compound is usually taken PO (or by direct IV injection).

Mechanism of Action: Synthetic CNS stimulant in the form of a free base hydrochloride salt, thus soluble in water; when burned, smoke contains the free drug. "Ice" is to methamphetamine what "crack" is to cocaine (see p. 455) with similar CNS effects; increased alertness, decreased fatigue and apetite, mood elevation, increased initiative and confidence levels, euphoria.

Elimination: When smoked, drug travels immediately to brain, thus resisting metabolism by hepatic enzymes, causing a more intense, less controllable "high."

Indications: Desoxyn (Abbott; see Chapter 23) available as schedule II drug for treatment of attention deficit disorder or (short term) for exogenous obesity.

Adverse Effects/Toxicity: Repeated administration causes long-lasting, possibly irreversible decreases in brain dopamine and serotonin levels. High drug levels can present as acute delusions, paranoid psychosis, and violent behavior that appears much sooner and persists longer (days to weeks) than with cocaine.

SUBSTANCE ABUSE

MARIJUANA

How Supplied: Flowering tops of *Cannabis sativa* hemp plant.
1. Hashish: dried resinous exudate of tops.
2. Bhang: dried leaves and flowering shoots (smaller amounts of active substance).
3. Ganja: Resinous mass from small leaves.

Administration: Typically smoked in cigarette form or via various pipelike apparatuses. Pharmacologic effects begin within minutes; plasma concentrations peak at 7–10 min; physiologic and subjective effects are greatest 20–30 min later.

Dose: Concentration of active agent tetrahydrocannabinol (THC) varies with plant strain, smoking technique, and amount altered by pyrolysis. A 1 gm cigarette containing 2% THC delivers up to 10 mg THC to lungs.

Mechanism of Action: Active ingredient THC; precise mechanism of action unclear but possibly related to decrease in activity of cholinergic neurons. Induces sense of well-being, relaxation, temporal disintegration (impaired memory-dependent goal-directed behavior), depersonalization (sense of strangeness and unreality about self), decreased balance, increased appetite, increased HR.

Indications: As an antiemetic in cancer chemotherapy. One synthetic cannabinoid, dronabinol (Marinol; Roxane), available in the United States for this sole indication.

Adverse Physiologic Effects: Anovulatory cycles, lowered serum testosterone levels, reversible inhibition of spermatogenesis; "amotivational syndrome"; bronchitis, asthma. Inadequate data on use in pregnancy, but a higher incidence of meconium staining and precipitate labor (<3 hr) has been reported.

Toxicity: Hallucinations, delusions, paranoia, accentuated depersonalization and altered time sense, anxiety to point of panic.

PSYCHEDELICS

How Supplied:
1. LSD: Lysergic acid diethylamide. Most potent.
2. Psilocin, psilocybin: Active ingredient of *Psilocybe mexicana*, Mexican hallucinogenic mushroom.
3. Mescaline: Active ingredient of the peyote cactus.

Administration: Typically PO.

Dose: Somatic symptoms perceived within minutes of 0.5–2 µg/kg dose. LSD 100 times more potent than psilocin and psilocybin and 4000 times as potent as mescaline.

Mechanism of Action: Actions at multiple CNS sites from cortex to spinal cord. Exact mechanism may involve agonistic action at 5–hydroxytryptamine prereceptor sites.

Mental Effects: Heightened awareness of sensory input with enhanced clarity but diminished control. Thought processes turn inward with a greater sense of "meaningfulness." Diminished capacity to differentiate boundaries of one object from another or of self from environment.

Somatic Effects: Largely sympathomimetic. Pupillary dilation, increased BP and HR, hyperreflexia, tremor, nausea, piloerection, muscle weakness, and increased body temperature.

Toxicity: Paresthesias, hallucinations, fear of self-fragmentation or disintegration, afterimages, overlapping perceptions, panic episodes. Effects of pure LSD on pregnancy and fetus unknown, but increased spontaneous abortion and fetal abnormalities after illicit LSD use are reported.

PHENCYCLIDINE

How Supplied: Crystalline powder for smoking or nasal inhalation ("snorting").

Administration: Well absorbed by all routes; considerable enterohepatic recirculation accounts for prolonged effects.

Mechanism of Action: Inhibits dopamine and norepinephrine uptake. Also known as "angel dust," "PCP." Originally developed for its anesthetic effect and now only legal use is as animal tranquilizer.

Dose: Average street "buy" can contain from 0.1 to over 160 mg.

Adverse Effects:
  1. Low dose (3–8 mg): Decreased perception and coordination, mind-body dissociations, numbness of extremeties, nausea.
  2. Larger doses: (10–20 mg): Emesis, flushing, drooling, indifference to pain, dysphoric numbness with sense of impending doom.
  3. High dose (>20mg): Seizures or coma lasting a week or more, intense fear, psychotic disorientation to time and place, catatonic muscle rigidity.

ETHANOL

Administration: PO; rapidly absorbed. Absorption delayed by presence of food in stomach, especially milk or fats.

Mechanism of Action: Primary continuous CNS depressant. Depression of inhibitory control mechanisms results in apparent stimulation, first involving those parts of the brain involved in the most highly integrated functions (e.g., with resultant increased reaction time, diminished fine motor control). Release of cortex from synthesized control allows for disorganization of thought processes and loss of self-restraint. With further intake, mood swings and emotional outbursts occur. Chronic excessive consumption leads to more marked CNS depressant effects, including brain damage and memory loss. Toxic effects resulting from formation of metabolites (acetaldehyde, acetate, increased NADH/NAD ratio) and membrane-disordering effects.

Elimination: Average rate of metabolization (in liver) = 30 ml (1 oz) in 3 hr; maximum 450 ml/24 hr. Rate varies with body weight, liver weight, and degree of tolerance (because of hepatic microsomal enzyme induction).

Toxicity: Threshold effects first noticeable at blood level 20–30 mg/dl; gross intoxication at 150 mg/dl; average fatality level around 400 mg/dl. Miscellaneous metabolic changes in chronic cases: peripheral polyneuropathies, pellagra, nutritional amblyopia, Wernicke's encephalopathy, Korsakoff's psychosis, fatty liver, cirrhosis.

Adverse Obstetric Effects:
1. Maternal: Associated malnutrition, polydrug abuse.
2. Fetal: Fetal alcohol syndrome (see below). Stillbirth abortion rate two to three times higher; perinatal death eight times more frequent. Neonate may experience withdrawal syndrome after birth.

Fetal Alcohol Syndrome: Ethanol effect: Inhibition of embryonic cellular proliferation in early gestation, leading to physical growth retardation beginning in utero and continuing after birth; CNS dysfunction (e.g., low IQ, microcephaly); characteristic facies (short palpebral fissures, hypoplastic upper lip, short nose, micrognathia).

Withdrawal Syndrome:
1. Early (within few hours after last drink): Tremulousness with nausea, weakness, anxiety, sweating; acute alcoholic hallucinosis.
2. Midphase (24–48 hr): Alcohol-related tonic clonic seizures.
3. Late (after 48 hr): Delirium tremens, with hyperthermia and CV collapse.

Interactions: Synergistic effect with sedatives, hypnotics, anticonvulsants, antidepressants, antianxiety agents, certain analgesics (e.g., opioids, propoxyphene). Possible disulfiram-like reaction with oral hypoglycemics, metronidazole, cephalosporins. Acute ingestion may delay phenytoin clearance (because of hepatic microsomal enzyme competition); chronic consumption may speed it (via enzyme induction).

SUBSTANCE ABUSE

NICOTINE

How Supplied: Tobacco, loose or as cigarettes; gum (see Nicotine Poliacrilex, below).

Administration: Smoked, chewed, or sublingual.

Mechanism of Action: Natural liquid alkaloid with both stimulant and depressant phases of action. Stimulates CNS and sympathetic ganglia, with short-term increased cognitive performance, alerting pattern on EEG, increased HR and BP, vasconstriction, nausea. Also has muscle relaxant effects, facilitates memory and attention, decreases appetite, and causes irritability.

Elimination: Multiexponential.

Chronic Toxicity: Dose-related increase in rates of pulmonary dysfunction, coronary artery and cerebrovascular disease, peripheral vascular disease; cancer of lung, larynx, oral cavity, esophagus, bladder, pancreas, and endometrium; earlier relative age of menopause; recurrent and spontaneous abortion; intrauterine growth retardation, perinatal mortality, abnormal bleeding during pregnancy, abruptio placenta, placenta previa (maternal hypoxia thought to account for decreased placental size, increased placental vascularity, thinning of placental vessel walls, and decidual necrosis at placental margin), premature rupture of fetal membranes, prematurity, low birth-weight infants, SIDS.

Withdrawal symptoms: Craving, nervousness, irritability, drowsiness, impaired concentration, increased appetite.

■ Nicotine Poliacrilex (Nicorette, Nicorette DS; Smith-Kline Beecham)

How Supplied: Nicotine bound to ion exchange resin in sugar-free flavored chewing gum base.

Dose: Contains 2 or 4 (DS) mg nicotine/piece. Usual dose 10–12 pieces/day; each piece should be chewed slowly and intermittently for 30 min.

Mechanism of Action: Nicotine released during chewing and absorbed via buccal mucosa (see Nicotine on p. 462).

Indications: Temporary aid to smoking cessation.

Contraindications: Recent MI, serious dysrhythmia, vasospastic disease, pregnancy, lactation. Use with caution in patient with hyperthyroidism, pheochromocytoma, insulin-dependent diabetes mellitus, peptic ulcer.

Adverse Effects: Hiccoughs, nausea, vomiting; dependence.

■ TRANSDERMAL NICOTINE PATCH (Habitrol; Basel. Nicoderm; Marion Merrell Dow. Nicotrol; McNeil Consumer. Prostep; Lederle)

How Supplied (various brands):
Patch:
    21, 14, 7 mg/day over 24 hr.
    22, 11 mg/day over 24 hr.
    15, 10, 5 mg/day over 16 hr.

Administration: Transdermal system provides systemic nicotine delivery for several hours after application to intact skin.

Mechanism of Action: See Nicotine on p. 462.

Dose: After complete cessation of cigarette smoking, begin with higher-dose patch × 6 (range 4–12) wks; then reduce dose q2–4 wk (start with lower dose or use 10-hour patch in patients with CV disease, weight 100 lb, or smoke 1/2 ppd). Entire course of nicotine substitution usually takes 14–20 wks.

Elimination: Mostly liver; some metabolism also in kidney and lung.

Indications: To treat nicotine withdrawal symptoms during smoking cessation.

Contraindications: Pregnancy; severe or persistent local skin reactions. Use with caution in patients with atopic or eczematous dermatitis, CHD (history of MI and/or angina), cardiac

SUBSTANCE ABUSE

dysrhythmia, vasospastic disease; hyperthyroidism; pheochromocytoma, IDDM (since nicotine causes catecholamine release from adrenal medulla); peptic ulcer (nicotine delays healing); accelerated HTN.

Adverse Effects: Diarrhea, dyspepsia, dry mouth, arthralgia, myalgia, sleep disturbance, insomnia; skin reactions.

Toxicity: Vomiting, tremor, mental confusion, hypotension, respiratory failure, convulsions.

CHAPTER 30

THYROID DRUGS

■ Thyroid   (Thyrar, Rhone Poulenc Rorer)

Obtained from bovine thyroid glands containing 35 µg levothyroxine (T₄) and 5 µg liothyronine (T₃) per grain thyroid.

How Supplied: 30, 60, 120 mg tablet, (1 grain = 60 mg).

■ Armour Thyroid, USP   (Forest Lab)

Obtained from porcine thyroid glands containing 38 mg levothyroxine (T₄) and 9 mg liothyronine (T₃) per grain thyroid.

How Supplied: 15, 300 mg tablets.

Dose: Usual starting dose 30 mg/day with individualization.

Indications:
1. As replacement or supplemental therapy in patients with hypothroidism.
2. To suppress pituitary TSH secretion.

Contraindications: Uncontrolled adrenal insufficiency or untreated thyrotoxicosis. Not for use in the therapy of obesity or female or male infertility unless there is a component of hypothyroidism.

Adverse Effects:
1. Hypermetabolic state.
2. Drug interactions with estrogenic hormones: estrogens tend to increase thyroxine-binding globulin, with theoretical decrease in free levothyroxine and need for increased thyroid dose.

■ Levothyroxine Sodium (Levothroid; Forest, Synthroid; Boots)

Synthetic T_4 produced by coupling of two molecules of diiodotyrosine.

How Supplied: Tablet, various doses from 25 to 300 µg.

Dose: Usual starting dose 50 µg/day with individualization.

Indications/Contraindications: See Thyroid on p. 465.

■ Liothyronine Sodium (Cytomel; Smith-Kline Beecham)

Synthetic L-triiodothyronine; 25 µg equivalent to 1 grain dessicated thyroid.

How Supplied: 5, 25, 50 µg tablet.

Dose: Usual starting dose 25 µg/day with individualization.

Indications/Contraindications:
See Thyroid on p. 465.

■ Liotrix (Thyrolar; Forest Lab)

Synthetic mixture of T_4 and T_3 in a 4:1 ratio.

How Supplied: 1/4, 1/2, 1, 2, 3 tablets, having various µg combinations of T_3 and T_4 per dose.

Dose: Individualized.

ANTITHYROID MEDICATIONS
■ Methimazole (Tapazole; Lilly)

How Supplied:
PO: 5, 10 mg tablets.

Administration: PO; readily absorbed; but possible delayed response if thyroid unusually large or iodine given beforehand.

Mechanism of Action: Inhibits thyroid hormone synthesis by interfering with iodine incorporation into tyrosyl residues; over time, results in depletion of stores or iodinated thyroglobulin as protein B hydrolyzed and hormones are released into circulation.

Dose: 15–60 mg/day divided tid.

Elimination: Excreted in urine.

Indications: Hyperthyroidism, either long-term to achieve disease remission or to ameliorate symptoms; e.g., during pregnancy, (but with caution; see adverse effects below); in preparation for subtotal thyroidectomy or radioactive iodine therapy.

Contraindication: Lactation; agranulocytosis, aplastic anemia, pancytopenia; exfoliative dermatitis; hepatitis (e.g., signified by transaminase level 3 × normal).

Adverse Effects: Urticarial papular rash; inhibition of myelo–poiesis, aplastic anemia, drug fever, lupuslike syndrome, insulin autoimmune syndrome, periarteritis, hypoprothrombinemia, crosses placenta and may induce goiter, cretinism or aplasia cutis in fetus.

Toxicity: GI distress, aplastic anemia or agranulocytosis; fulminant hepatitis with fatal liver necrosis and encephalopathy; nephrotic syndrome; neuropathies; CNS stimulation or depression.

Monitor: Bone marrow function; LFTs; PT; TSH.

■ Propylthiouracil (Lederle)

How Supplied: *PO:* 50 mg tablets.

Administration: *PO.*

Mechanism of Action: See Methimazole on p. 466.

Dose: 100 mg tid.

Elimination: See Methimazole on p. 466.

THYROID

Indications/Contraindications: See Methimazole on p. 466.

Adverse Effects/Toxicity: See Methimazole on p. 466. However, no reports of scalp defects caused by aplasia cutis with propylthiouracil, so may be preferrable when treatment is required in pregnancy.

CHAPTER 31

TOCOLYTICS

ß-SYMPATHOMIMETICS
■ Ritodrine HCl   (Yutopar; Astra)

How Supplied:
PO: 10 mg tablets.
Parenteral:
    50 mg (10 mg/ml), 5 ml vial and ampule.
    150 mg (15 mg/ml), 10 ml vial and syringe.

Administration:
PO: rapidly but incompletely (30%) absorbed.
    Parenteral: IV, by controlled infusion for appropriate dose titration, with patient in left lateral position to avoid hypotension. D_5W as diluent preferred to saline solutions in most cases to minimize risk of pulmonary edema; limit total fluid intake to 2 L/24 hr.

Dose:
    Initially: 0.1 mg/min; increase by 0.05 mg/min q10min until labor is controlled or max of 0.35 mg/min is reached.
    Usual effective dose: 0.15–0.35 mg/min; continue for 12 hr after contractions cease.
    Maintenance: 10 mg PO 30 min before discontinuing IV infusion, then 10 mg q2h for first 24 hr. Subsequently, 10–20 mg q4h depending on uterine activity and side effects; max 120 mg/24 hr.
    Recurrence of preterm labor: Return to IV therapy.

Mechanism of Action: Selective β_2–receptor agonist and thus inhibits uterine smooth muscle contractility and decreases intensity and frequency of uterine contractions. Other β_2 actions include lowered diastolic BP with a widened pulse pressure, and reflex tachycardia and increased cardiac output. Metabolic effects include enhanced renin secretion, which decreases renal excretion of sodium, water, and potassium and may contribute to potential volume overload; also, hyperglycemia; transient hypokalemia caused by net intracellular movement of potassium.

Elimination: 50% of IV dose and 90% of PO dose excreted in urine as inactive conjugates; half-life 1.7–2.6 hr.

Indications: Preterm labor between 20 and 36 wk gestation.

Contraindications: Pregnancy less than 20 wk gestation; any condition in which continuation of pregnancy may be hazardous to mother or fetus, such as antepartum hemorrhage (vasodilation may exacerbate), severe pregnancy-induced hypertension, intrauterine fetal death, chorioamnionitis, maternal cardiac disease, pulmonary hypertension, hyperthyroidism, uncontrolled diabetes mellitus (may precipitate ketoacidosis). This includes maternal conditions potentially adversely affected by β–mimetics, such as hypovolemia, cardiac dysrhythmias associated with tachycardia or digitalis intoxication (reflex tachycardia may aggravate), uncontrolled hypertension, pheochromocytoma, and bronchial asthma already treated by β-mimetics or steroids. Ruptured membranes are considered a relative contraindication because of risk of infection.

Side Effects:

Common (80%–100%): Maternal and fetal tachycardia (adjust dose to keep maternal pulse <140; see later discussion), widened pulse pressure; transient elevation of blood glucose and insulin valves (return toward normal in 48–72 hr); hypokalemia, not usually requiring treatment.

Frequent (10%–50%): Palpitations, tremor, nausea, headache.

Infrequent (1%–3%): Cardiac symptoms and dysrhythmias; impaired liver function. Sensitivity to metabisulfite (more common in asthmatic patients) may evoke anaphylactic symptoms or asthmatic episodes.

Neonatal effects (rare): Hypoglycemia, ileus, hypocalcemia, hypotension.

Toxicity: Potentially fatal pulmonary edema, sometimes even after delivery; more often in patients also on steroid therapy.

May be complicated by myocardial ischemia and necrosis, and dysrhythmias (e.g., tachydysrhythmias, premature beats, bundle branch block). Suspect if persistent maternal tachycardia >140 or chest pain or tightness occurs. Discontinue drug immediately and obtain ECG. Excessive β–stimulation may also manifest as hypotension, dyspnea, or vomiting.

Monitor: Baseline ECG to rule out occult maternal heart disease; values for serial glucose, electrolytes, and CBC (may indicate state of hydration).

Interactions: Corticosteroids potentiate risk of pulmonary edema. Cardiovascular effects, especially dysrhythmia and hypotension, may be potentiated by magnesium sulfate, diazoxide, meperidine, and potent general anesthetics. Parasympatholytics (e.g., atropine) may exacerbate systemic hypertension. Concurrently administered sympathomimetics have an additive effect; β–adrenergic blockers counteract ritodrine actions.

TERBUTALINE

See Chapter 27. Not FDA-approved for use as a tocolytic. Indicated for preterm labor only as part of specific research protocols under controlled conditions at academic institutions.

■ Magnesium Sulfate (Magnesium Sulfate Injection, USP; Astra)

How Supplied:
Parenteral:
    10% solution (9.9 mg Mg/ml); 20, 50 ml vial.
    50% solution (49.3 mg Mg/ml): 2, 10, 20 ml vial; 5, 10 ml additive syringe.

Administration: Constant IV infusion preferable to IM (painful); plasma levels vary depending on route of administration, renal function, and individual patient metabolic physiology.

Dose: Protocols vary, depending on institution and indication for use.

IM: 10 gm loading dose (may add 4 gm IV over 5–15 min for severe PIH), then 5 gm q4h.

IV: 4–6 gm loading dose over 15–20 min, then 1–3 gm/hr.

Titrate dose to maintain therapeutic Mg plasma level 4–8 mg/dl (3.3–6.6 mEq/L).

Mechanism of Action: Blocks neuromuscular transmission: Competes with calcium at neuromuscular junction and inactivates calcium ATPase system, thus decreasing intracellular calcium, inhibiting actin-myosin binding and antagonizing calcium-dependent acetylcholine release and end-plate sensitivity. Also, blocks the release of catecholamines from the adrenal gland, resulting in further uterine relaxation and peripheral vasodilatation, with decreased BP and increased uteroplacental blood flow. Other effects include CNS depression and a mild osmotic diuresis.

Elimination: Renal: Glomerular filtration with resorption in proximal renal tubules.

Indications: Preterm labor; pregnancy-induced hypertension (PIH).

Contraindications: Not for use as a tocolytic in conditions where continuation of pregnancy is hazardous to mother or fetus (e.g., hemorrhage of uncertain cause, intrauterine fetal death, chorioamnionitis, fetal malformation incompatible with life, abruptio placentae, severe intrauterine growth retardation). Relative contraindications to tocolysis include fetal distress, cervical dilation >4–5 cm. No contraindications to use in PIH unless evidence of toxicity (see below) or renal output <25 ml/hr.

Side Effects: Flushing, feeling of warmth, headache, lethargy, nausea; decreased TPR, increased CO and HR, widened pulse pressure; hypocalcemia. Neonates may exhibit respiratory depression and decreased muscle tone.

Toxicity:

mg/dl	mEq/L	Clinical Signs
Plasma Mg:		
10–12	8–10	Loss of deep tendon reflexes (patellar reflex)
16–18	13–15	Respiratory depression
18–25	15–20	Cardiac conduction defects (prolonged P-R + QRS intervals, peaked T waves)
25–30	20–25	Cardiac arrest in diastole

Monitor: Deep tendon reflexes, urine output (minimum 25–30 ml/hr), serial plasma Mg levels.

Antidote: 1 gm calcium gluconate IV (may not completely reverse effect; ventilatory support may be required).

Interactions: Potentiates depolarizing and nondepolarizing neuromuscular blocking agents. Use with ritodrine may improve chances for successful tocolysis and allow for lower doses of ritodrine; however, risk of untoward cardiovascular side effects increase, especially myocardial ischemia.

TOCOLYTICS

CHAPTER 32

UROLOGIC AGENTS

ANALGESICS

■ **Phenazopyridine HCl** (Azo-Standard; PolyMedica. Prodium; Zeneca. Pyridium; Parke-Davis)

How Supplied:
PO: 95, 100, 200 mg tablet.

Administration: PO, well-absorbed.

Dose: 200 mg tid pc × 2 days.

Mechanism of Action: Exerts topical analgesic effect on urinary tract mucosa as excreted in urine; exact mechanism unknown.

Elimination: Renal excretion.

Indications: Relief of pain, urgency, and frequency because of lower urinary tract mucosal irritation from infection, trauma, surgery, or instrumentation.

Contraindications: Drug hypersensitivity; renal insufficiency. Inadequate data on use in pregnancy and lactation.

Adverse Effects: GI upset (10%); headache; rash; pruritus. Stains body fluids orange-red, including urine and aqueous humor.

Toxicity: Methemoglobinemia, hemolytic anemia, renal or hepatic toxicity.

STIMULANTS: CHOLINERGICS
■ **Bethanechol Chloride** (Myotonachol; Glenwood. Urecholine; Merck)

How Supplied:
PO: 5, 10, 25, 50 mg tablet.
Parenteral: 5 mg/ml; 1 ml vial.

Administration:
PO: Requires 60–90 min for maximum effect; duration 1 hr.
SC injection: More intense bladder action than PO form.

Dose:
PO: Initially 5–10 mg; repeat q1h until satisfactory response or max (total) 50 mg. Usual dose 10–50 mg tid–qid.

SC: Initially 0.5 ml (2.5 mg), repeat q15–30 min until satisfactory response or maximum total 2 ml (10 mg). Maintain on minimum effective dose tid–qid.

Mechanism of Action: Cholinergic agonist, with predominantly muscarinic effects. Increases detrusor muscle tone to contract sufficiently to initiate micturition and bladder emptying. Also stimulates gastric motility, increases gastric tone, and improves peristalsis. Not destroyed by cholinesterase.

Indications: Nonobstructive urinary retention and inadequate bladder emptying, including acute postoperative and postpartum retention, chronic hypotonic, myogenic, neurogenic bladder. Use SC form for acute cases and oral form for chronic cases until voluntary or automatic voiding begins, then taper.

Contraindications: Hyperthyroidism, peptic ulcer, asthma, significant bradycardia or hypotension, vasomotor instability, coronary artery disease, epilepsy, parkinsonism. Also, bladder neck obstruction, recent GI resection and anastomosis, and peritonitis (hypermotility may be harmful). Inadequate data on use in pregnancy and lactation.

Toxicity: Nausea, diarrhea, bronchoconstriction, miosis, flushing, urgency, detrusor-like dyssynergia, hypotension with reflex tachycardia. Accidental IM or IV injection may produce cholinergic overstimulation with cardiovascular collapse.

UROLOGIC

Antidote: Atropine 0.6 mg q2h.

Interactions: Use with ganglionic blocking agents (e.g., mecamylamine, trimethaphan) may result in significant hypotension.

ANTISPASMODICS: ANTICHOLINERGICS
■ **Oxybutynin Chloride** (Ditropan; Marion Merrell Dow)

How Supplied:
PO:
    5 mg tablet.
    5 mg/ml syrup.

Administration: PO, well-absorbed.

Dose: 5 mg bid–tid; max 20 mg/day.

Mechanism of Action: Anticholinergic, predominantly antimuscarinic effect. Direct antispasmodic effect on smooth muscle increases bladder capacity, diminishes frequency of uninhibited detrusor contractions and sensation of urgency in both incontinent episodes and voluntary urination.

Indications: Unstable bladder voiding symptoms as seen in uninhibited neurogenic or reflex neurogenic bladder.

Contraindications: Increased intraocular pressure (e.g., glaucoma) with angle closure (anticholinergics may aggravate); GI tract obstruction (may mask symptoms), paralytic ileus, intestinal atony in the elderly or debilitated, megacolon, severe colitis, myasthenia gravis, obstructive uropathy, unstable cardiovascular status in acute hemorrhage. Inadequate data on use in pregnancy and lactation.

Adverse Effects: Urinary hesitancy and retention, constipation, nausea, rash, amblyopia, impotence, suppressed lactation; heat prostration (fever and heat stroke caused by decreased sweating).

Toxicity: CNS excitation with tremor, convulsions, delirium, tachycardia, and coma.

■ Hyoscyamine (Cystospaz; PolyMedica. Levsin, Levsinex; Schwarz)

How Supplied:
PO:
    0.15, 0.125 mg tablets.
    0.375 mg timed-release capsule.
    0.125 mg/5 ml elixir.
Parenteral:
    0.5 mg/ml 1 ml ampule.

Administration: PO or sublingual, best before meals and without antacids. Subcutaneous, IM or IV, undiluted.

Mechanism of Action: See Oxybutynin on p. 476. Also inhibits GI motility and decreases gastric acid and respiratory tract secretions.

Dose:
PO: T–TT tab prn or max qid; or T capsule bid.
Parenteral: 0.25–0.5 mg single dose or q4 h prn; 0.125 IV intraoperatively.

Indications: To control lower urinary tract spasm and hypermotility. Also as adjunctive therapy in peptic ulcer and irritable bowel syndrome, acute enterocolitis to control gastric secretions and spasm; biliary and renal colic. Also used intraoperatively to reduce drug-induced bradycardia.

Contraindications: See Oxybutynin on p. 476.

Adverse Effects: See Oxybutynin on p. 476.

Toxicity: Severe dryness of skin and mucous membranes, hyperpyrexia, dilated pupils, CNS irritability, tremors, convulsions, respiratory failure and death.

Interactions: Additive anticholinergic effects with other antimuscarinics; e.g., amantadine, haloperidol, phenothiazines, MAO inhibitors, tricyclic antidepressants, some antihistamines. Antacids may decrease absorption.

■ Flavoxate HCl   (Urispas; Smith-Kline Beecham)

How Supplied: *PO:* 100 mg tablets.

Administration: *PO.*

Mechanism of Action: Teritiary amine antimuscarinic; counteracts urinary tract smooth muscle spasm.

Dose: T–TT tid–qid.

Indications: Symptomatic relief of dysuria, urgency, nocturia, suprapubic pain, frequency and incontinence as in cystitis and urethritis.

Contraindications: Any obstructive conditions of the lower GI or urinary tract; glaucoma. Avoid use in pregnancy, lactation.

Adverse Effects: Dry mouth, GI distress, mental confusion, tachycardia, reversible leukopenia, increased ocular tension, blurred vision.

COMBINATION AGENTS

Table 32-1.

Table 32-1.
COMBINATIONS AGENTS*

Azo Gantanol (Roche):	500 mg sulfamethoxazole
	100 mg phenazopyridine hydrochloride
Azo Gantrisin (Roche):	500 mg sulfisoxazole
	50 mg phenazopyridine hydrochloride
Urobiotic 250 (Roerig):	250 mg oxytetracycline
	250 mg sulfamethizole
	50 mg phenazopyridine hydrochloride

*See also Agents to treat Urinary Tract Infections, Chapter 3.

UTERINE STIMULANTS

OXYTOCICS

■ **Oxytocin** (Oxytocin; Wyeth-Ayerst. Pitocin; Parke-Davis. Syntocinon; Sandoz)

How Supplied:
Parenteral:
   5 units/0.5 ml ampule.
   10 units/1 ml ampule and disposable syringe.
   10 units/ml, 10 ml multiple dose vial.
   Nasal spray: 40 units/ml; 2, 5 ml squeeze bottle.

Administration: Promptly absorbed in all parenteral forms. Onset of action 3–7 min IM, within 1 min IV. Use IV form via controlled infusion only; add 10–40 units to 1000 ml 0.9% NaCl or Ringer's lactate.

Dose:
1. Induction or augmentation of labor:
   a. IV: Initially 1–2 mU/min, increase by 1–2 mU/min q15 min until adequate contraction pattern is established. (Specific protocols in academic institutions that start or increment at higher intervals are designed for highly controlled use within specific clinical settings.)
2. Cervical ripening: Begin at 1 mU/min IV and increase as in no. 1a until contractions occur q2–3 min at 40–60 mm Hg × 6–8 hr.
3. OCT: Begin at 1 mU/min IV and increase as above until 3 contractions/10 min without decelerations. Usual dose required is <10 mU/min.
4. Postpartum uterine bleeding:
   a. IV: 10–40 units in 1 L nonhydrating diluent; maximum rate 100 mU/min.
   b. IM: 10 units × 1 after delivery of placenta.

5. Incomplete or inevitable abortion: 10 units in 500 ml 0.9 NS or D$_5$W at 20–4 gtt/min.

6. To assist postpartum milk ejection reflex: One spray into one or both nostrils 2–3 min before nursing or pumping breasts.

Mechanism of Action: Selectively stimulates frequency and force of uterine smooth muscle tone, with a particular increase in uterine responsiveness near term, during labor, and immediately postpartum. Does not contain the same amino acids as vasopressin, so there are fewer and less severe CV effects. Also causes smooth muscle contraction of the myoepithelial elements of breast alveoli, thus forcing milk into larger ducts for easier ejection.

Elimination: Short half–life. Rapidly metabolized by oxytocinase in placenta and uterus, then removed from plasma by kidney, liver, and lactating mammary gland and excreted in urine.

Indications:

1. OCT (CST).
2. Augmentation or induction of labor.
3. Cervical ripening before induction of labor.
4. Adjunctive therapy in incomplete or inevitable abortion.
5. Control of uterine atony and postpartum hemorrhage.
6. Nasal spray: To assist postpartum milk ejection once milk formation has commenced.

Contraindications:

1. Any contraindication to vaginal delivery, such as severe CPD, unstable fetal lie or malpresentation (e.g., incomplete breech), obstetrical emergency where surgical intervention would be more favorable for mother or fetus (e.g., fetal distress or severe PIH), cord prolapse, placenta or vasa praevia.
2. Uterine hypertonus.
3. Previous vertical cesarean section scar or myomectomy scar into uterine cavity.

Toxicity:

1. Maternal: Anaphylaxis, postpartum hemorrhage, cardiac dysrhythmia, PVCs, fatal afibrinogenemia, nausea, vomiting, uterine hypertonicity, tetany, and uterine rupture (with excessive doses), H$_2$O intoxication with convulsions and coma (ADH–like effect and excess glomerular H$_2$O reabsorption; more common at extremely high doses), death caused by

hypertension and subarachnoid hemorrhage, hypotension with bolus administration.
2. Fetal and neonatal: Bradycardia, PVCs and other dysrhythmias, CNS damage (from induced uterine motility), jaundice.

Interactions:

Hypotension, maternal sinus bradycardia and abnormal atrioventricular rhythms with cyclopropane, severe hypertension with vasoconstrictors used prophylactically with caudal block anesthesia.

■ Methylergonovine Maleate (Methergine; Sandoz)

How Supplied:
PO: 0.2 mg tablet.
  Parenteral: 0.2 mg/ml, 1 ml ampule.

Administration:
PO: Slowly and incompletely absorbed.
  IM: Effective dose is 10% of oral dose, but absorption is also slow (≤24 min latent effect).
  IV: Effective at 50% IM dose (uterine response within 5 min); however, must be given slowly (no faster than 1 ml/min) to avoid sudden hypertension or CVA (thus IV route indicated only as lifesaving measure).

Dose:
IM, IV: 0.2 mg after delivery of anterior shoulder or placenta or in puerperium; repeat prn q2–4h.
PO: 0.2 mg q6–8h × 1 wk max in puerperium.

Mechanism of Action: Amide derivative of D–lysergic acid; acts directly on uterine smooth muscle to increase tone, rate, and amplitude of contractions, thus inducing a rapid and sustained tetanic uterotonic effect that shortens the third stage of labor and decreases blood loss.

Elimination:
1. Metabolized by liver; excretion partially renal and partially hepatic.

2. Exercise caution in patients with sepsis, obliterative vascular disease, hepatic or renal dysfunction.

Indications: Routine labor management after delivery of placenta, postpartum atony or hemorrhage, subinvolution.

Contraindications: Hypertension, pregnancy-induced hypertension, pregnancy.

Toxicity: Hypertension with seizures, headache; hypotension; transient chest pain; numbness; nausea and vomiting.

Interactions: Exercise caution with other vasopressors (e.g., dopamine, epinephrine, other ergot alkaloids).

PROSTAGLANDINS
■ **Dinoprostone** (Prostin E2; Upjohn. Prepidil Gel; Upjohn. Cervidil; Forest Labs)

How Supplied: Prostin E_2 vaginal suppository containing 20 mg of dinoprostone. Store in freezer and bring to room temperature before use.

Cervidil vaginal insert containing 10 mg dinoprostone in hydrogel insert within polyester retrieval system.

Prepidel Gel in syringe applicator contains 0.5 mg PGE_2.

Administration:

Prostin Vaginal Suppositories: Insert one suppository high in vagina. Repeat in 3–5 hours.

Cervidil vaginal insert: Insert into posterior fornix of vagina transversely.

Prepidel Gel: Insert one syringeful into cervical canal, according to instructions supplied by manufacturer. Repeat dose at 6 hrs, if necessary. Maximum recommended dose is 3 inserts (1.5 mg of dinoprostone) over 24 hrs.

Mechanism of Action: Dinoprostone is the naturally occurring form of prostaglandin E_2 and stimulates the smooth muscle of the uterus and gastrointestinal tract, and in large doses, the smooth muscle of arterioles.

Prostin E_2 suppository.

Indications:
Termination of pregnancy from the 12th through 20th week of gestation.

Incomplete or missed abortion.

Evacuation of intrauterine fetal death up to 28 weeks.

Evacuation of nonmetastic gestational trophoblastic benign tumor.

Contraindications:
Hypersensitivity to dinoprostone.

Acute pelvic inflammatory disease.

Women with active cardiac, pulmonary, renal or heptic disease.

Adverse Effects:
Vomiting and elevated temperature, headache.

Myocardial infarction reported in patients with preexisting heart disease.

Cervidil Vaginal Insert.

Prepidil Gel.

Indications: Induction of labor by cervical ripening.

Contraindications:
Hypersensitivity to dinoprostone.

Suspicion of fetal distress.

Unexplained vaginal bleeding during this pregnancy.

Suspicion of cephalopelvic disproportion.

Patients in whom oxytocin is contraindicated.

Multipara with 6 or more term pregnancies.

Nonvertex presentation.

Ruptured membranes.

Vaginal delivery is contraindicated.

Caution in patients with previous uterine scar (vertical uterine incisions), previous myomectomy.

Caution in women with asthma.

Adverse Effects:
Uterine hypertonicity/hyperstimulation.

May cause sustained uterine contraction with possible fetal distress.

See above for other effects.

CHAPTER 34

VULVOVAGINAL PREPARATIONS

ANTIINFECTIVES

ANTIFUNGALS

See Chapter 4.

BACTERIOSTATIC CREAMS AND SUPPOSITORIES

■ **Sulfanilamide** (AVC Cream, Suppositories; Marion Merrell Dow)

■ **Sulfathiazole, Sulfacetamide** (Sulfabenzamide, Sultrin Triple Sulfa Cream, Vaginal Tablets; Ortho. Trysul; Savage)

How Supplied: Vaginal cream, suppository, tablet.

Dose: 1 applicatorful (cream), suppository, or tablet qhs or bid, × 4–10 days.

Mechanism of Action: Topically bacteriostatic; also lowers pH to encourage potential Döderlein's bacillus growth.

Indications:
Sultrin: Hemophilis vaginalis vaginitis.
AVC: Candida albicans vaginitis.

Contraindications: Hypersensitivity to sulfonamides. (Sultrin also not for use in kidney disease, pregnancy at term, and lactation.)

Toxicity: Local irritation, allergy.

BACTERIOSTATIC DOUCHES

■ **Povidone-Iodine Vaginal Douche** (Massengil Medicated Disposable Douche; Smith-Kline Beecham)

How Supplied: Single povidine-iodine vial with sanitized fluid bottle and intravaginal nozzle.

Administration: Intravaginal.

Dose: Qhs, × 1–7 nights.

Mechanism of Action: Povidine-iodine: Broad-spectrum microbicide.

Indication: Symptomatic relief of vaginitis caused by *C. albicans, Trichomonas,* and *Gardnerella vaginalis.*

Contraindication: Pregnancy.

VULVAR DYSTROPHY AGENTS

TOPICAL STEROIDS
    See Table 34-1.

■ **Topical Testosterone** (2% Testosterone in White Petrolatum)

How Supplied: Each prescription must be mixed in the pharmacy using testosterone powder or suspension.

Table 34-1

STEROID CREAMS FOR VULVAR HYPERPLASTIC DYSTROPHIES

Chemical Name	*Brand Name (Mfg)	How Supplied	Usual Dose/Administration†
Halcinonide	Halog (Westwood-Squibb)	Cream 0.1%	Rub in gently bid–tid
	Halog-E‡ (Westwood-Squibb)	Ointment, Topical solution 0.1%	Apply thinly bid–tid
		Cream 0.1%	Rub in gently qhs–tid
Flucinonide	Lidex (Syntex)	Cream, gel, ointment, topical solution 0.05%	Apply thinly bid–qid
	Lidex E§(Syntex)	Cream 0.05%	Apply thinly bid–qid
Triamcinolone Acetonide	Aristocort-A‖ (Fujisawa)	Cream 0.025%, 0.1%, 0.5%	Apply thinly tid–qid
		Ointment 0.1%	Apply thinly tid–qid
Fluocinolone Acetonide	Synalar (Syntex)	Cream 0.025%, 0.1%	Apply bid–qid
		Ointment 0.025%	Apply bid–qid
		Topical solution 0.01%	Apply bid–qid
	Synalar-HP¶ (Syntex)	Cream 0.2%	Apply bid–qid
	Synemol§ (Syntex)	Cream 0.025%	Apply bid–qid

Table 34-1

STEROID CREAMS FOR VULVAR HYPERPLASTIC DYSTROPHIES–Cont'd

Chemical Name	*Brand Name (Mfg)	How Supplied	Usual Dose/Administration†
Bethamethasone Valerate	Betatrex (Savage)	Cream, ointment, lotion 0.1%	Cream, ointment: Apply qhs–tid Lotion: Rub in few drops bid–tid; qhs after improvement.
Hydrocortisone	Hytone (Dermik)	Cream, lotion, ointment 1%, 2.5%	Apply thinly bid–qid
	Synacort (Syntex)	Cream 1%, 2.5%	Apply thinly bid–qid
Crotamiton#	Eurax (Westwood)	Cream, lotion 10%	Steroic cream adjunct

*Listed in decreasing order of potency.
†Expect clinical response within 2 weeks; longer for very thick hyperplastic lesions.
‡In hydrophilic vanishing cream base.
§In water-washable aqueous emollient base.
‖In Aquatain hydrophilic or special ointment base.
¶In water-washable aqueous base.
#Not a steroid, but often added to decrease pruritus (e.g., 7 parts betamethasone to 3 parts crotamiton).

Administration: Massage thoroughly into affected skin.

Dose:
    Initial therapy: 0.5 gm (kidney bean–sized amount = 8–10 mg testosterone) bid-tid first 6 wk.
    Maintenance therapy: 0.5 gm qhs or qod.
    Recurrence prevention: 0.5 gm 1–2 times/wk.

Mechanism of Action: Trophic hormone; acts locally to stimulate skin growth in disorders characterized by lack of growth.

Indication: Adult lichen sclerosus.

Contraindications: Childhood lichen sclerosus; vulvar ulcerations.

Toxicity: Clitoral hypertrophy, increased libido, excess facial hair growth. Skin ulceration from too vigorous massage best managed by substituting testosterone preparation with corticosteroid cream for 1 wk until healed, then alternate corticosteroid and testosterone cream qod.

ACIDIFYING AGENTS
■ Therapeutic Vaginal Jelly   (Aci-Jel; Ortho)

How Supplied: 85 gm tube and applicator.

Administration/Dose: 1 applicatorful intravaginally bid.

Mechanism of Action: Nonirritating water-dispersible buffered acid jelly that restores and maintains normal vaginal acidity.

Indication: Adjunctive therapy where acidic vaginal pH must be maintained.

Contraindication: Inadequate data on use in pregnancy and lactation.

Toxicity: Local stinging.

CERVICITIS THERAPY

■ Cervical Cream   (Amino-Cerv; Milex)

How Supplied: 2¾ oz tube and applicator.

Administration/Dose: 1 applicatorful qhs × 2–4 wk.

Mechanism of Action: Amino acid (methionine and cystine), urea, and inositol cream formulated to aid wound healing, epithelialization, and debridement of sloughing tissue.

Indication: Cervicitis, postpartum cervical tears, postcauterization, postcryosurgery, postconization.

LUBRICANTS

Table 34-2.

Table 34-2.
■ VAGINAL LUBRICANTS*

Brand Name (Mfg)	How Supplied	Usual Dose/Administration
Astroglide (Biofilm)	Water-soluble liquid	1/16 oz. (1/2 tsp) prn
Gyne-Moistrin Vaginal Moisturizing Gel (Schering-Plough Health Care)	Water-based gel	Use externally or with internal applicator prn
K-Y Jelly (Johnson & Johnson)	Water-soluble jelly	Prn
Lubrin (Upsher-Smith)	Water-soluble vaginal inserts (liquefy after insertion)	10 min before coitus (effects last several hours)
Ortho Personal Lubricant (Ortho)	Water-soluble jelly	Prn
Replens† (Warner Wellcome)	Vaginal gel	Intravaginally 3 times per week

*Not spermicidal.
†Primarily indicated for postmenopausal vaginal dryness.

ANTICONDYLOMA MEDICATIONS
■ Podofilox (Condylox; Oclassen)

How Supplied: Topical liquid: 0.5% solution 95% alcohol, 3.5 ml bottle.

Dose/Administration: Apply bid × 3 days with cotton-tipped applicator; then withhold use × 4 days; Limit to 10 cm² of wart tissue and 0.5 ml/day. Consider alternative treatment if no response in 4 wk.

Mechanism of Action: Antimiotic; results in necrosis of visible wart tissue.

Indication: Topical treatment of external condyloma acuminatum. Not indicated for perianal and mucous membrane lesions. Biopsy if diagnosis in doubt (to rule out squamous cell cancer).

Contraindications: Avoid use in pregnancy and lactation.

Toxicity: "Burn" is due to overexposure (treat with cold wet 1:40 Burow's solution dressing bid–tid, antibacterial corticosteroid preparation). Atypical histologic changes seen on biopsy of podofilox-treated skin may mimic carcinoma in situ (alert pathologist to history of treatment). Desquamative vaginitis when used intravaginally, with potential systemic drug absorption and neurotoxicity (treat with irrigation, debridement, corticosteroid cream).

■ Trichloroacetic Acid

How Supplied: Topical solution.

Administration: Protect surrounding normal skin with petroleum jelly; apply to wart and keep area dry for 12–24 hr.

Dose: qwk × several wk.

Mechanism of Action: Halogenated acetic acid; denatures all proteins on contact.

Indication: Vulvar and perineal condyloma acuminatum.

Contraindication: Vaginal and cervical condyloma; pregnancy. Inadequate data on use in lactation.

Toxicity: Local burning. Systemic absorption with fatal neurotoxicity reported after use in pregnancy.

■ 5-Fluorouracil   (Efudex; Roche)

How Supplied:
   Topical cream: 5%, 25 gm tube.

Administration: Protect vulva with layer of petroleum jelly, then insert high into vagina. Systemic absorption = 6% of topical dose. Wash hands immediately afterward.

Dose: 1/2 applicatorful qhs × 5–7 days; or T applicator/wk hs × 6 wk.

Mechanism of Action: Pyrimidine analog antineoplastic antimetabolite; interferes with thymidylic acid metabolism, thus preventing normal DNA (and to some extent, RNA) synthesis, especially in rapidly multiplying cells, resulting in intracellular thymine deficiency, unbalanced growth and death of the cell.

Indication: Vaginal condyloma acuminatum (Sometimes also used for vulvar carcinoma in situ and recurrent Paget's disease of vulva; multiple actinic or solar keratoses).

Contraindication: Pregnancy. No data on use in lactation.

Adverse Effects: Local pain, burning, vaginal discharge, edema.

RISK CATEGORY FOR DRUGS IN PREGNANCY

The FDA has established five categories to indicate the potential of a drug to cause birth defects. Category differentiation depends on reliability of documentation.

Category A—Adequate studies in pregnant women have not demonstrated a risk to the fetus in the first trimester, nor is there evidence of risk in later trimesters.

Category B—Animal studies have not demonstrated a risk to the fetus, but there are no adequate studies in pregnant women. Or, animal studies have shown an adverse effect, but adequate studies in pregnant women have not demonstrated a risk to the fetus in the first trimester, and there is no evidence of risk to the fetus in later trimesters.

Category C—Animal studies have shown an adverse effect on the fetus, but there are no adequate studies in pregnant women. Benefits for the use of the drug by pregnant women may outweigh the potential risks.

Category D—There is positive evidence of human fetal risks, but the benefits may outweigh the potential risks to the fetus.

Category X—Studies in animals and humans demonstrated fetal abnormalities. The risks to the fetus clearly outweigh any possible benefit to the pregnant woman.

SOME EXAMPLES OF DRUGS BY RISK CATEGOIRES

DRUG OR CLASS	PREGNANCY RISK CATEGORY
Antibiotics	
Acyclovir	C
Cephalosporins	A
Erythromycin	A
Gentamicin	A
Kanamycin	D
Lincomycin	A
Metronidazole	B
Miconazole	C
Nitrofurantoin	B
Penicillin	A
Rifampin	C
Streptomycin	D
Sulfonamides	B
Tetracycline	D
Tobramycin	A
Anticoagulants	
Heparin	C
Warfarin	D
Anticonvulsants	
Diphenylhydantoin	D
Phenobarbital	D
Trimethadione	D
Valproic Acid	D
Antiemetics	
Chlorpromazine	C
Meclizine	B
Prochlorperazine	C

Antihypertensives

Hexamethonium	C
Hydralazine	C
Propanolol	C
Reserpine	D

Antineoplastics

Actinomycin-D	D
Aminopterin	X
Busulfan	D
Chlorambucil	D
Cyclophosphamide	D
5-Fluorouracil	D
6-Mercaptopurine	D
Thiotepa	D
Vinblastine	D
Vincristine	D

Diuretics

Furosemide	C
Spironolactone	D
Thiazides	D

Hormones

Androgens	X
Clomiphene	X
Corticosteroids	D
Diethylstilbestrol	X
Estrogens	X
Insulin	B
Progestins	X
Propylthiouracil	D
Thyroid	A

Pain Relievers

Acetaminophen	B
Aspirin	C
Codeine	C
Ibuprofen	B
Indomethacin	B
Narcotics	B
Naproxen	B

Psychotropics

Alcohol	D
Amphetamines	C
Barbiturates	D

Bromides	D
Cocaine	C
Chlordiazepoxide	D
Diazepam	D
Haloperidol	C
Lithium	D
LSD	C
Marijuana	C
Meprobamate	D
Phencyclidine (PCP)	X
Tricyclic Antidepressants	D
Miscellaneous	
Aminophylline	C
Ammonium Chloride	B
Caffeine	B
Cyclamate	C
Digitalis	C
Etretinate (retinoid)	X
Griseofulvin	D
Guaifenesin	C
Iodine compounds	D
Quinacrine	C
Ranitidine	B
Ritodrine	B
Senna	C
Simethicone	C
Terbutaline	B
Theophylline	C

DRUG ENFORCEMENT ADMINISTRATION SCHEDULES OF CONTROLLED SUBSTANCES

The controlled substances that come under jurisdiction of the Controlled Substances Act are divided into five schedules. Examples of controlled substances and their schedules are as follows:

SCHEDULE I SUBSTANCES

The controlled substances in this schedule are those that have no accepted medical use in the United States and have a high abuse potential. Some examples are heroin, marijuana, LSD, peyote, mescaline, psilocybin, THC, methaqualone, dihydromorphine, and others.

SCHEDULE II SUBSTANCES

The controlled substances in this schedule have a high abuse potential with severe psychic or physical dependence liability. Schedule II controlled substances consist of certain narcotic, stimulant, and depressant drugs, including: opium, morphine, codeine, hydromorphone. Also in Schedule II are amphetamine and methamphetamine, phenmetrazine, methylphenidate, amobarbital, pentobarbital, secobarbital, fentanyl, and phencyclidine.

SCHEDULE III SUBSTANCES

The controlled substances in this schedule have an abuse potential less than those in Schedules I and II and include compounds containing limited quantities of certain narcotic drugs and nonnarcotic drugs such as derivatives of barbituric acid except those that are listed in another schedule, glutethimide, methyprylon, nalorphine, benzphetamine, phendimetrazine, and paregoric. Any suppository dosage form containing amobarbital, secobarbital, or pentobarbital is in this schedule.

SCHEDULE IV SUBSTANCES

The controlled substances in this schedule have an abuse potential less than those listed in Schedule III and include such drugs as: barbital, phenobarbital, mephobarbital, chloral hydrate, ethchlorvynol, ethinamate, meprobamate, paraldehyde, methohexital, fenfluramine, diethylpropion, phentermine, chlordiazepoxide, diazepam, oxazepam, clorazepate, flurazepam, clonazepam, prazepam, lorazepam, alprazolam, temazepam, triazolam, dextropropoxyphene, and pentazocine.

SCHEDULE V SUBSTANCES

The controlled substances in this schedule have an abuse potential less than those listed in Schedule IV and consist of preparations containing limited quantities of certain narcotic drugs generally for antitussive and antidiarrheal purposes.

BIBLIOGRAPHY

American Medical Association: *Drug evaluations,* ed 7, Chicago, 1993, AMA.

Anderson HF, Hopkins M: Postpartum hemorrhage. In Sciarra JJ, editor: *Gynecology and obstetrics,* vol 2, Philadelphia, 1989, Harper & Row.

Baker RJ: Blood component therapy and transfusion reactions. In Condon RE, Nyhus LM, editors: *Manual of surgical therapeutics,* Boston, 1993, Little, Brown.

Barton JR, Hiett AK, Conover WB: The use of nifedipine during the postpartum period in patients with severe pre-eclampsia, *Am J Obstet Gynecol* 162:788, 1990.

Barton JR, Sibai BM: Acute life-threatening emergencies in pre-eclampsia-eclampsia, *Clin Obstet Gynecol* 35:402, 1992.

Bassuk EL, Schoorover SC, Gelenberg AJ, editors: *The practitioner's guide to psychoactive drugs,* New York, 1983, Plenum Publishing.

Becker KL, editor: *Principles and practice of endocrinology and metabolism,* Philadelphia, 1995, JB Lippincott.

Beeson PB, McDermott W, Wyngaarden JB, editors: *Cecil textbook of medicine,* Philadelphia, 1993, WB Saunders.

Belfort MA et al: The use of nimodipene in a patient with eclampsia: color flow Doppler demonstration of retinal artery relaxation, *Am J Obstet Gynecol* 169:204, 1993.

Benitz WE, Tatro DS: *The pediatric drug handbook,* ed 2, St Louis, 1988, Mosby.

Berkowitz RL, Coustan DR, Mochizuki TK: *Handbook for prescribing medications in pregnancy,* Boston, 1986, Little, Brown.

Bhorat IE et al: Malignant ventricular arrhythmias in eclampsia: a comparison of labetalol with dihydralazine, *Am J Obstet Gynecol* 168:1292, 1993.

Boehm JJ: Resuscitation of the newborn and prevention of asphyxia. In Sciarra JJ, editor: *Gynecology and obstetrics,* vol 3, Philadelphia, 1987, Harper & Row.

498

Brater DG: *Drug use in clinical medicine,* Indianapolis, 1993, Improved Therapeutics.

Briggs GG, Freeman RK, Yaffe SJ: *Drugs in pregnancy and lactation,* ed 3, Baltimore, 1990, Williams & Wilkins.

Centers for Disease Control: *Tuberculosis and human immunodeficiency virus infection,* Recommendations of the Advisory Committee for the Elimination of Tuberculosis, *MMWR* 38:236, 1989.

ACOG Committee Opinion: *Cocaine abuse: implications for pregnancy,* Committee on Obstetrics: Maternal and Fetal Medicine, American College of Obstetrics and Gynecology, Washington, DC, March 1990, no 81.

Condon RE, Nyhus LM, editors: *Manual of surgical therapeutics,* Boston, 1993, Little, Brown.

Considine T: Principles of blood replacement. In Sciarra JJ, editor: *Gynecology and obstetrics,* vol 3, Philadelphia, 1985, Harper & Row.

Costrini NV, Thomson WW, editors: *Manual of medical therapeutics,* Boston, 1977, Little, Brown.

Creasy RK, Resnik R, editors: *Maternal-fetal medicine: principles and practice,* Philadelphia, 1994, WB Saunders.

Davis JM et al: Changes in pulmonary mechanics after the administration of surfactant to infants with respiratory distress syndrome, *N Engl J Med* 319:476, 1988.

DeBacker NA, Shoichet SH, Webster JR: Pulmonary diseases in pregnancy. In Sciarra JJ, editor: *Gynecology and obstetrics,* vol 3, Philadelphia, 1993, Harper & Row.

Drug information for the health care provider, ed 7, vol 1, Pharmacopeial Convention, Rockville, Md, 1987.

Fredriksen MC: Labor inhibition. In Sciarra JJ, editor: *Gynecology and obstetrics,* vol 3, Philadelphia, 1989, JP Lippincott.

Friedrich EG: *Vulvar disease,* Philadelphia, 1983, WB Saunders.

Goodman LS et al, editors: *The pharmacological basis of therapeutics,* ed 8, New York, 1993, Macmillan.

Hoeprich PD, Jordan MC: *Infectious diseases,* Philadelphia, 1989, JB Lippincott.

Horn EH et al: Widespread cerebral inschemia treated with nimodipine in a patient with eclampsia, *Br Med J* 301:794, 1990.

Keith LG, MacGregor SN, Sciarra JJ: Substance abuse in pregnancy. In Sciarra JJ, editor: *Gynecology and obstetrics,* vol 3, Philadelphia, 1993, Harper & Row.

Mabic WC, Gonzalez AR, Sibai BM: A comparative trial of labetalol and hydralazine in the acute management of severe hypertension complicating pregnancy, *Obstet Gynecol* 70:328, 1987.

Magann EV, Martin JN: Compliated postpartum pre-eclampsia-eclampsia, *Obstet Gynecol Clin N Am,* 22(2):337, 1995.

McDonald JS: Anaesthesia and the high-risk fetus. In Sciarra JJ, editor: *Gynecology and obstetrics,* vol 3, Philadelphia, 1993, JP Lippincott.

Niebyl JR: Drugs and related areas in pregnancy. In Sciarra JJ, editor: *Gynecology and Obstetrics,* vol 2, Philadelphia, 1987, Harper & Row.

Papper S, Williams GR, editors: *Manual of medical care of the surgical patient,* Boston, 1990, Little, Brown.

Physicians gen rx 1995, St Louis, Mosby, 1995.

*Physicians desk reference 1995,*New Jersey, 1995, Medical Economics.

Physicians desk reference for generics, Medical Economics Publishers, 1995, New Jersey.

Prescribing reference for obstetricians and gynecologists, vol 5, no 2. New York, Prescribing Reference, Fall-Winter 1994-1995.

Rakel RE, editor: *Conn's current therapy,* Philadelphia, 1986, WB Saunders.

Rayburn WF, Zuspan FP: *Drug therapy in obstetrics and gynecology,* ed 3, New York, 1992, Appleton-Century-Crofts.

Schwartz RH: Crack use in pregnancy, *Postgrad Obstet Gynecol* 10(6), 1990.

Seltzer V, Sall S: Nutritional support in patients with gynecologic malignancy. In Sciarra JJ, editor: *Gynecology and obstetrics,* vol 4, Philadelphia, 1987, Harper & Row.

Thurnau GR: Immunologic disorders specifically associated with pregnancy. In Sciarra JJ, editor: *Gynecology and obstetrics,* vol 3, Philadelphia, 1993, JB Lippincott.

US Department of Health and Human Services: *Transfusion alert—indications for the use of red blood cells, platelets and fresh frozen plasma,* National Blood Resource Education Program, National Institutes of Health, 1989, Bethesda, Md.

Usta IM, Sibai BM: Emergency management of puerpal eclampsia, *Obstet Gyn Clin N Am* 22(2):315, 1985.

Wilson JD et al, editors: *Harrison's principles of internal medicine,* ed 12, New York, 1991, McGraw-Hill.

Zatuchni, GI: *Female contraception in principles and practice of endocrinology and metabolism,* Philadelphia, 1995, JB Lippincott.

Zatuchni, GI: *Known and potential complications of steroidal contraception in principles and practice of endocrinology and metabolism,* Philadelphia, 1995, JB Lippincott.

Zuspan FP, Quilligan EJ: Current therapy in obstetrics and gynecology, Philadelphia, 1994, WB Saunders.

INDEX